MEDICAL
MICROBIOLOGY

MEDICAL MICROBIOLOGY

Myra Wilkinson MSc, MA, FIBMS, CSci, CIBiol

Principal Lecturer, School of Pharmacy and Biomedical Sciences,
University of Portsmouth

With contributions from

Ron Cutler MSc, PhD, FIBMS, FBiol, CIBiol, CSci

Deputy Director of Biomedical Science, School of Biological and Chemical Sciences,
Queen Mary, University of London

Scion

© Scion Publishing Ltd, 2011
First edition published 2011

ISBN 978 1904842 61 3

A CIP catalogue record for this book is available from the British Library.

Scion Publishing Limited
The Old Hayloft, Vantage Business Park, Bloxham Road, Banbury, OX16 9UX, UK
www.scionpublishing.com

Important Note from the Publisher

The information contained within this book was obtained by Scion Publishing Limited from sources believed by us to be reliable. However, while every effort has been made to ensure its accuracy, no responsibility for loss or injury whatsoever occasioned to any person acting or refraining from action as a result of information contained herein can be accepted by the authors or publishers.

Although every effort has been made to ensure that all owners of copyright material have been acknowledged in this publication, we would be pleased to acknowledge in subsequent reprints or editions any omissions brought to our attention.

Readers should remember that medicine is a constantly evolving science and while the authors and publishers have ensured that all dosages, applications and practices are based on current indications, there may be specific practices which differ between communities. You should always follow the guidelines laid down by the manufacturers of specific products and the relevant authorities in the country in which you are practising.

Typeset by Phoenix Photosetting, Chatham, Kent, UK
Printed by Charlesworth Press, Wakefield, UK

Contents

Preface

'May you live in interesting times.'

A curse or a blessing? This phrase, widely believed to be of Chinese origin, is enigmatic in its use of the word 'interesting' – exciting, challenging, changing, turbulent, insecure? The word can conjure a multitude of descriptors and contexts. The study of microbiology and its place as a key discipline in the delivery of modern pathology services is certainly interesting at all levels. During the writing of this book there have been significant changes in the organization of clinical microbiology laboratories, led by both innovation and economics. From discrete laboratories within a hospital, using conventional culture techniques, to amalgamated laboratories, automated systems and the introduction of mass spectrometry, the practice of microbiology is constantly evolving and changing. Microorganisms themselves are never static; emerging pathogens are a constant reminder of this, able to adapt to changing environmental pressures, to acquire genetic characteristics and cause severe disease.

This book is intended for all students studying microbiology at university and in the laboratory. The first chapters provide sufficient theoretical underpinning of the subject for readers to be able to appreciate the practice of microbiology within pathology. These chapters include a brief history as well as information about nomenclature, the microorganisms, host–pathogen relationships, and basic microscopy. They also include a description of the identification techniques used within later chapters and an overview of the organization of a typical microbiology laboratory. These early chapters do not set out to provide a detailed study of genetics, biochemistry and antibiotic structure. Further chapters then describe the most likely pathogens and their diagnosis and treatment from a range of clinical specimens and body sites, and from food and water. At the end of each chapter I have included self-assessment questions, and many chapters include case studies related to the subject area.

You will notice that the book is black and white – this has been done deliberately to keep the price of the book down for students; however, lots of colour images are available on the website that supports the book (see below) and, of course, via the readily-accessible Google Images!

Web material

The website that accompanies the book (www.scionpublishing.com/medmicro) features:

- Detailed answers to all the self-assessment questions in the book
- Answers to the case study questions
- Colour photographs of microorganisms, equipment, typical results – some of these images are reproduced in the book in black and white, but others are new images that should help with understanding or recognition

This material can all be found at www.scionpublishing.com/medmicro and will be updated as useful material and images become available.

When I was a student and as a biomedical scientist I have always wanted to know 'why?' and 'how do they do that?' and I've never lost that passion for microbiology and awe of the microorganisms involved. The 'why?' and 'how?' questions continue to focus research into disease mechanisms, pathogenesis and genetics. Students continue to ask questions and this book is dedicated to all the students past and present who have inspired and refined my teaching and have reinforced my passion for the subject. I have been fortunate to have spent several years as a biomedical scientist before making the transition to lecturing, teaching both undergraduate and postgraduate students. Because of the nature of the part-time and integrated undergraduate degree programmes I have been able to maintain close associations with the excellent laboratories in my geographical area and I am grateful to them for their continued support in my writing of this book, keeping my ideas focused and current.

I hope you will enjoy reading this book and that it will help you to understand the ways in which disease is caused, transmitted, diagnosed and treated. I would also like to think that, more than just reading the facts in the chapters, you begin to develop a fascination and respect for all the bacteria, viruses and eukaryotic microorganisms and the many ways in which they interact with us in health and disease.

Myra Wilkinson
July 2011

Acknowledgements

I am grateful to Ron Cutler from the School of Biological and Chemical Sciences at Queen Mary, University of London for his contributions to some of the chapters. I must also thank Andy Tuck and Sue Jones at the HPA Southampton, and to the staff of the microbiology laboratories in Portsmouth and Winchester for their help checking practical procedures and the provision of images.

I would also like to thank Jonathan Ray and Clare Boomer of Scion Publishing Ltd for their expertise and constant support.

Abbreviations

ACC	aerobic colony count
AFB	acid-fast bacilli
AIMS	immunomagnetic bead separation
APC	aerobic plate count
API	Analytical Profile Index
ATP	adenosine triphosphate
Aw	available water
BAL	broncho-alveolar lavage
BCYE	buffered charcoal yeast extract
CCDC	Consultant in Communicable Disease Control
CCHF	Crimean Congo haemorrhagic fever
CFT	complement fixation test
CFU	colony-forming units
CHI	Community Health Index
CJD	Creutzfeldt–Jakob disease
CLED	cystine, lysine, electrolyte deficient
CMV	cytomegalovirus
CNS	central nervous system
CRS	congenital rubella syndrome
CSF	cerebrospinal fluid
CSU	catheter samples of urine
DCA	deoxycholate citrate agar
DIC	disseminated intravascular coagulation
DNA	deoxyribonucleic acid
EBV	Epstein–Barr virus
EDTA	ethylenediaminetetraacetic acid
ELISA	enzyme-linked immunosorbent assay (sometimes known as EIA or enzyme immunoassay)
EM	electron microscopy
ESBL	extended spectrum β-lactamase
FRET	fluorescence resonance energy transfer
GABA	γ-aminobutyric acid
GALT	gastric-associated lymphoid tissue
GDH	glutamate dehydrogenase
GI	gastrointestinal
GUM	genitourinary medicine
GVPC	glycine vancomycin polymixin cycloheximide
HAART	highly active anti-retroviral therapy
HACCP	hazard analysis critical control points
HAV	hepatitis A
Hib	*Haemophilus influenzae* type B
HPA	Health Protection Agency
HSE	Health and Safety Executive
HSV	herpes simplex virus
HUS	haemolytic uraemic syndrome
IF	immunofluorescence
IM	infectious mononucleosis
ISO	International Organization for Standardization
IUCD	intrauterine contraceptive device
KDO	2 keto-3-deoxy-octanate
LED	light-emitting diode
LEE	locus of enterocyte effacement
LOS	lipo-oligosaccharide
LPS	lipopolysaccharide
MALDI-TOF-MS	matrix-assisted laser desorption time-of-flight mass spectrometry

MALT	mucosa-associated lymphoid tissue	PFGE	pulsed-field gel electrophoresis
MBC	minimum bactericidal concentration	PID	pelvic inflammatory disease
MBL	mannose-binding lectin	PPD	purified protein derivative
MHC	major histocompatibility complex	PPE	personal protective equipment
MHRA	Medical and Healthcare products Regulatory Agency	PPV	pneumococcal polysaccharide vaccine
MIC	minimum inhibitory concentration	PVL	Panton–Valentine leukocidin
MKTTn	Muller-Kauffmann tetrathionate novobiocin	RNA	ribonucleic acid
		RSV	respiratory syncytial virus
MPN	most probable number	RT	reverse transcriptase
MRD	maximum recovery diluents	RVS	Rappaport Vassiliadis soya peptone
MRSA	methicillin-resistant *Staphylococcus aureus*	SEM	scanning electron microscopy
MSSA	methicillin-sensitive *Staphylococcus aureus*	SOP	standard operating procedure
MSU	midstream urine	SPA	suprapubic aspirate
NAAT	nucleic acid amplification technique	STD	sexually transmitted disease
		STI	sexually transmitted infection
NAD	nicotinamide–adenine dinucleotide	TEM	transmission electron microscopy
NEQAS	National External Quality Assurance Schemes	THP	Tamm–Horsfall protein
		TMA	transcription-mediated amplification
NNRTI	non-nucleoside reverse transcriptase inhibitor	TVC	total viable count
NPA	naso-pharyngeal aspirate	UKAS	United Kingdom Accreditation Service
NRTI	nucleoside reverse transcriptase inhibitor	URT	upper respiratory tract
		UTI	urinary tract infection
OD	optical density	VCA	virus capsid antigen
ONPG	*o*-nitrophenyl-β-D-galactopyranoside	vCJD	variant Creutzfeldt–Jakob disease
PAF	platelet-activating factor	VHF	viral haemorrhagic fever
PAMP	pathogen-associated molecular pattern	VNC	viable non-culturable state
		VP	Voges–Proskauer
PBS	phosphate buffered saline	VZV	varicella-zoster virus
PCR	polymerase chain reaction	WHO	World Health Organization
PCV	pneumococcal conjugated vaccine	XLD	xylose lysine decarboxylase
		ZN	Ziehl–Neelsen

Introduction to medical microbiology

Learning objectives
After studying this chapter you should confidently be able to:

- **Discuss the evolution and diversity of microorganisms and describe the difference between prokaryotes and eukaryotes**
  Microorganisms have been in existence ever since the earth began to cool. They were instrumental in creating the oxygen-rich environment which supports human, animal and plant life. Bacteria and archaea did not evolve beyond the microbial stage, but have developed into a widely diverse group of prokaryotic microorganisms. Bacteria include all the environmental and human-associated commensal and pathogenic bacteria; archaea include the prokaryotes continuing to live in extreme environments in high levels of acid, alkali, salt and temperatures. Eukaryotic cells continued to evolve and developed membrane-bound nuclei, mitochondria and chloroplasts. They include protozoa, fungi, algae and helminths. Whereas prokaryotes remained single cell organisms, eukaryotes formed the cells of macroorganisms in humans, plants and animals.

- **Demonstrate an understanding of the ways in which microorganisms are classified and named**
  Microorganisms are classified and named either by using evidence gained from observed, phenotypic characteristics or from analysis of the genome. They are classified into families, genera and species. The genera and species are written in italics to denote their Latin origin. In medical microbiology it is important to distinguish between species, as one species may be harmless to man, whereas another may cause serious disease.

- **Discuss the impact of historic events on the development of modern microbiology**
  The development of the early microscope allowed a view of the microscopic world previously unknown to man. Gradually through observation and experiment the link between living microorganisms and human disease was established. The identification of bacteria became possible as culture and staining methods developed. Once the causes of disease were established, appropriate treatment strategies were developed. The discovery of the molecular structure of microorganisms in the twentieth century continues to provide new information and treatment options.

- **Outline Koch's postulates and discuss their application to current clinical diagnosis of infectious disease**
  In the late nineteenth century Robert Koch produced a set of criteria, known as postulates, to be used to establish whether a microorganism was the cause of a particular disease. He said that the suspected causal organism must be present in every case of the disease, but absent from healthy people. This causal organism must then be isolated in pure culture and then re-inoculated into a fresh susceptible host. This host must then develop the same disease, and specimens taken from them must grow the same microorganism in pure culture. While this is true of some diseases and their associated microbial

causes, it has limitations in others, which even Koch realized. Opportunistic infections, infection by pathogens of low virulence or part of the host's normal bacteria, are now an important consideration in the interpretation of results from clinical samples from patients with compromised immune systems. Host–pathogen relationships are a complex balance between the health of the host and the threat posed by the potential pathogen.

■ **Describe the scope of medical microbiology**
Microbiology is the study of microscopic organisms (microbes) such as bacteria, viruses, protozoa and fungi. Medical microbiology involves the isolation, identification and treatment of microorganisms isolated from relevant clinical specimens. It is important that the appropriate specimen is obtained from the patient and then appropriate investigations can be carried out.

Microbiology is the study of microbes or microorganisms and their interaction with other living organisms. Microbes are single-cell organisms which are beyond the range of the human eye (with the exception of the larger roundworms). Bacteria, protozoa, yeasts, fungi and the eggs of intestinal worms are visible using a light microscope as they are greater than 0.3 µm (1 µm =1/1000 mm), whereas viruses (ranging from 0.01 µm to 0.3 µm) can only be seen using an electron microscope. One of the important and interesting facts about microbiology is the sheer number and diversity of microorganisms. For this reason there are different areas of microbiology dealing with a range of aspects: environmental, soil, plants, diverse and extreme environments, water and waste management; veterinary; pharmaceutical, ensuring that products intended for human treatment are safe and sterile; the development of antimicrobial therapies; microbiology laboratories specializing in food testing; plus research and development for all these areas of interest.

Medical or clinical microbiology is one of the principal pathology disciplines specializing in the diagnosis, treatment and research into microorganisms known to cause human disease. The number of bacteria, viruses, fungi, protozoa, helminthic worms and flukes involved in human infection represents a small proportion of the total population of microorganisms. However, past pandemics and current global infection levels demonstrate the fact that their diagnosis, treatment and control are significant and defining factors in determining the lifespan, health and well-being of the worldwide population.

The purpose of this first chapter is to provide a background and framework for the rest of the book, to introduce the theory and practice of medical microbiology through its history, conventions and context in the diversity of microbiology.

1.1 EVOLUTION AND DIVERSITY

The earliest fossil evidence for the existence of microorganisms is believed to be between 3.3 and 3.5 billion years old, soon after the surface of the earth cooled sufficiently to allow the formation of water. They had the world to themselves and adapted to extreme conditions, ice ages, volcanic activity, collisions with meteors and oceans without oxygen. Without their contribution the earth and its atmosphere would not have been transformed sufficiently to support plant and animal life. Oxygen was first introduced to the atmosphere by cyanobacteria as they used the light from the sun and split water molecules to produce oxygen in the process of photosynthesis. The gradual increase in the levels of oxygen led to the oxidation of minerals and the establishment of a different, more hospitable environment. An ozone layer was formed around the earth, enabling life forms to survive outside the water without the threat of radiation from the sun. Eukaryotic microorganisms are thought to have developed 2 billion years ago from the combination of a non-photosynthetic cell and a bacterial cell; fungi appeared in the last several hundred million years, and may have co-evolved with plants. Bacteria, algae and fungi have all been identified in 220 million-year-old pieces of amber (fossilized tree resin). The evolution of viruses is less straightforward; as they rely on their hosts for replication, they could only have evolved when there were susceptible bacterial, plant and animal hosts to infect.

Because microorganisms have been in existence for so long they have had time to evolve and diversify. With bacterial generation times being as short as 20–30 minutes (compared with at least 20 years for humans), bacteria continually mutate in response to pressures. For example, if susceptible bacteria are treated with antibiotics the majority will die, but a small proportion of spontaneous mutations could survive. If they were to carry on reproducing, resistance to the antibiotic may be achieved.

Prokaryotes and eukaryotes

Bacteria and archaea did not evolve beyond the microbial stage and are classified as prokaryotes, 'pro' denoting 'early' or 'primitive'. Considerable diversification of the genotypic (DNA composition) and phenotypic (observed structure and biochemical reactions) characteristics have taken place, forming the basis of bacterial taxonomy and classification.

Eukaryotes, however, continued to evolve, developing mitochondria, chloroplasts and membrane-bound nuclei. Eukaryotic microorganisms include protozoa, fungi, algae and helminths. They also form the cells of macroorganisms, humans, plants and animals.

Prokaryotes include bacteria and archaea. Bacteria, sometimes referred to as eubacteria, include all the known disease-causing bacteria and most of the environmental bacteria found in soil, water, animals and other environments. Some of the environmental bacteria are restricted to specific species of plants and animals; others have adapted to human hosts and can be transmitted from one host to another to cause human infection. Other bacteria are strict human pathogens and are incapable of causing infections in other species.

Archaea are mostly anaerobes (able to survive without oxygen) and thrive in extreme environments including hot springs, freezing water, extremely acidic and alkaline environments and in the presence of high levels of salt.

One of the principal differences between prokaryotes and eukaryotes is the presence of membrane-bound organelles in eukaryotes and their absence in prokaryotes, as shown in *Table 1.1*.

Other important differences are the methods of reproduction, the structure of the cell wall and the size of the ribosomes used for protein synthesis. Because of the differences, particularly between bacterial and human cells, it has been possible to develop antimicrobial drugs to target cell walls, protein synthesis, DNA replication and the super-coiling of bacterial nuclear material, with minimal damage to human cells. This is called selective toxicity, and can be harder to achieve when the target cells

Table 1.1 Differences between prokaryotes and eukaryotes

Prokaryotes	Eukaryotes
Size – less than 5 μm	Larger cells greater than 10 μm
Single cells	Often multicellular
DNA not enclosed in membrane, circular and supercoiled	Discrete nucleus with nuclear membrane
DNA not associated with histones and proteins	DNA linear, high histone content and associated with non-histone proteins to form chromatin
Cell division by binary fission	Cell division by mitosis or meiosis
Asexual reproduction	Asexual or sexual reproduction
No organelles	Membrane-bound organelles
No cytoskeleton	Always have cytoskeletons
Complex cell wall	Simple cell wall if present
Variety of metabolic pathways	Common metabolic pathways
70S ribosomes	80S ribosomes
Ability to form biofilms	No biofilm formation
Motile genera have rotating flagellae composed of flagellin	Motility by flexible waving cilia or flagellae composed of tubulin

are eukaryotes, because there are fewer differences between the cells, and host cells are more likely to be destroyed along with the eukaryotic pathogens. The structure and reproduction of prokaryotes and eukaryotes associated with human disease are explored in *Chapter 2*.

Microbial populations

In nature, populations of related cells live in a habitat or niche in association with other microorganisms, to form a microbial community and their own ecosystems. Within these ecosystems there is often extensive cooperation; one group of bacteria may break down large molecules and use them as nutrients, and another group are then able to use the waste products as their nutrients. The interaction between populations can also be competitive in relation to nutrients and niches, or even antagonistic, with the production of toxins and antibiotic substances. Microbial populations form the microflora of their particular habitat. This is also true within the human body where a diverse range of bacteria (and in some areas of the body, yeast cells) cohabit as part of the normal microflora. The human body is covered with bacteria on all mucous surfaces communicating with the outside world and the skin. In fact the normal flora outnumbers the cells of the body (10^{14} microorganisms and 10^{13} cells); a large number, particularly considering that many of the deeper tissues and organs do not have any bacteria associated with them. In terms of normal human flora the relationship is mutualistic, with benefits for the host and microorganisms. The normal microbial flora is an important factor in medical microbiology as it is protective, but can also be the source of infection. Furthermore, knowledge of the presence or absence of normal flora must be taken into account when looking at culture plates grown from clinical specimens. The composition and presence of normal flora at particular body sites is discussed further in *Chapter 3*.

Bacteria and fungi fulfil very important roles in nature, as many are saprophytic –

breaking down, decaying and recycling organic material, plants, trees and animals. If the world were devoid of microorganisms the earth's surface would be miles deep in waste, and totally uninhabitable.

- Different genera of bacteria play an important role in agriculture where they are involved in fixing nitrogen from the atmosphere, using the enzyme nitrogenase, into a form that can be used by the plants to build amino acids and proteins. Note that nitrogen is abundant in the atmosphere but not in a form that is readily available to plants.
- Other bacteria are involved in cycling nitrogen from organic material in the soil.
- Bacteria are used in the dairy industry for making yoghurt and cheese, and it is the addition of bacteria that gives blue cheeses their distinctive flavour and appearance.
- Naturally occurring antibiotics produced by fungi and bacteria are exploited and produced on an industrial scale. Biological washing powders contain enzymes called subtilisins, produced by an environmental bacterium, *Bacillus licheniformis.*
- Bacteria are also a valuable source of vitamins and amino acids, while yeasts are a key ingredient in brewing and bread making.

1.2   CLASSIFICATION AND NOMENCLATURE

Taxonomy is the scientific study of classification that allows microorganisms to be placed into categories. The categories of the most recent taxonomic hierarchy (1990) are:

- domain
- class
- order
- family
- genus
- species.

When bacteria are isolated and identified from clinical specimens they are reported as genus and species. The species is important, as some species of a genus cause more serious infections than another; for example, within the genus *Yersinia*, *Yersinia pestis* is the causative organism in bubonic plague, whereas *Yersinia enterocolitica* causes an intestinal infection which sometimes mimics appendicitis. Within the genus *Bacillus*, *Bacillus anthracis* causes anthrax, whereas *Bacillus megaterium* is found harmlessly in the environment. *Table 1.2* shows the full classification for the bacterium *Escherichia coli.*

The genus and species are named using the Latin binomial system, developed by the Swedish botanist Carolus Linnaeus in the mid 18th century. This system applies equally to plants, animals and microorganisms. Because they are Latin names, bacterial nomenclature follows the convention of writing the genus and species in italics. The genus is often shortened to one letter, for example *E. coli*. However, this can be confusing if there is more than one genus beginning with the same letter, such as *Staphylococcus* and *Streptococcus*. For the sake of clarity, full names for bacteria, viruses and fungi are used throughout this book. The names of families, for example

Table 1.2 Hierarchy of taxonomical classification, using *Escherichia coli* as an example (from National Centre for Biotechnology Information (NCBI))

Taxonomic hierarchy	Example
Super kingdom	Bacteria
Phylum	Proteobacteria
Class	Gamma proteobacteria
Order	Enterobacteriales
Family	Enterobacteriaceae
Genus	*Escherichia*
Species	*E. coli*

Enterobacteriaceae, Staphylococcaceae and Streptococcaceae are not italicized but have a capital letter.

Taxonomic systems

Taxonomy has a direct impact on medical microbiology, because the correct identification of a microbe may affect the treatment, control and potentially the spread of any infection. It is important, therefore, to understand the basis of current taxonomic systems, their apparently continual state of change and the impact this can have on clinical microbiology. The two main taxonomic systems are based either on the phenotypic or physical characteristics of the microbes, or on their genetic or phylogenic characteristics. In reality, clinical laboratories depend mainly on the definition of physical characteristics to determine the identification of isolates. However, more and more genetic identification systems, based on the amplification of key sequences of the genome, are being introduced. Comparison of the genetic similarities and differences made possible by these systems has a direct impact on the epidemiological study and control of nosocomial (hospital-acquired) infection outbreaks. Such genetic checks enable you to see whether there is one predominant outbreak strain, more suggestive of a single source, or whether there are several genetic strains circulating, more indicative of transfer of strains from the community into the hospital or between hospitals.

Before the advent of techniques for determining the genetic composition, classification was based solely on phenotypic characteristics. The system obviously worked well, because there have not been a large number of changes since the advent of molecular (genetic) based techniques.

■ **Phenetic system.** Organisms are grouped using phenotypic characteristics, which may or may not match evolutionary groupings.

Characteristics such as response to Gram stain, cell shape, motility, size, aerobic/anaerobic capacity, nutritional capabilities, cell wall structure and chemistry, and immunological characteristics (for example, presence of specific antigenic structures on the cell surface) are determined. A small number of specific biochemical tests can often provide discrimination between genera. Biochemical test systems such as the API (analytical profile index) incorporate 10 or 20 tests, including enzyme reactions and sugar reactions, to produce a numerical profile for identification of a range of species of bacteria. The use of all these techniques is the subject of *Chapter 6*.

■ **Phylogenetic system.** Organisms are grouped by shared evolutionary heritage. This can be achieved by sequencing either RNA or DNA. DNA sequencing shows the genetic code of the bacterial genome, by sequencing the guanine and cytosine (G–C) and adenine and thymine (A–T) pairings. Amplification of either the 16 S or 18 S ribosomal RNA is also commonly used. The unit 'S' denotes Svedberg units, which relate to sedimentation. 16 S is the small RNA subunit of prokaryotic cells; 18 S is the smaller ribosomal subunit of eukaryotic microorganisms. The sequences of a number of genomes are compared using a computer program. Changes in the sequence of the 16 S or 18 S RNA, DNA or protein sequences give an idea of the phylogenetic relationship, or common ancestry, between strains of bacteria. This is explained in *Figure 1.1*. It is the standard method for identifying the family, genus and species of microorganisms. Toxins, protein structures exported from cells to cause specific damage to other cells (for example destroying red or white blood cells or cells in the gastrointestinal tract), can also be analysed by sequencing the proteins in their structure to see how closely related they are. Some toxins are quite closely related, sharing a large percentage of their structure; if, for example, the structure of toxin A is 50% the same as toxin B, they are said to share 50% homology.

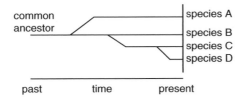

Figure 1.1
This theoretical evolutionary diagram is based on the genetic analysis of four species derived from a common ancestor. Over a period of time the four species have changed by diversification and from the acquisition of DNA from other bacteria. The result is an accurate picture of how and when organisms diverged from common ancestors over time.

Throughout the study of microbiology the terms 'species', 'strain', 'serovar' and 'isolates' are used, and although bacteria are used to describe the terms here, the definitions also apply to eukaryotes and viruses:

■ **Species.** A species of bacteria is a population of cells that share similar characteristics. A collection of strains that share certain properties can be called the same species even if they differ by up to 30% at the DNA level. Knowledge of a bacterial species has a practical use in identification and diagnosis of disease.

■ A **strain** is a subset of a bacterial species descended from a single organism. Clinical isolates, for example, may be of the same species but are different strains; they often have slight differences in virulence, biochemical reactions and/or antibiotic susceptibility.

- The **type strain** is usually the first strain isolated or best characterized. It is kept in culture collections (the NCC (National Culture Collection) in the UK, or the ATCC (American Type Culture Collection) in the USA). Type strains are often used as control strains in the laboratory for controlling identification and antibiotic susceptibility tests.

- **Serovars** are strains differentiated from one another by serological means (by the presence of different cell surface antigens). Salmonella bacteria have over 2000 different serovars, determined by using specific antibodies to detect a range of antigens on their cell surfaces.

- An **isolate** is a species of bacteria isolated in pure culture from a clinical specimen containing a mixed wild population of microorganisms.

1.3 THE IMPACT OF HISTORY

The practice of microbiology has a long and interesting history, with several seminal discoveries that have shaped the detailed knowledge and diagnostic methods used today.

- Understanding that infectious disease is caused by living microorganisms.
- The development of first the light microscope and later the electron microscope, enabling their presence to be seen and described.
- The development of staining methods to distinguish between major groups of bacteria.
- The development of asepsis and control of infection methods.
- The development of culture media and successful *in vitro* culture methods to visualize the growth of bacteria from a single cell into a visible colony.
- Control of infectious disease by vaccination.
- The discovery and advent of effective antimicrobial chemotherapy.
- The development of genetic methods to give detailed information on the genetic structure of microorganisms and improve diagnosis.

Abiogenesis versus biogenesis – recognition of the role of microorganisms in infectious disease

Abiogenesis, the formation of life from non-living matter, was the commonly held belief prior to the invention and use of microscopes, which led to the discovery of microbes. Biogenesis, on the other hand, is the formation of life from living matter. Aristotle (384–322 BC) and others believed that living organisms arose from non-living materials and this doctrine of 'spontaneous generation' was accepted for centuries until the Renaissance. The idea that infectious diseases could be transferred between individuals was hypothesized by Fracastorius in 1530. He suggested that syphilis and other diseases could be transmitted through direct contact with an infected person, contaminated materials, or even through breathing infected air.

Over a century later in the Great Plague of London of 1665, some physicians still believed that 'miasmata' of poisonous air floated around, infecting those who inhaled them. Because of this, people often wore nosegays (sweet smelling posies) containing petals and sometimes medicinal herbs to protect themselves. It was over 200 years later that the causative agent *Yersinia pestis* and its mode of transmission in the fleas of rats were identified.

Francesco Redi (1688) rebutted the theory of abiogenesis in relation to insects. He demonstrated that rotten meat, if kept isolated from flies, did not spontaneously develop maggots. It was not, however, until almost two centuries later, in 1861, that Louis Pasteur's experiments showed that microorganisms were not spontaneously generated but were carried in dust and air.

Although Fracastorius in the sixteenth century was amongst the first to recognize that disease could be spread between individuals, it was not until 1835 that Bassi de Lodi published the first description of a microorganism causing disease; he reported a fungus that infected a silk worm. He also theorized that many plant, animal and human diseases could be caused by animal or vegetable parasites; this theory predated both Pasteur's and Robert Koch's proposals of a germ theory of disease.

Pasteur, whose name is synonymous with the development of microbiology, proposed his 'germ theory' of disease in 1857, developed techniques for the safe preservation of food and milk (pasteurization), and was also responsible for the development of early vaccines.

Development of the microscope and staining techniques

From theories regarding the diagnosis and spread of disease, advances in microscopy were the next stage in the development of microbiology. Robert Hooke was the first person, in 1653, to demonstrate the use of a compound microscope with three lenses in anatomical research, but it was Anton van Leeuwenhoek (1632–1723) who is credited as the first person to see microbes using a simple microscope.

One of the problems with examining bacteria under a microscope was that most bacterial cells are not coloured and are difficult to see. The visualization of bacteria and their shapes was improved through the development of staining techniques. The most famous and most widely used staining technique, the Gram stain, was developed in 1884 by Christian Gram. Initially it had been designed to identify bacteria in tissue, but today the differentiation between Gram-positive and Gram-negative bacteria remains an essential determinant in the laboratory diagnosis of bacterial infection.

Development of aseptic techniques and control of infection

Any form of early surgery was a risky business, not only because of the lack of anaesthetic, but also because the risk of post-operative infection was so high. In Hungary in 1847 Semmelweis began to investigate the high numbers of deaths from infection amongst women who had just given birth. He discovered that doctors were moving directly from dissecting dead bodies to treating the women without washing their hands. Simple changes in practice dramatically reduced the death rate. Hand washing with either soap or alcohol gel remains a basic tenet of control of infection practice for anyone in contact with a patient; it is simple, cheap and very effective. In 1865 Joseph Lister, a professor of surgery in Glasgow, read of Pasteur's work on the microbial souring of wine in relation to the spread of infection, and introduced the use of the first antiseptic (in this case carbolic antiseptics (phenol) in soap and sprays) into surgery and in so doing significantly reduced post-operative infections.

The final experimental proof of the relationship between infection by microorganisms and disease came in 1884 when Koch published his *Postulates* (see *Section 1.4*). These postulates laid out a procedure that demonstrated cause and effect.

Microbial culture and isolation

One of the main problems with establishing that a microbial pathogen causes a disease is the same today as it was in Pasteur's and Koch's era: the microorganism has to be isolated and identified. As was recognized even in van Leeuwenhoek's time, the world is full of microorganisms, although in the main these are harmless to man and in many cases are beneficial.

Pasteur initially grew bacteria in liquid culture, relying on selective agents to aid isolation and discriminate between bacteria; however, there were difficulties in distinguishing one kind of bacteria from another using this method. In 1881, Koch developed a method for growing bacteria on solid gelatine medium and this allowed researchers to pick out individual colonies from mixed cultures and purify them for testing. This method was improved by Walther and Angelina Hesse the following year when gelatine (which often melted in the heat and was degraded by gelatinases produced by some bacteria) was replaced by agar (from the Malay word for jelly, *agar-agar*), a gelatinous material extracted from the cell walls of red algae and used successfully by Frau Hesse to set her jam. Agar is still the mainstay of solid microbiological media. Eventually, bacterial cultures were prepared in a special glass dish devised by Richard Julius Petri (1852–1921); today sterile plastic Petri dishes are a standard laboratory consumable.

Once methods had been developed to isolate and identify microbial pathogens, other methods were required to identify novel antimicrobial agents and new therapies were needed to treat these microbial infections. Two main areas of research were pursued: immunization and antimicrobial therapy.

Immunization and treatment of infection

At first, immunization was used to treat viral infections; this was long before the existence of viruses had been recognized. Variolation (inoculating fluid or crusts from smallpox lesions into the skin or mucosal surfaces) was used before the germ theory of disease was understood (see *Box 1.1*). This technique usually produced mild illness without complications and conferred life-long immunity, but between 1 and 2% of patients died because of infection. Variolation was practised successfully for centuries in India, Persia and China, but it was not until 1720 that Mary Wortley Montagu introduced it to the UK.

In a search to find a safer method than variolation, Edward Jenner, a physician, used local traditional knowledge to find a substitute. It was known that dairymaids infected with cowpox (a less virulent disease than smallpox) were immune to smallpox. In 1796, Jenner injected an eight-year-old boy with pus from cowpox blisters. He subsequently exposed him to smallpox; the boy did not contract the disease. Jenner repeated the experiment on other children, including his son; he concluded that vaccination with cowpox provided immunity to smallpox without the risks involved in variolation, and he published these findings in 1798.

Box 1.1 From variolation to vaccination

The history of vaccination has its origins in the fight against the viral disease smallpox. The last outbreak was in Yugoslavia in 1972 where 35 people died. The first epidemic of smallpox occurred in 1350 BC and spread from Africa to India and China via traders, reaching Europe between the fifth and seventh century. Millions died worldwide and the infection was rife in all European cities in the eighteenth century. Infection taken by the Spaniards to Mexico wiped out a large proportion of the native Aztecs and Incas. With a mortality rate of around 30%, 300 million people died worldwide in the twentieth century. If patients recovered, they were left with terrible scars from the pustules, but it was also realised that they were protected from the disease for the rest of their lives.

The first attempts to protect the population from the disease involved variolation, a practice recorded in China in the eleventh century. A Buddhist nun is credited with grinding up the scabs from an infected person and then blowing it into the nostrils of a non-infected person. Other practices included injecting the infected pus under the skin and in India, children were wrapped in the clothing of infected patients. Variolation was not without its risks, and about 2% died of variolated smallpox, a risk worth taking compared with the high mortality rate from the full-blown disease. Lady Mary Wortley Montagu, wife of the British Ambassador in Constantinople, had her own children inoculated and when she returned to Britain in 1718, eventually persuaded the Prince of Wales to have his children inoculated. The breakthrough came when Edward Jenner and others observed that cows suffered from a similar, but milder pustular disease, 'variolae vaccinae' and that the milkmaids who contracted the milder disease maintained their good complexions and were immune to smallpox. In 1796, Jenner inoculated James Phelps with fluid from cowpox pustules (the need for ethical approval was still a long time in the future). The boy recovered from cowpox and was subsequently inoculated with smallpox, which Jenner called the 'speckled monster'. No reaction occurred on that occasion, or when he was subsequently re-inoculated with smallpox a few months later.

Jenner's findings were initially rejected by the Royal Society. However, following the publication of his work in 1798, inoculation with cowpox was introduced. The word vaccination came into use and a series of laws between 1840 and 1871 made vaccination compulsory and free. The compulsion was withdrawn in 1948 and routine smallpox vaccination was administered until the 1970s. The last sporadic case was recorded in Somalia in 1977 and the disease was declared globally eradicated in 1980.

It was Pasteur who first developed methods for immunizing against bacterial infections and these were based on the ability to isolate and grow cultures in the laboratory and manipulate them. In 1885 Pasteur weakened bacteria by producing aged (old) cultures, and transferring them regularly to new culture media, a process called passaging. He used these 'attenuated' cultures to vaccinate animals against infections such as anthrax and rabies. Although at the time no one was aware of the viral nature of rabies, Pasteur managed to attenuate virus containing clinical tissue by air-drying the spinal marrow of 'rabid' rabbits. This material was eventually used to vaccinate animals, and finally human volunteers, previously bitten by rabid dogs. These developments also, remarkably, preceded detailed scientific understanding of the immune system. Today, vaccination using attenuated, killed or extracted fragments of pathogens is common practice in the control and prevention of disease. The UK vaccination programme ensures that children are vaccinated against the most serious infectious diseases. Global surveillance and cooperation in the development and implementation of vaccines has eradicated some of the most dangerous diseases, yet the challenge of tuberculosis, malaria and HIV, among others, still remains.

Development of antibiotics

Early in the twentieth century there were few treatments to fight bacterial infections. Prevention and, in a few cases, immunization were the main means of control. Researchers were constantly looking for effective antimicrobial agents, and one of these researchers was Paul Ehrlich, director of the newly formed Royal Institute of Experimental Therapy in Frankfurt. Ehrlich initially specialized in the differential staining of bacteria and from that work he speculated that chemicals may selectively target bacteria. He developed the discipline of chemotherapy (where therapeutic agents are derived from chemical reactions rather than being produced by natural agents), and in 1909 produced Salvarsan, an agent derived from arsenic and effective against syphilis. However, it was only in 2005 that the true structure of Salvarsan was established. Ehrlich's work on chemotherapeutic agents was very important because it stimulated research leading to the development of sulfa-drugs, penicillin and other antibiotics.

In 1928 Alexander Fleming discovered an antibacterial factor in the exudate of the *Penicillium notatum* mould and in the 1930s sulphonamide drugs were discovered. These sulphonamide drugs offered a wide range of antibacterial activity. It was not, however, until 1941 that penicillin, purified by Howard Florey and Ernst Chain, was tested on humans. Driven by a need for a potent antimicrobial agent to treat troops in World War II, the mass production of penicillin took place in 1943.

In 1941, Selman Waksman was first to use the term 'antibiotic' to describe antibacterial drugs that were derived from living organisms. In 1944, Waksman's group discovered streptomycin, the first aminoglycoside antibiotic; this is produced naturally by the soil organism *Streptomyces griseus*. Streptomycin's main importance at the time was that it was the first anti-tuberculous drug. Other novel antibiotics such as chloramphenicol and tetracycline followed in the late 1940s, heralding a new age for antibiotic discovery.

The methods eventually used to test for antibiotic activity had been established before the discovery of antibiotics, as they had been developed to test for disinfectant activity. This followed the success of Lister and Pasteur in convincing surgeons of the importance of hygiene and disinfectants in reducing post-operative infections. Pasteur, Koch and others had already described methods for determining *in vitro* antibiosis (the antagonistic association between organisms where one of the organisms is killed, or between one organism and a chemical produced by another). They had developed the use of test tubes containing broth for determination of growth inhibition, tests for measuring the loss of motility, and animal protection studies. This was all before the discovery of antibiotics. The now commonly used agar diffusion test was first described by Beijerinck in 1889. In this test, the antimicrobial agent is placed on a lawn of newly inoculated bacteria, the plate incubated overnight and then examined for a zone of inhibition or clearing around the agent. Beijerinck was studying the effect of different auxins (plant growth regulators) on bacterial growth and in these first tests a trough or well was cut into the agar and filled with the agent. In 1940 Heatley introduced the use of filter paper discs carrying varying antimicrobial concentrations; the 6 mm filter paper discs still used today were first described by Bondi and co-workers in 1947.

Significant dates in the history of microbiology are shown in *Table 1.3*.

Table 1.3 Significant dates in the history of microbiology

Developments in medical microbiology	Date
Theory of spontaneous generation	350 BC–1500 AD
Direct spread of infection – syphilis	1530
Microscopy – Hooke and van Leeuwenhoek	1650
Theory of spontaneous generation rebutted in relation to flies	1688
Beginnings of vaccination – Jenner and cowpox	1796
First description of a microbe-causing disease	1835
Lister and antiseptics	1870
Pasteur's germ theory refutes spontaneous generation for microbes	1857
Koch's isolates – pure bacterial cultures	1877
Koch's postulates	1884
Ehrlich lays ground for chemotherapy – dyes kill bacteria	1885
Beijerinck first showed viruses may be infective agents	1899
Ehrlich discovers Salvarsan for treating syphilis – first chemotherapeutic agent (arsenic base)	1910
Fleming discovers an antibacterial factor from penicillium mould	1928
Waksman discovers streptomycin and first uses the term 'antibiotic'	1941–44
Luria shows bacteria can produce spontaneous mutations – beginnings of molecular microbiology	1943
New antibiotics introduced, including streptomycin, chloramphenicol and tetracycline, and the age of antibiotic chemotherapy	1940–1950
First penicillin-resistant staphylococci detected	1946

1.4   KOCH'S POSTULATES AND APPLICATION TO MODERN PATTERNS OF INFECTION

Koch's postulates are summarized in *Box 1.2*. Koch had been working on TB as well as anthrax and cholera; the work that led to the publication of the postulates in 1884 was based on anthrax, caused by *Bacillus anthracis*. The disease mainly affects grazing animals in endemic countries after they ingest the anthrax spores from the grass – the spores vegetate into bacteria and release lethal toxins. Anthrax is transmitted to humans by contact with spores from an infected animal or animal product, for example skin or hide. Humans can contract the disease by inoculation, inhalation or ingestion. Koch was able to demonstrate that bacteria taken from the infected animal

---

Box 1.2 Koch's postulates

1. The suspected causal organism must be present in every case of the disease and absent in healthy individuals.
2. The suspected causal organism must be isolated in pure culture from an infected animal and grown in artificial media.
3. When a healthy susceptible host is inoculated with the pathogen from pure culture the same or a similar disease must develop.
4. The same pathogen must be re-isolated in pure culture from animals infected under experimental conditions.

The first three rules for experimental proof of the pathogenicity of an organism were presented in 1883 by Robert Koch; the fourth was added by E.F. Smith (1905).

could be isolated in pure culture. Bacteria taken from the pure culture and inoculated into a susceptible host produced the symptoms of the disease. Furthermore, bacteria taken from the second host could again be isolated in pure culture.

Even in the late nineteenth century, Koch realized some limitations of his postulates, particularly the first one. For example, although he could isolate *Vibrio cholerae* from both sick and healthy people, he could not culture the bacteria that caused leprosy, although the symptoms were obvious. The culture of *Mycobacterium leprae* remains a challenge, and no medium has yet been developed to culture *Treponema pallidum*, the causative agent of syphilis. Other limitations of the postulates include:

- Asymptomatic carriage of pathogenic bacteria in healthy individuals.
- Viruses do not cause symptomatic infection in everyone who is infected.
- Nucleic acid based methods detect the presence of agents not yet cultured *in vitro*, for example ribosomal RNA analysis of mouth flora indicates many as yet unidentified bacteria.
- Some infections are polymicrobial; a deep abscess for example, containing species of anaerobic bacteria that are interdependent and difficult to grow as pure cultures.

Probably the most significant limitation encountered today is the recognition of opportunistic infection, where a bacterium, virus, fungus or protozoan pathogen is completely harmless to one individual but may cause serious and life-threatening disease in another, usually because the latter has some degree of suppression of their immune system.

Opportunistic infections do not fulfil Koch's postulates and are often caused by low pathogenicity microorganisms from the patient's own resident population of normal flora. The relationship between potential infectious disease-causing microorganisms and the host is important, as this host–pathogen relationship is dynamic and a small shift in the status of either can affect the outcome. From the pathogen's viewpoint the advantage can be gained if there is unexpected access to tissues that were not previously available, via a cut, a bite or the entrance site of a plastic tube for the administration of drugs, or by the sheer numbers present. The host will have an advantage against infectious agents if they have a well functioning immune system, and if that immune system has been primed against the agent by vaccination or by previous infection. If the hosts are hospitalized, undergoing treatment with toxic drugs (for example chemotherapy), have underlying serious illness or have had an operation or traumatic injury, they are more vulnerable to infection from the external environment as well as their own flora.

Host–pathogen relationships and the development of symptomatic infectious disease are developed further in *Chapter 4*.

1.5   THE SCOPE OF MEDICAL MICROBIOLOGY

The majority of interactions between hosts and potential pathogens are uneventful and do not result in symptomatic illness. The number of these interactions is, of course, impossible to assess, but can be likened to an iceberg. Because of previous encounters, strong immune reactions, or small numbers of pathogens, the broad base of the iceberg represents non-symptomatic or previously immune patients. Then there are those who are infected, suffer self-limiting mild infection and recover. The tip of the iceberg represents the individuals who have symptomatic disease that causes them to seek clinical advice. Clinical specimens are then sent to the hospital laboratory for microbiological diagnosis.

The investigations selected to identify a pathogen are guided by the clinical information given by the requesting doctor and the type of specimen received. The range of specimens is relatively broad; it could be sputum for a lung problem, blood to test for antibodies, a urine or stool specimen, or pus from an abscess, all of which will have been collected in sterile, specialized swabs or containers and sent to the laboratory. Whole blood, which, in a healthy person, should be devoid of microorganisms, can also be tested for the presence of bacteria or fungi by culturing the blood in specialized media bottles using an automated continuous monitoring system over a period of days, to investigate the possibility of systemic infection and septicaemia. Similar types of specimens are grouped together and tested in a specialized area of the laboratory, as described in *Chapter 7*.

- Depending on the type of specimen it may be appropriate and informative for microscopic examination to be performed and/or a macroscopic description to be recorded. If culture is requested, the specimen is inoculated onto appropriate selective and non-selective media.
- For investigations into the presence of antibodies to a specific antigen, the serum is separated from the cells and tested. Individual investigations are detailed and explained throughout the following chapters.
- For all specimens requiring bacterial culture, differential and selective media are used, to supply the correct nutrients for the bacteria of interest to grow into visible colonies, and various chemical agents within the media will differentiate and distinguish any pathogens from the normal body flora.
- Normally after overnight incubation, the specimen plates are examined and a provisional identification made.
- At this point further identification tests may be carried out (Gram stain, biochemical tests for sugar utilization, tests for enzyme production, and genetic or immunological tests). These are normally carried out in conjunction with antimicrobial susceptibility tests to guide treatment options. Once an appropriate antimicrobial is identified, patient treatment is commenced or reassessed on the basis of the laboratory results.

The initial bacterial cultures may not always identify a significant cause of the patient's symptoms. If their symptoms persist, further samples are taken and retested for the initial pathogens and/or further investigations are requested to assist the diagnosis.

SUGGESTED FURTHER READING

Brooks, G.F., Carroll, K.C., Butel, J.S., & Morse, S.A. (2007) *Jawetz, Melnick, & Adelberg's Medical Microbiology*, 24th edn. McGraw-Hill Medical.

Goering, R., Dockrell, H., Zuckerman, M. & Wakelin, D. (2007) *Mims' Medical Microbiology*, 4th edn. Mosby.

Winn, W., Allen, S., Janda, W. *et al.* (2005) *Koneman's Color Atlas and Textbook of Diagnostic Microbiology*, 6th edn. Lippincott Williams and Wilkins.

Full taxonomy on most species can be found at http://www.ncbi.nlm.nih.gov/sites/entrez?db=Taxonomy

SELF-ASSESSMENT QUESTIONS

1. Infectious disease was a common cause of early death for many centuries, but its origin and modes of transmission were not understood. Briefly discuss the discoveries that helped to finally link microorganisms to disease.
2. Outline five differences between prokaryotic and eukaryotic cells.
3. Given that Salmon discovered the genus *Salmonella*, Neisser, *Neisseria* and Pasteur, *Pasteurella*, how would a bacterium discovered by you be named? There are several species of these bacteria; one species affects the blood, another causes enteric infection and a third species only infects the skin. Suggest some Latin species names for them.
4. Describe some simple phenotypic tests that can be carried out easily within the laboratory to attempt to identify an unknown bacterium growing on a culture plate.
5. Define species and strains in relation to microorganisms.

Answers to self-assessment questions provided at:
www.scionpublishing.com/medmicro

Structure and physiology of microorganisms associated with human disease

Learning objectives
After studying this chapter you should confidently be able to:

■ **Discuss the structural similarities and differences between the major groups of prokaryotic and eukaryotic microorganisms associated with humans**
Bacteria are prokaryotic single cell microorganisms ranging from 0.1 to 2 µm in diameter and up to 10 µm in length, with cell walls that can be distinguished by the Gram stain. They can be further classified by their shape and cellular arrangements, their ability to move, the presence of a capsule and the production of endospores and toxins. Bacteria are visible by light microscopy, whereas viruses are visible only by electron microscopy because of their small size, 0.03–0.3 µm. Eukaryotic cells (which range in size from 10–100 µm diameter), including human cells, have membrane-bound organelles and a nuclear membrane. Eukaryotes associated with human infection include some protozoa and fungi, and also helminths (worms and flukes).

■ **Discuss the physiological processes of bacteria, protozoa, fungi and helminths in relation to their ability to survive and grow in natural environments and adapt to life within human hosts**
Bacteria display characteristic cell growth and reproduction cycles, as well as protein synthesis, anabolic and catabolic processes, depending upon the nutrients available in the environment. Some bacteria have the ability to form endospores when resources are limited. Within the human body they are often stressed by nutrient availability and by the pressure of the immune system, yet adapt and survive through the expression of gene products used for protection, for example capsules and toxins. Protozoa often have life cycles that include human and other hosts, e.g. mammals and mosquitoes, in addition to environmentally safe cyst forms. The protozoa responsible for malaria and sleeping sickness are transmitted by mosquitoes and flies and examples of the latter are the cysts of *Cryptosporidia* and *Giardia lamblia*. The life cycles of parasitic helminths are often complex and can involve several hosts for the larval and developmental stage and a final host for the adult parasite. In some infections, man is an accidental host as a result of eating infected meat, e.g. tapeworms, or through environmental contact, for example water containing snails infected with schistosomes, leading to bilharzia.

■ **Explain how knowledge of microbial physiology and growth requirements has enabled the development of a range of *in vitro* diagnostic methods**
Knowledge and understanding of bacterial growth curves, temperature, atmosphere, nutrients and metabolic pathways have led to the development

of *in vitro* culture media to provide all these requirements. The presence of surface antigens enables specific serology tests to be carried out. Protozoa can often be diagnosed from blood films, by the use of specific stains, e.g. cysts present in faeces, urine or tissue. Characteristic fungal growth can be observed on specific culture media and identification of fungal structure achieved by microscopy. Helminths can be diagnosed by the presence of adult forms either within, or when expelled from, humans, e.g. the identification of ova from faeces, urine or biopsy material. Knowledge of the genomes of all these microorganisms has led to the application of specific diagnostic molecular methods.

■ **Discuss how knowledge of structure, function and physiology informs the development of a range of therapeutic options to treat human infections caused by bacteria, protozoa and helminths**
Bacterial structure and to some extent fungal structure provides sites of selective toxicity. The principle is that pathogenic cells are targeted, with minimal effect on human tissue. A relatively wide range of antibacterial drugs are available compared to antiviral therapy. Knowledge of the life cycle, structure and physiology aids in the development of protozoan treatments; however, not all have a treatment option. Similarly, treatment for helminth infections is guided by an understanding of the life cycle of the individual pathogen.

The purpose of this chapter is to explain why it is important to develop an understanding of the ways in which the structure and physiology of microorganisms affect not only their ability to survive and reproduce in human hosts, but how they influence the development of the methods used to isolate them and subsequently treat the infections they cause. Without this knowledge and understanding diagnostic microbiology would be ineffective and it is so embedded in practice that it is rarely questioned. Questions that may be asked include, 'Why do cultures for *Campylobacter* species need to be incubated in micro-aerophilic conditions?'; 'Why are gonococci so fastidious and why do *Haemophilus influenzae* prefer chocolate agar?', and 'What is it that makes some cultures of pneumococci look so glossy and others look dry?'

Despite all the advances in culture media development, one of the oldest human bacterial pathogens, the causative agent of syphilis, *Treponema pallidum,* cannot be cultured, and detection relies on the measurement of the body's antibody response to infection, or visualization of the bacteria from the primary lesion. New pathogens are constantly emerging and the challenge to understand them and develop accurate diagnostic and treatment options is ongoing. At the same time a greater understanding of the genetic code of microorganisms has enabled highly specific molecular methods to be brought into current practice. It is beyond the scope of one chapter to describe all the structural aspects, growth and physiology of the major groups of microorganisms in detail, but it is possible to contextualize these aspects in relation to the diagnostic microbiology discussed in further chapters. The prokaryotes include bacteria and archaea; since the latter are only found in extreme environments and not as human pathogens, they are not covered.

Viruses infect all types of organisms from animals and plants to bacteria and archaea. They rely on living host cells for their replication, as their simple structures include only their nucleic acid, a protein coat and in some cases, an envelope.

They are considerably smaller than bacteria, ranging in size from 20 to 300 nm (1 nm = 10^{-3} μm), and are beyond the resolution of the light microscope. They are obligate intracellular parasites, relying on their host cells for the ribosomes on which to reproduce their proteins and host raw materials to reproduce their genetic material and proteins. Viruses contain either RNA or DNA and this provides one of the criteria by which they are classified. Replication of their genomic material takes place in either the nucleus or cytoplasm of the host cell: RNA in the cytoplasm, DNA in the nucleus. *Chapter 3* describes their structure, replication, diagnosis and treatment in detail. Viruses, in common with other microorganisms, are the cause of disease in a variety of different body sites, as they are tropic for specific cell types.

2.1 PROKARYOTES: BACTERIA

Bacteria form a group of diverse and well adapted single-cell organisms that evolved over three billion years ago as the earth's surface cooled and water formed. Bacteria, sometimes referred to as eubacteria, contain all the human disease-causing bacteria and most of the bacteria found in soil, water, animals and other environments. They are prokaryotes: single-cell organisms that lack a nucleus and membrane-bound organelles within the cytoplasm.

Bacterial cells are remarkably versatile cells. They can respond and adapt to external environmental changes such as temperature, pH and oxygen levels. They have the ability to transport macromolecules across their cell membrane, break them down into smaller components and use them to create new bacterial cell components. Furthermore they are able to adapt from their natural environment to the very different conditions they encounter within a human host. They are abundant in nature and have essential roles in agriculture, sewage breakdown, the food industry and the pharmaceutical and chemical industries. In nature, groups of related bacteria live in specific niches and habitats and can associate with other microbial communities where they form ecosystems for their mutual benefit. There is also competition for nutrients and relationships can be antagonistic, involving the production of toxins and antibiotics. The appearance of humans expanded the habitats and many bacteria now live in microbial communities on the mucosal surfaces of the human body, forming the normal flora. For others, their encounter with a human host is not of mutual benefit and infection and disease result.

Shape, size and cell structure

Bacteria are the smallest free-living organisms, ranging in size from 0.1 to 10 μm (there are 1000 μm in 1 mm) and visible using light microscopy. Cells can be viewed either stained or unstained, but generally as part of the identification process they are stained prior to viewing under the ×100 oil immersion lens. The Gram stain, described further in *Chapter 5*, is commonly used because it distinguishes not only shape and size but gives an indication of the cell wall structure by the retention or not of the first stain, crystal violet. Gram-positive cell walls retain the crystal violet as their structure is less porous and contains more peptidoglycan than the Gram-negative cell walls.

The shape of the cells can be spherical or slightly ovoid, called coccus (singular) or cocci (plural). They can also be straight or slightly curved rods or bacilli (bacillus in the singular). Sometimes the bacteria form very short rods and are called coccobacilli. Fusiform bacilli have tapered ends. Other bacteria are curved and can be short curved rods or bacilli, for example the *Vibrio* species that cause cholera. Spiral shaped bacteria are spirilla (spirillum in the singular) if they are rigid cells, and spirochaetes if they are flexible and capable of movement. *Figure 2.1* shows these shapes, with examples of relevant bacteria.

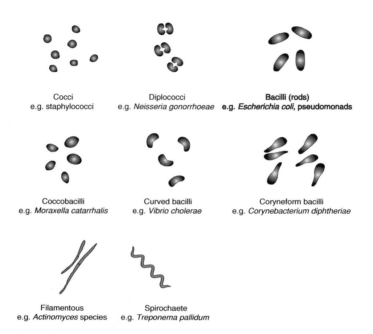

Cocci	Diplococci	**Bacilli (rods)**
e.g. staphylococci	e.g. *Neisseria gonorrhoeae*	**e.g. *Escherichia coli*, pseudomonads**

Coccobacilli	Curved bacilli	Coryneform bacilli
e.g. *Moraxella catarrhalis*	e.g. *Vibrio cholerae*	e.g. *Corynebacterium diphtheriae*

Filamentous	Spirochaete
e.g. *Actinomyces* species	e.g. *Treponema pallidum*

Figure 2.1
Different shapes of bacteria. Bacteria can be visualized by light microscopy, usually in Gram-stained preparations. The morphology (shape) of the cells, along with the Gram reaction, can give some indication of the identity of the cells. Staphylococci are Gram-positive cocci, as are streptococci. *Escherichia coli* are Gram-negative rods, while *Neisseria* species are Gram-negative diplococci. The spirochaete *Treponema pallidum* would only be seen directly from clinical samples because no culture medium has been developed that would support its growth. *Campylobacter* species are examples of spirilla.

When individual bacteria divide they sometimes stay together in pairs, chains or clusters and so form larger cell arrangements. Because many Gram stain preparations are made from colonies formed on solid culture media these arrangements can be disrupted as they are spread on to the glass slide, whereas preparations made from liquid cultures require less manipulation and will often demonstrate the arrangements more clearly, particularly in the case of streptococcal chains. Examples of these arrangements are shown in *Figure 2.2*.

A typical bacterial cell consists of:

■   the cell wall
■   a variety of structures external to the cell wall (which are present in some bacteria but not all), such as flagellae, pili, fimbriae and capsules

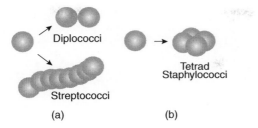

Figure 2.2
Cellular arrangements of two characteristic Gram-positive cocci. (a) shows division of streptococci in a single plane as they divide into diplococci and then continue to divide along the same plane to form chains. (b) shows staphylococci dividing in two planes to form tetrads. As they carry on dividing they form clumps resembling bunches of grapes. These arrangements are more readily observed when the bacteria are growing in liquid culture medium and have not been disrupted when the Gram stain is prepared from solid culture medium.

■ the structures inside the cell wall such as the plasma membrane and the cytoplasm containing the bacterial chromosome
■ any additional genetic material such as plasmids, along with ribosomes and storage granules.

Additionally, some bacteria are capable of forming spores and these may be visible within the cell.

Cell walls

Bacterial cell walls are either thick and made up of many layers of peptidoglycan or much thinner, comprising a more complex membrane structure. This difference is exploited by the Gram stain and so this often provides the first clues to the identification of an unknown bacterium isolated from a clinical specimen. This is particularly the case when the bacteria are in a liquid, such as a blood culture or joint fluid, and so there are no visible bacterial colonies on a culture medium to aid identification. The principal component in the Gram stain is crystal violet, and this is retained in the Gram-positive cell wall but washed out of the Gram-negative cell wall (see *Chapter 5*). A counterstain is then used to provide Gram-negative cells with a pink colour for easy microscopic identification. The retention, or not, of the stain is directly related to the structure and permeability of the bacterial cell walls: Gram-positive cell walls tend to be thick and contain many layers of peptidoglycan, whereas Gram-negative cell walls are thinner but more complex in structure. Some of the major differences between the two types of cell walls are summarized in *Table 2.1*.

Gram-positive cell walls. Peptidoglycan has a basic structure of two sugar derivatives, *N*-acetyl glucosamine and *N*-acetyl muramic acid. Together they form a repeating structure called a glycan tetrapeptide, linked by β1–4 linkages (see *Figure 2.3*). These linkages can be broken down by the enzyme lysosyme present in human tears and other secretions, providing some protection against Gram-positive bacteria. The layers are further cross-linked with tetrapeptides, which are characteristic for different bacteria, in order to form a rigid mesh-like structure around the cell. In

Table 2.1 A summary of the differences between Gram-positive and Gram-negative cell walls

Component/characteristic	Gram-positive cell wall	Gram-negative cell wall
Peptidoglycan	Thick layer	Thin layer
Teichoic acid and lipoteichoic acid	Present	Absent
Lipids	Very little	Lipopolysaccharide (LPS) containing lipid A
Outer membrane	Absent	Present
Toxins	Exotoxins excreted from cell	Endotoxin component of cell wall + exotoxins excreted from cell
Periplasmic space	Not significant	Site of β-lactamase activity + breakdown of macromolecules
Susceptibility to antibiotics	More susceptible, with exceptions e.g. MRSA	Generally less susceptible to antibiotics and disinfectants
Survival	Survive well in dry environments	Survive well in moist environments and within the human digestive system

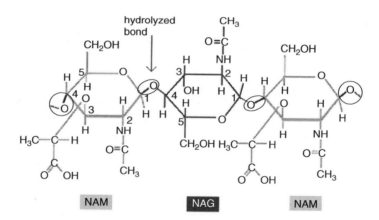

β (1➔4) glycosidic bonds circled

Figure 2.3
The structure of peptidoglycan, joined by β1–4 glycosidic bonds. NAG, *N*-acetyl muramic acid; NAM, *N*-acetyl glucosamine.

Gram-positive bacteria the cross-linking involves a peptide interbridge; for example, in *Staphylococcus aureus* this bridge consists of five molecules of the amino acid glycine connected by peptide bonds.

The thick layer of peptidoglycan in Gram-positive cell walls provides rigidity and prevents the bacteria rupturing during changes in osmotic pressure; it is also porous enough to allow diffusion of molecules in and out of the cell. It protects the cell within the human body because, in conjunction with other structural components, it can interfere with phagocytosis of the bacteria by neutrophils. The thick layer of peptidoglycan makes it harder for the membrane attack complex formed by the complement proteins to penetrate the cell wall. At the same time it stimulates the immune system and is pyrogenic (causes a rise in body temperature). The structure of the Gram-positive cell wall is shown in *Figure 2.4*. Lipoteichoic acid and teichoic acid, glycerol-containing acids, protrude outwards from the cell wall beyond the peptidoglycan layer, and help bacteria attach to host cells. Teichoic acid goes some way into the peptidoglycan layer, whereas lipoteichoic acid links to lipids in the plasma membrane.

The plasma membrane, a phospholipid bilayer, provides a semi-permeable barrier between the cell wall and the cytoplasm of the cell. Proteins are also present in the cell wall and plasma membrane and are involved in transport of molecules, enzymic activity and, on the cell surface, specific proteins may have a pathogenic role. Examples of this are found in the M proteins of Group A streptococcus and protein A on the surface of *Staphylococcus aureus*.

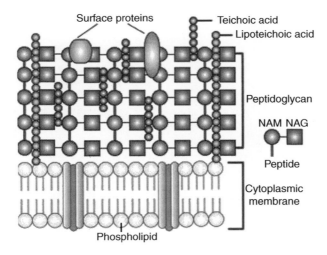

Figure 2.4
The structure of the Gram-positive cell wall. It consists of a cytoplasmic membrane, a thick layer of peptidoglycan containing teichoic acid and lipoteichoic acid. The outer surface also contains proteins. NAM, *N*-acetyl muramic acid; NAG, *N*-acetyl glucosamine.

Gram-negative cell walls. The Gram-negative cell wall, shown in *Figure 2.5*, has two membranes, the inner and outer membranes, a thin layer of peptidoglycan and a periplasmic space. The peptidoglycan is anchored to the outer membrane by lipoproteins. The outer membrane of Gram-negative cells and the periplasmic space are important features as they determine some of the pathogenic effects on host cells and the susceptibility of these bacteria to antibiotics. The outer membrane forms a permeability barrier to large molecules, such as lysozyme, and provides protection from adverse conditions, such as those found in the human digestive system. The

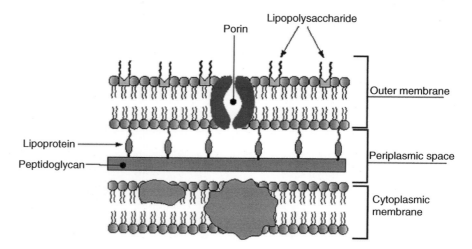

Figure 2.5
The structure of the Gram-negative cell wall, consisting of an inner and outer membrane. The outer membrane has lipopolysaccharide embedded into its structure. When the cell dies, lipid A is released from the LPS and has a toxic effect upon the human host. The periplasmic space contains the peptidoglycan layers and enzymes for the breakdown of macromolecules before they cross the inner cell membrane.

principal bacterial pathogens of the human gastrointestinal system are Gram-negative (see *Chapter 9*).

The outer membrane is a phospholipid membrane with a characteristic outer layer consisting of an amphipathic lipopolysaccharide (LPS) molecule called endotoxin. The presence of endotoxin in the host is a powerful stimulator of the immune response, leading to fever and, if present in large quantities, septic shock and multi-organ failure. LPS has three structural components, shown in *Figure 2.6*:

■ lipid A, embedded in the membrane and protruding from the cell
■ the core oligosaccharide which is branched and contains 9–12 sugars including the unusual sugar 2 keto-3-deoxy-octanate (KDO); this core region is constant for a species of bacteria

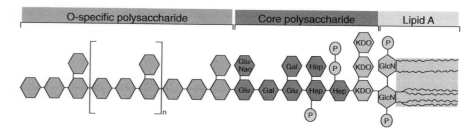

Figure 2.6
The structure of lipopolysaccharide. The lipid A is embedded in the outer membrane of the Gram-negative cell wall. The O specific polysaccharide varies in length in different genera of bacteria, and is antigenic. Different types of O antigen can be identified by using specific antisera.

■ the outer part of LPS, which is a long linear polysaccharide containing 50–100 repeating saccharide units of 4–7 sugars per unit. This is known as the O antigen and can be used to serotype bacterial species (*Salmonella* bacteria have up to 2000 different serotypes; the typing and significance of this are discussed in *Chapter 8*).

When bacteria die the lipid A is released from the cells as they lyse, and has toxic effects upon the host. Humans are very sensitive to the presence of lipid A and respond by releasing chemical messengers called cytokines that raise the body temperature and facilitate the movement of effector cells such as neutrophils to the site of infection by allowing them to move from the blood vessels to the tissues to engulf (phagocytose) the bacteria. The complement protein cascade is also stimulated to attack the bacterial cell membranes. This is the normal immune response to infection. However, these activities can become harmful to the host if large amounts of lipid A are present and the immune system becomes overstimulated with high levels of circulating cytokines. The relaxed blood vessels allow egress of immune cells to the extent that they are no longer able to maintain their usual tension, resulting in a situation called hypovolaemic shock. If vital organs are deprived of oxygen and nutrients for a period of time, multi-organ failure and death may occur (see *Chapter 12* in relation to septic shock). This underlines the importance of diagnosing Gram-negative septicaemia in the laboratory as quickly as possible and also the importance of a good antibiotic prescribing policy to ensure that the treatment is targeted and effective.

Porin proteins are present as channels in the outer membrane, with up to 10^5 per cell, allowing selective transport of metabolites across the membrane. They are more permeable to hydrophilic molecules and less permeable to hydrophobic molecules. Many antibiotic molecules are hydrophobic in nature and thus less effective in Gram-negative bacteria. Additionally, the bacteria can alter the shape of the porin channels and use efflux pumps to eliminate antibiotic molecules. Thus, Gram-negative bacteria are less susceptible to antibiotics than many Gram-positive cells. Braun's lipoprotein links the outer membrane to the peptidoglycan in the periplasmic space.

The periplasmic space contains periplasm (a gel containing the peptidoglycan) and a range of enzymes including proteases, phosphatases, lipases, nucleases and carbohydrate-degrading enzymes for the breakdown of macromolecules prior to their transfer across the inner membrane to the cell cytoplasm. There are also components of chemotaxis sytems used to sense the environment outside the cell. The periplasmic space of pathogenic bacteria also contains virulence factors, enzymes to break down tissue, and often enzymes called β-lactamases, which are used to break down the structure of the β-lactam ring found in penicillin. If antibiotic molecules containing the β-lactam structure are to be effective in the majority of Gram-negative bacteria, they need to be protected by additional chemical structures.

Acid-fast cell walls. These are so called because they contain high levels of wax and resist decolorization with acid alcohol during the acid-fast staining procedure. The acid-fast staining technique uses carbol fuchsin as the initial dye. This is retained, giving positive cells a red appearance. In addition to Gram-positive and Gram-negative cell walls there are a group of bacteria, notable among them being the Mycobacteria (the causative organisms of tuberculosis and leprosy) that have variable amounts of a waxy lipid called mycolic acid in their cell walls. Mycobacteria are classified as Gram-positive, but the lipid-rich cell wall makes the bacteria hydrophobic and resistant not only to laboratory stains but also to disinfectants. The cell wall structure is also responsible for the slow growth characteristics of these bacteria and their resistance to many antibiotics. For this reason, careful consideration must be given to the choice of disinfectant used in areas of the laboratory where contamination with Mycobacteria species is a possibility. The structure of the cell wall is shown in *Figure 2.7*.

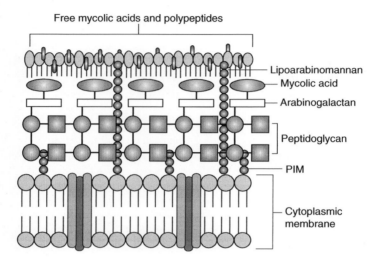

Figure 2.7
The structure of an acid-fast cell wall. The extra layers of mycolic acid, lipoarabinomannan and arabinogalactan in the Gram-positive cell wall structure make the cell wall less permeable to nutrients, and consequently slower-growing. Acid-fast (ZN) or fluorescent stains are used to distinguish these bacteria.

Bacterial cells without walls. *Mycoplasma* and *Ureaplasma* bacteria are the smallest free-living bacteria and are unique because they do not have a cell wall. The absence of a cell wall means that they are resistant to any of the antibiotics that target the cell wall. Their cell membranes contain sterols and they can be cultured on special culture media containing animal sterols. In contrast, L forms (named after the Lister Institute, where early work was carried out on L forms) or spheroplasts are bacterial cells without walls which are, however, capable of forming cell walls under appropriate growth conditions. L form bacteria can either be unstable, with the ability to revert to the production of a cell wall, or stable and unable to revert. L forms can be generated in the laboratory; for example, *Escherichia coli* or *Bacillus subtilis* can be treated with antibiotics that remove the cell wall, and then they can be maintained in an isotonic solution. The role of the L forms *in vivo* is not fully understood; however, it is believed that L forms produced in response to cell wall antibiotic treatment could live inside cells of the immune system, particularly macrophages, and lead to chronic infection.

The glycocalyx – capsules and slime layers
The glycocalyx is found on the outside of the cell wall and is a sticky, sugary layer composed of polysaccharides or polypeptides produced within the cytoplasm and

secreted to the outside of the cell. If these molecules are loosely attached to the cell they are called a slime layer; if they are attached to the cell surface to produce a tight fitting structure around the cell, this is called a capsule. A capsule/slime layer offers protection from the host immune system and also provides a means of attaching to host cells. Because they are hydrophilic (water-loving), capsules also protect the cell from drying out and act as a barrier to hydrophobic molecules. The slime layer can allow bacteria to adhere to the conditioning pellicle, a biofilm already present on the surface of teeth, composed of salivary proteins and bacterial products. Other bacteria then attach to the first layer until there is a complex mixture of bacteria on the tooth surface. If this is not regularly removed by brushing, there is a build-up of plaque and subsequent tooth decay. The expression of the glycocalyx is under genetic control and is influenced by signals from outside the cell, so it is not necessary to express the structures all the time and resources can be preserved.

Capsules are associated with virulence and successful pathogens such as *Staphylococcus aureus* and *Streptococcus pyogenes*, which cause a wide range of infections in a variety of body sites, and *Neisseria meningitidis,* the cause of meningitis, all express a capsule during the infection process. Early experiments demonstrated that the bacteria commonly associated with pneumonia, *Streptococcus pneumoniae*, was only able to cause the disease in mice if they were injected with the capsulated (smooth) form rather than the non-capsulated (rough) form. Without the capsule the bacteria could not survive in the presence of the components of the immune system. When grown on culture media in the laboratory, capsulated organisms will have a shiny, glossy appearance, whereas those not expressing the capsule will be drier in appearance. After growing safely on laboratory media for some time there is no need to express the capsule. Some bacteria such as *Streptococcus pneumoniae* and *Klebsiella* species have very thick capsules, giving them a very obvious capsulated presence, whereas the microcapsules of other bacteria are much thinner. Capsules can be visualized under the light microscope – either by using a negative stain such as nigrosin, which stains the background and shows the capsules as haloes around the cells (see *Section 5.4*), or a Gram stain when they are seen as clear areas around the cell after staining. Because the capsules do not take up any stain, using Indian ink to stain the background and crystal violet to stain the cells demonstrates the clear area of the surrounding capsule well.

Because capsules are such effective virulence factors and stimulate the host immune response, they make excellent vaccines. They are known as subunit vaccines because the relevant antigens of the capsule are extracted from the cells and then incorporated into the vaccine formulation. Successful examples of this are the *Haemophilus influenzae* vaccine (Hib), the pneumococcal vaccine and the meningitis C vaccine, all of which are included in the UK childhood vaccination schedule. There are exceptions, where capsular constituents are present on human cells and therefore are not seen as foreign. Before the advent of antibiotic treatment, patients frequently developed rheumatic fever after Group A streptococcal infections, because antibodies raised against the hyaluronic acid in the capsule cross-reacted with and damaged heart muscle.

Pili and fimbriae
Pili (singular pilus) and fimbriae are hair-like filaments, composed of the protein pilin, located on the surface of many Gram-negative bacteria. They are involved in

adherence of the bacterium to host cell surfaces, where they bind to lectins such as mannose, and they play an important role in the infection process. Fimbriae are crucial in the adhesion of *Neisseria gonorrhoeae* to epithelial cells. Good adhesion is vital in the establishment of urinary infection with *Escherichia coli* to avoid the flushing action of the urinary flow.

Pili have several functions, including adhesion, evasion of the immune system, movement and transfer of genetic material. Pili can be expressed during the process of an infection. The pathogenic *Escherichia coli* O157 expresses bundle-forming pili which attach to intestinal epithelial cells prior to forming a secretion system that injects proteins into the cell. Pili on cell surfaces allow a gliding or twitching movement across the surface of the cells after initial contact, by retracting the pili. The pili of *Neisseria gonorrhoeae* have the capability to change their antigenic expression by gene rearrangement and protein expression. This means that antibodies raised by the immune system to the pilin protein are no longer effective against the newly expressed proteins and the process of developing antibodies has to start again.

Flagellae

Flagellae are long thin appendages that originate from the cytoplasmic membrane and extend through the cell wall into the surrounding medium. They allow bacterial movement; bacteria possessing flagellae are described as motile and are able to move towards nutrient sources by a process called chemotaxis. They are also able to move away from harmful substances by repulsion. Bacteria are further described by the position of their single flagellum or multiple flagellae, whether they are at one end of the cell, at both ends or covering the cell (see *Figure 2.8*). Flagellae are composed of a protein called flagellin which is transported from inside the cell through the filament to the end of the flagella. The structure and movement of flagellae are remarkable in terms of design and effect, enabling movement of the single-cell bacterium at a rate of up to 60 lengths a second, which is faster than the movement of a cheetah. Each flagellum consists of three sections: the motor, called the basal body, the hook

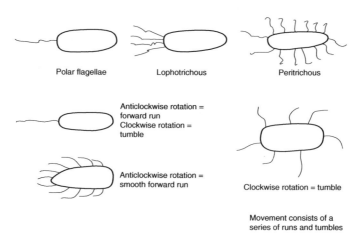

Figure 2.8
Position and movement direction of flagellae in motile bacteria.

and the filament. The basal body is anchored in the cytoplasmic membrane and cell wall and consists of a rod passing through a series of rings, three in Gram-negative bacteria (LPS, peptidoglycan and cytoplasmic membrane) and two in Gram-positive bacteria because there is no LPS. Proteins on either side of the basal body drive the motor and act as switches. The energy that drives the motor is provided by proton motive force, in which protons are moved across the membrane into the cytoplasm, 1000 protons being required for each rotation of the filament. If the flagellae are at the ends of the bacterium the resultant movement will be spinning in a clockwise or anticlockwise action. Bacteria covered with flagellae (called peritrichous bacteria) can move in a tumbling way, with clockwise rotation, which takes them in a straight line, or smooth swimming with anticlockwise rotation of the flagellae. Movement is usually made up of a random number of runs and tumbles.

The flagellae can also be involved in pathogenesis, allowing bacterial movement towards a surface for attachment, and also enabling them to cross hostile areas. *Helicobacter pylori* are Gram-negative curved bacteria with polar flagellae, now recognized as the cause of stomach ulcers. The bacteria need to survive in the acidic environment of the stomach and move through the mucous layer of the stomach lining to attach to the gastric cells below. The use of flagellae and the release of an enzyme called urease to break down urea and raise the pH are both employed during early infection as part of the pathogenic process.

The flagellin protein is antigenic, referred to as the H antigen, and along with the O antigen (described earlier in relation to the LPS of Gram-negative bacteria) allows for the serotyping of bacteria. In addition to O and H antigens, capsular antigen K can also be identified using specific antisera.

Endospores

Endospores are spherical or oval structures containing the cell's genetic material in an environmentally hardy form (see *Box 2.1*). They are produced by spore-forming bacteria in response to restricted nutrients or adverse environmental conditions. The bacterium then dies, leaving this tough, environmentally hardy form of its genetic material, which is able to vegetate into a new cell if conditions improve and there are sufficient nutrients. Two bacterial genera of clinical importance form these highly resistant endospores, and both are Gram-positive rods. *Bacillus* species are aerobic (able to live in normal oxygen levels) and *Clostridia* are anaerobic (cannot live in the presence of oxygen). Members of the *Bacillus* and *Clostridia* species are responsible for several serious and life-threatening diseases – *Bacillus anthracis* causes anthrax, *Clostridium tetani*, tetanus, *C. perfringens*, gas gangrene, *C. botulinum*, botulism, and *C. difficile* is the cause of antibiotic-associated diarrhoea and pseudomembranous colitis. When the bacteria are cultured, the spores can be seen within the cells as they age and the position of the spores can be characteristic for a particular species of bacteria. Some are at the end of the cell, in a terminal position, and others central to the cell, as demonstrated in *Figure 2.9*. For this reason, Gram-positive spore-forming rods often appear as a mixture of Gram-positive and Gram-negative when stained, because as the cell walls break down, they do not take up the stain and appear Gram-negative. The dense spores do not take up the stain at all and appear as clear areas within the cells.

Endospores contain the genetic material of the bacterium and during their formation become coated with a thick protective spore coat. Because the spores

Box 2.1 Spores in the environment

The natural environment of the spore-forming bacteria is soil, where the spores can remain for many years and then cause infection if they come into contact with animals or humans. Anthrax, for instance, is an animal disease caused primarily when the spores are ingested by grazers. Humans come into contact with the spores in infected animal products such as skins and wool. Although largely controlled by stringent regulations on imported products, sporadic cases do still occur in the UK. Gangrene caused by *Clostridium perfringens* was a problem on battlefields when the spores entered soldiers' wounds along with cannon balls and the tips of spears and swords. This was well before the advent of antibiotics and amputation was the method of control. Tetanus, *Clostridium tetani*, leading to a rigid paralysis, is a disease associated with soil and animals. The disease is controlled in the UK by a vaccination programme, but neonatal tetanus continues to cause up to half a million deaths a year in countries without vaccination and where the spores enter the umbilical cord as it is cut. Food-borne disease caused by *Clostridium botulinum* is also a rare occurrence in the UK and results from spores entering food from the environment. This is often in canned food because it is cooled in water after the canning process. There has, however, been a rise in cases of clostridial infections of the skin and soft tissues as the result of spores entering the skin during intravenous drug use. Symptoms of all these diseases are caused by production of powerful bacterial toxins attacking specific host cells.

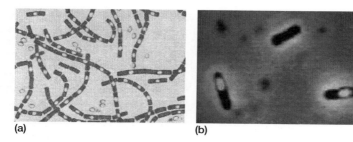
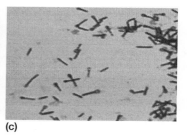

(a)   (b)   (c)

Figure 2.9
Spores can be present in different positions within the cell. (a) shows a central spore, as seen in *Bacillus cereus*, (b) shows a sub-terminal spore, as seen in *Bacillus subtilis* and (c) shows the large terminal spore position of *Clostridium tetani*.

are so well equipped to live in the environment, they are resistant to many of the methods used in laboratories to control them, and this includes some disinfectants. Therefore careful consideration must be given to the choice of chemicals used for the cleaning of equipment used in the processing of specimens and for the safe disposal of culture media after the bacteria have been grown. Chemical disinfectants must be used at the concentration known to kill spores. Autoclaving, the process of using moist heat at a high temperature and under pressure, is used to dispose of culture plates after use and also in the preparation of sterile equipment and media prior to use. Quality control has to demonstrate that the sterilizing conditions will destroy spores. Spores also move freely in the air and therefore pose a threat to the purity of bacterial growth on culture media, thus necessitating aseptic techniques (see *Chapter 6*) to protect both the environment and the person carrying out the work.

Bacterial chromosome and ribosomes

Bacteria are prokaryotic microorganisms and therefore do not have a nucleus. The genetic material is in the form of a single circular chromosome and is referred to as the nucleoid or nuclear region. All the genetic information is contained in this region, containing up to 4000 genes, which is tightly coiled like a wound-up rubber band. When the cell divides into two during binary fission the DNA uncoils for replication and is then re-coiled by an enzyme called DNA gyrase.

Some bacteria contain extrachromosomal DNA carried on a circular plasmid. The plasmid can vary in size from 0.1 to 10% of the chromosome and a bacterium can contain more than one plasmid. Plasmids are important because they often contain genes that code for toxins and resistance to antibiotics. Furthermore these resistance plasmids can be horizontally transferred from one cell to another by sex pili.

The genes are translated into proteins on bacterial ribosomes; a single bacterial cell may contain up to 25 000 ribosomes. Bacterial ribosomes, in common with eukaryotic cells, are composed of two subunits, but the subunits are of a different size. The 70 S ribosome in bacteria comprises two subunits, called the 50 S and 30 S. The S (Svedberg units) refers to the rate of sedimentation during centrifugation rather than size, and explains why the two separate figures do not add up to 70.

Bacterial growth

Bacterial growth is achieved through binary fission, a process involving the replication of the genetic material and the development of two cells from one parent cell. The process of cell division is described in *Figure 2.10*. Each division is a generation and the interval between divisions is called the generation time. This may be as little as 20 minutes or over 20 hours in the case of slow-growing bacteria like Mycobacteria, where nutrient intake is slower because of the waxy nature of the cell wall. The material for creating new cells has to be obtained through the breakdown of macromolecules taken into the cell, a process known as catabolism, and then built into new cellular components by a process called anabolism or biosynthesis.

Bacteria are classed as chemoheterotrophs, meaning that they obtain energy by breaking down organic compounds. For bacteria to reproduce successfully they have to obtain sufficient nutrients from the environment and break them down using

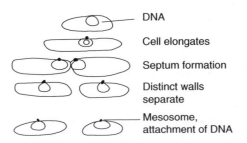

Figure 2.10
The process of cell division in a rod-shaped bacterium. During cell division the cell elongates and the DNA replicates. A septum forms between the two cells; the cells then separate to form two daughter cells.

metabolic pathways to create energy in the form of ATP (adenosine triphosphate) by respiration or fermentation. In respiration, energy is produced by the transfer of electrons along a chain with exogenous (external) final receptors. If the respiration is aerobic, this terminal receptor will be oxygen; if anaerobic, nitrate or sulphate. In fermentation processes, electrons are passed to an endogenous (internal) receptor. Bacteria are also classified as fermenters and non-fermenters depending on whether they break down sugars by fermentation: *Escherichia coli,* which ferments sugars including lactose, is a fermenter, whereas *Pseudomonas aeruginosa* is a non-fermenter.

The energy produced by respiration and fermentation is used to build new molecules and cellular components. The source of nutrients can be the natural environment, an artificially created environment such as culture medium, or the rather restricted nutrient environment bacteria often have to face within the human host. All the components for creating new cell walls described earlier have to be synthesized, along with new genetic material and numerous proteins. Proteins are synthesized on the ribosomes located in the cytoplasm of the cell. The reproduction of cellular DNA, as in humans, is achieved by the copying of each strand of the original DNA.

The metabolic pathways and nutrients used by bacteria are important as they provide a means of classifying bacteria and form the basis of the methods used to cultivate and confirm the identity of unknown isolates in the laboratory. Different types of culture media are used to produce visible colonies of bacteria for the purpose of recognition, identification and diagnosis. Culture media provide all the essential nutrients needed for growth *in vitro* and are buffered to absorb waste products such as hydrogen ions produced when carbohydrates are broken down into acidic products (see *Chapter 6*). The metabolic pathways also influence the conditions in which the cultures are incubated during the growth period.

Some bacteria have very exacting growth requirements and could be missed in clinical samples if appropriate culture media are not used. *Haemophilus influenzae* cannot extract haem (X factor) and NAD (nicotinamide–adenine dinucleotide, V factor) from the blood cells in blood agar, resulting in poor growth. If chocolate agar, where the blood has been heated to release these X and V factors, is used, growth is enhanced.

The growth curve

When bacteria are inoculated into a liquid culture medium or spread on to solid medium containing sufficient nutrient sources, they will adjust to the new environment and then go through the phases of a typical growth curve, shown in *Figure 2.11*. If the new growth environment is very different from the previous conditions bacteria will display a lag phase, where new constituents are synthesized (see *Box 2.2*). Cells may need to recover from stress or damage imposed by their previous environment and they may need to synthesize new enzymes.

An exponential (logarithmic) phase follows the lag phase and is the time of optimum growth where bacteria are growing and dividing at a constant maximum rate. This phase is described as logarithmic because a graph of the logarithm of the number of bacterial cells against time produces a straight line (see *Figure 2.11*). Exponential means that the number of bacteria double at each successive generation: 1 becomes 2, 2 become 4, 4 become 8, etc. It is during this phase that colonies of bacteria can be observed on culture media between 18 and 24 hours after inoculation. Most cultures

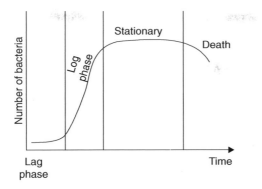

Figure 2.11
A typical bacterial growth curve. The first phase, which is not always present, is the adaptation
of the bacteria to a new medium. The bacteria then grow in an exponential phase where the
increase in the number of cells is logarithmic. When the nutrients become less available and toxic
products build up, growth is stationary (an equal number of bacteria are dying and reproducing).
In the death or decline phase, the number dying exceeds replication.

Box 2.2 Food preservation – prolonging the lag phase

One of the principles of food preservation is to prolong the lag phase, indefinitely if possible, so that
conditions for growth are never favourable and any bacteria present are kept in low numbers. Bacteria
need water, nutrients, a suitable acid/base balance, and an optimum temperature and atmosphere in
which to grow. These conditions can be artificially manipulated so that the combination of growth
conditions is never achieved. Freezing, boiling, salting, smoking, chilling, vacuum packing, the addition
of vinegar and drying are all examples of successful preservation methods. Two or more parameters
are sometimes used together, to create a combined, hurdle effect; if the bacteria can survive one stress
they cannot overcome the combined effect, for example of freeze drying, chilling and vacuum packing.

taken from clinical samples are observed for growth after 24 hours of incubation
and again at 48 hours to check for bacteria that may have been stressed or are slower
growing. Cultures incubated in anaerobic conditions are checked at 24 hours but
allowed up to 48 or 72 hours of total incubation. Each single colony represents the
exponential growth of one original bacterium. Methods of measuring growth are
discussed in *Chapter 6*. Bacteria in this phase are at their most metabolically active
and most sensitive to antibiotics.

The stationary phase occurs when nutrient levels begin to fall and the level of waste
products rises. The number of cells dying is roughly equal to the number of cells being
produced, showing as a plateau on the growth curve. Dead cells also provide a source
of nutrients to the remaining bacteria. The death or decline phase is again exponential
and represents the decline of the cell population as the nutrients run out and the toxic
waste products increase. During the death phase the cells experience starvation and
may enter a state where they maintain minimal cell activity and although viable, would
not form colonies on a culture medium. This viable non-culturable state (VNC) is
observed in the natural environment as a means to preserve the cell population until
nutrient availability and temperatures are more favourable. An example is the survival
of the bacteria that cause cholera, *Vibrio cholerae*, which exist in this form in water

during colder seasons where nutrients are also less readily available. However, when bacteria are grown *in vitro* in a clinical microbiology laboratory, bacterial isolates of interest and those requiring further tests for identification would be transferred to a new culture plate and the growth process would begin once more. If a culture, for example of a control organism, is kept alive by transferring a single colony to a new culture plate, this is called passaging. After a set number of passages it is advisable to take a new sample from the original stock culture to ensure that the characteristics have not changed during the passaging process. Passaging over a length of time can be used to render pathogenic bacteria less harmful, as they stop expressing some of their virulence factors or changes occur in their genetic make-up. This method is also called attenuation and has been successfully used in the production of live attenuated bacteria and viruses for vaccine production. It is not, however, without risks, because the bacteria or viruses could revert to a pathogenic form, especially if given to someone whose immune system is impaired. The pathogen can also be attenuated by passaging through animals to render it less likely to infect human hosts. One of the most successful bacterial attenuated vaccines has been the BCG, using a strain of *Mycobacterium bovis* passaged over a very long period in glycerol-soaked potato slices to which ox bile had been added.

The effect of temperature and pH on growth

Across the spectrum of microbial growth there are microorganisms which can survive over an extreme range of temperatures, from bacteria living in frozen seas at −22°C to those living in hot sulphur springs at temperatures over 100°C. Adaptation to temperature is achieved through changes in the composition of the fatty acids in the cell membrane. Most bacteria infecting human host are classed as mesophiles, with a temperature range between 25 and 40°C. The majority of culture plates are incubated at human body temperature, 35–37°C. However, cultures specifically inoculated to isolate *Campylobacter* species cultures are often incubated at 40–42°C because the bacteria will still grow at this temperature but some of the other bacteria present in the faecal sample are discouraged.

The optimum pH for bacterial growth from human hosts is around 7, although in the environment there are bacteria capable of surviving extremely low pH values (acidophiles) and others which live in very high alkaline environments.

The effect of the growth atmosphere

This is a very important aspect of bacterial growth and is used as a method to classify bacteria and to design appropriate growth conditions in the laboratory. The ability to grow in the full oxygen tension of air (about 21% oxygen) is determined by the presence or absence of bacterial enzymes capable of processing toxic oxygen molecules produced during metabolism and respiration by flavoproteins. In aerobic respiration oxygen is the final electron acceptor in the electron transport chain, but toxic superoxide free radicals and hydrogen peroxide are also created. These can be enzymatically modified to produce harmless water and oxygen. Obligate aerobes and facultative anaerobes contain the enzyme superoxide dismutase which catalyses the reaction of superoxide radicals and hydrogen ions to form hydrogen peroxide and oxygen. Hydrogen peroxide is also toxic to the cells and can be further neutralized by either catalase, which converts the hydrogen peroxide to water and oxygen, or peroxidase, which converts the hydrogen peroxide to water. The presence or absence of catalase is used as part of identification tests to distinguish between two important groups of Gram-positive cocci: *Streptococci* species are catalase negative, *Staphylococci* species catalase positive. The equations are:

$$2O_2^- + H_2O \xrightarrow{\quad SOD \quad} H_2O_2 + O_2$$

$$2H_2O_2 \xrightarrow{\quad catalase \quad} 2H_2O + O_2$$

$$Or\ H_2O_2 + 2H^+ \xrightarrow{\quad peroxidase \quad} 2H_2O$$

Aerobic respiration is more efficient and produces more ATP than anaerobic. In anaerobic respiration the terminal electron receptor is nitrate or sulphate rather than oxygen.

Bacteria, however, do not divide neatly into either aerobes or anaerobes. While some bacteria are strictly aerobic and others strictly anaerobic, some are able to use oxygen and nitrate in aerobic *or* anaerobic respiration:

- Strict or obligate aerobes can only grow in the presence of oxygen. Because of this they will not be found in deeper areas of the body where oxygen is limited. Micrococci, for instance, are Gram-positive cocci found only on the skin.
- Facultative anaerobes, as the name suggests, are able to grow in the presence or absence of oxygen. Aerobic respiration is more efficient and so facultative anaerobes grow better in oxygen. Bacteria such as *Escherichia coli* can grow in a wide range of body sites; they thrive on moist areas of the skin with abundant oxygen but also within the colon where conditions are anaerobic.
- Aerotolerant anaerobes can grow in the presence of oxygen, but do not use it in metabolism. Some members of the genus *Clostridia*, including *C. histolyticum*, fall into this category.
- Micro-aerophilic bacteria are aerobic but require lower oxygen levels than air. *Campylobacter* species are grown on specialized culture media in artificially lowered levels of oxygen.
- Capnophilic bacteria prefer an environment where the carbon dioxide is higher than normal. This enhanced growth is a feature of *Neisseria gonorrhoeae*, *Neisseria meningitidis*, *Haemophilus influenzae* and *Streptococcus pneumoniae*.
- Obligate anaerobes are killed by the presence of oxygen so if their presence is suspected in a clinical sample they must be cultured on appropriate media and incubated in anaerobic conditions immediately. Strict anaerobes are found in deeper sites of the body. *Clostridium perfringens* causes infections within tissue and can also create its own anaerobic environment by breaking down tissue by excreting protein toxins, leading to gangrene.

Figure 2.12 illustrates the relative positions of the growth of aerobic and anaerobic bacteria in test tubes.

The list above demonstrates that some types of bacteria will not be able to grow in some areas of the body, whereas others are able to grow in a range of oxygen levels and are therefore able to cause infection in a wider range of sites and tissues. Other factors including where bacteria are able to find attachment sites influence the establishment of infection (see *Chapter 4*) and contribute to the knowledge about which types of pathogens are likely to cause specific infections (see *Box 2.3*).

Capped tubes

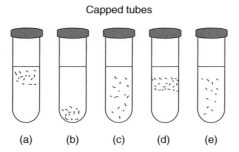

(a)   (b)   (c)   (d)   (e)

Figure 2.12
Demonstration of the growth requirements of bacteria. Oxygen only reaches the upper area of
the tube, creating a variable environment with the most anaerobic conditions (least oxygen) at
the base of the tube. (a) Obligate aerobes grow where there is the greatest level of oxygen. (b)
Anaerobes grow where there is least oxygen. (c) Facultative anaerobes grow in the presence or
absence of oxygen and therefore spread throughout the medium. (d) Micro-aerophilic bacteria
prefer the area where oxygen is reduced. (e) Aerotolerant anaerobes can grow with or without
oxygen and are therefore able to grow throughout the medium.

One area of the body where obligate anaerobes live alongside aerobes is the
oral cavity. The environments vary from the aerobic areas of the tongue and tooth
surfaces to the very anaerobic niches found in the crevices between the base of the
tooth and the gum. Bacteria with very different requirements for oxygen are able to
form micro-environments where the aerobic members use up the oxygen and allow
the obligate anaerobes to survive.

Obligate intracellular bacteria, chlamydia and rickettsia
The Chlamydiaceae are dependent on host cells for replication because although they
contain DNA, RNA and ribosomes and synthesize their own proteins and nucleic

---

Box 2.3 Isolation and identification of *Neisseria gonorrhoeae*

The isolation of bacteria from clinical samples requires a combination of knowledge of the morphology
of the bacteria, specific characteristics and growth requirements as illustrated by *Neisseria gonorrhoeae*:
Neisseria gonorrhoeae are aerobic Gram-negative diplococci, the causative agent of the sexually
transmitted infection gonorrhoea. They are strictly human pathogens requiring warmth and moisture
and they are killed easily if allowed to dry. The specimen must be taken from the correct site, based on
knowledge of where the bacteria infect, for example the columnar epithelial cells of the female cervix
rather than vaginal epithelial cells. They also have fastidious growth requirements, are inhibited by fatty
acids and trace metals in some laboratory media and may be present in small numbers amongst the
normal bacteria found on mucosal surfaces. They are therefore a challenge for culture media, requiring a
medium that is selective (suppressing the growth of commensal bacteria by the addition of antibiotics)
and also contains growth factors. Several specialized culture media are available, for example GC
medium and Thayer–Martin. Culture plates are often inoculated in the clinic as soon as the specimen is
taken. At the same time a Gram stain is prepared from the patient sample to demonstrate the presence
of the bacteria directly. After isolation the identity of the bacteria can be confirmed by testing for the
presence of the enzyme cytochrome oxidase (part of the electron transport chain in some bacteria) and
a series of biochemical tests including specific sugar fermentations.

acid, they cannot make their own ATP. They are classified as Gram-negative bacteria because they have an inner and outer membrane and LPS, but no peptidoglycan layer. *Chlamydia trachomatis* causes sexually transmitted infections while other serovars infect the conjunctiva, causing ocular trachoma. *Chlamydophila* (formerly *Chlamydia) pneumoniae* and *Chlamydophila* (formerly *Chlamydia*) *psittaci* infect the human respiratory tract. *Chlamydophila pneumoniae* is passed from person to person in respiratory secretions whereas *Chlamydophila psittaci* is a zoonotic disease passed from infected birds to humans.

Chlamydia bacteria exist in two distinct forms:

- *Elementary bodies* are metabolically inert rigid structures, 0.3 µm in size, able to exist in harsh environments. They are the infectious form of the cells and are spread from person to person or bird to human.
- *Reticulate bodies* are the fragile, non-infectious replicative form of the bacteria. They are 1 µm in diameter and found intracellularly.

The elementary bodies attach to columnar epithelial cells of the host and are internalized within endocytic vesicles. Within the first hours of infection the elementary bodies start to change and more diffuse reticulate bodies are formed. These replicate by binary fission, using host ATP as their energy source. The reticulate bodies then change back into elementary bodies and are released from the cell to begin a new round of infection and replication. There is evidence that *C. pneumoniae* also infect polymorphs and macrophages attracted to the site in respiratory infections. In chronic infections with *C. pneumoniae* the organism enters a persistent state with diminished metabolic processes, and are called cryptic bodies.

Rickettsia are Gram-negative aerobic coccobacilli with a typical cell wall. They are obligate intracellular parasites found in either the cytoplasm or nucleus of the host cell. They are often transmitted by arthropod vectors and cause diseases such as epidemic typhus (*Rickettsia prowazekii*) and Rocky Mountain spotted fever (*Rickettsia rickettsii*).

In vitro diagnostic methods

The structure, physiology, genetics and growth patterns of bacteria provide many characteristics that can be used to isolate and accurately identify bacterial pathogens from clinical specimens (these methods are described in more detail in *Chapter 6*). The size, shape arrangement and Gram stain reaction provide a starting point, either directly from a clinical specimen or from a colony on a culture plate. Bacteria can be selectively grown from single cells to visible colonies through the use of carefully formulated media that contain appropriate nutrients. The bacteria may only grow on particular culture media and may grow better aerobically or anaerobically. The colonial morphology is often characteristic for a particular genus of bacteria and further identification tests can be carried out. These tests, based on the presence or absence of various enzymes and biochemical reactions, can be performed singly or incorporated into a commercial product to produce a profile that is distinctive for a particular genus or species.

Genome mapping of bacteria, where a specific gene can be probed for and amplified, has led to the development of molecular based techniques. For example, the presence of a specific resistance gene can be used to distinguish between methicillin-resistant *Staphylococcus aureus* (MRSA) and methicillin-sensitive *Staphylococcus aureus* (MSSA) (see *Chapter 6*).

Selective toxicity

Prokaryotic cells have several important structural and physiological differences when compared with human eukaryotic cells. The principle of selective toxicity is that aspects of the bacterial cell can be targeted by chemotherapeutic agents with minimal effect on the host cells. The cell walls and membranes provide an excellent target for drugs and there are several classes of antibiotics directed towards them. Other classes of antibiotics target the ribosomes and protein synthesis pathways. Replication is targeted via DNA gyrase and DNA-dependent RNA polymerase enzymes. *Figure 2.13* shows the target sites used in selective toxicity and gives examples of the antibiotics used at these sites.

Other characteristics of bacterial cell structure and growth provide clues about the problems associated with the development and use of antibiotics. Bacteria can divide every 20–30 minutes and a large population of dividing bacteria pressurized by the presence of antibiotics will develop spontaneous mutations and thus develop resistance by several methods:

- changing the target site so that there is a lowered affinity for the drug
- altered access to the target site. This can be achieved by decreasing the permeability of the cell wall, or actively pumping out the drug

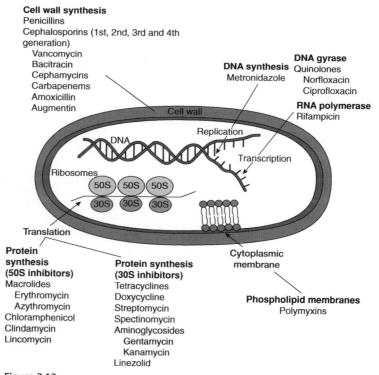

Figure 2.13
Target sites used in selective toxicity and examples of the antibiotics used at these sites.

- expression of enzymes that either modify or destroy the drug, e.g. β-lactamases, aminoglycoside modifying enzymes
- acquisition of resistance genes via plasmids from another bacterium.

2.2   EUKARYOTIC MICROORGANISMS

The major groups of eukaryotic microorganisms encountered in human infections include fungi, protozoa and helminths.

Fungi

Fungi belong to the kingdom Eumycota and are ubiquitous in nature. There are an estimated 100 000 species but only about 100 are associated with human disease. In common with bacteria they are chemoheterotrophs, using carbon sources for nutrition. Many are saprophytic and obtain their nutrients from the enzymic degradation of decaying organic matter, performing a valuable role in nature. Fungi are important in many commercial processes, for example yeast for brewing, and fungi in the ripening of cheeses and the manufacture of antibiotics. The few fungi that cause disease in humans are principally opportunistic in nature, ranging from skin lesions and yeast (thrush) infections to life-threatening systemic infections in severely immuno-compromised individuals. They do not generally cause acute infections like bacteria do; fungal infections are more likely to be subacute or chronic. These are described further, in the context of laboratory diagnosis, in *Chapter 13*. The study of fungi is called mycology, and the diseases they cause are termed mycoses.

Classification
The principal fungi associated with human infections are caused either by yeasts (single cells) or filamentous moulds, which are multicellular. Moulds form a mycelium, composed of hyphae, whereas yeasts are single cells that reproduce by budding. There are four divisions of the Eumycota: the Ascomycota, Basidiomycota, Zygomycota and Chytridiomycota. Most of the fungi of medical importance are Ascomycetes, with a few Basidiomycetes and Zygomycetes. While most of the fungal infections encountered in a microbiology laboratory are either yeasts or moulds, there are some genera that are described as dimorphic, displaying either yeast-like morphology at environmental temperatures but growing as moulds within the human body or vice versa. The switch between the two forms is the result of temperature change or adaptation to life within a human host. *Table 2.2* summarizes the division and genera of fungi likely to be isolated from clinical specimens and indicates whether these infections are most likely to be opportunistic or the cause of systemic infection.

Cell structure
Fungi have all the features of eukaryotic cells and therefore differ from bacterial cells in several important ways. Fungi have a nucleus, with single chromosomes and nucleoli. Cells contain an actin cytoskeleton and have membrane-bound organelles including the nucleus, mitochondria, endoplasmic reticulum and Golgi bodies. The plasma membrane differs from bacteria in that it contains the sterol ergosterol, which helps to make it stronger (note that human membranes contain cholesterol).

Fungal cell walls are also different in structure from bacterial cells, consisting of

Table 2.2 The classification of the principal fungal pathogens isolated in clinical specimens

Division	Genus and species	Type of infection	Typical growth	Presence of hyphae	Disease
Ascomycota	Aspergillus	Opportunistic pathogen	Mould	Yes	Allergic Aspergillosis Aspergilloma
	Blastomyces dermatidis	Systemic	Dimorphic, inhaled as mould, changes to yeast form in body	Yes	Blastomycosis, a chronic infection with lesions anywhere on the body
	Candida albicans, C. glabrata, C. kefyr and others	Opportunistic pathogen, can be systemic	Yeast form on mucous membranes, mould when invasive	Yes	Vaginal and oral thrush, candidiasis, meningitis
	Coccidioides immitis	Systemic	Dimorphic, inhaled as mould, changes to yeast form in body	Yes	Coccidioidosis
	Histoplasma capsulatum	Systemic	Dimorphic, inhaled as mould, changes to yeast form in body	Yes	Histoplasmosis (pulmonary or systemic disease)
	Pneumocystis jirovecii	Opportunistic pathogen	Cysts	No	Pneumocystis pneumonia
	Sporothrix schenckii	Subcutaneous	Dimorphic	Yes	Sporotrichosis, chronic infection of skin and subcutaneous tissue
	Arthroderma – Trichophyton, Epidermophyton Microsporum	Dermatophytes			Superficial skin lesions, ringworm of hair, nails and skin
Basidiomycota	Cryptococcus neoformans	Systemic	Yeast	No	Cryptococcoccal pneumonia, meningitis
	Malassezia furfur	Superficial, skin	Yeast	No	Pityriasis, known as tinea versicolor Pale or dark skin patches
Zygomycota	Mucor, Rhizopus	Opportunistic pathogens	Mould	Yes	Zygomycosis in immunosuppressed people

the polysaccharides mannan, glucan and chitin. Mannan is found on the cell surface and in the wall matrix, where it is attached to proteins. The antigenic determinants of the cell wall are made up of the mannan proteins. Some of the glucans, polymers of glucose, form fibrils and these, in conjunction with chitin, increase cell wall strength. Chitin is composed of long unbranched polymers of *N*-acetyl glucosamine. Fungi have the ability when they are growing to form strong aerial hyphae, and it is the chitin that gives them the strength to achieve this.

Fungal growth

Fungi are mostly obligate aerobes with a few facultatively anaerobic forms, but unlike bacteria, there are no obligately anaerobic fungi. Fungi break down organic compounds as nutrients, use glycolysis, and are mesophilic, growing at temperatures between 5 and 40°C. They normally occupy acidic damp environments and will therefore tolerate *in vitro* culture conditions that are more acidic than those formulated for bacteria. Some of the filamentous moulds causing infections of hair, skin and nails grow only on keratinized cells, using an enzyme called keratinase to degrade the keratin.

Fungi can undergo both asexual and sexual reproduction. The mould form, asexual reproduction, where mitotic division takes place, involves conidia which are formed on the hyphae. Hyphae themselves are extensions of the cell cytoplasm that form tube-like structures with thick parallel walls. Hyphae can either have cross walls (septate) or form a continuous tube (non-septate). All hyphae have many nuclei. The hyphae can form an interwoven mat called a mycelium. The microscopic appearance of the hyphae and the conidia (macro- and microconidia) are characteristic for particular genera and species of fungal moulds. As the cells grow on culture media or in nature, the mycelium penetrates the nutrient medium, allowing aerial hyphae to push upward. Fungal growth can be relatively fast or, as seen in the dermatophyte genera, it can be up to 3 weeks before significant macroscopic growth is seen. The resultant growth is also characteristic, in the colour of the colonies and the nature of the surface, whether powdery or dusty. Fungi use spores for sexual reproduction, called ascospores, basidiospores and zygospores depending on the division represented. Haploid nuclei or two cells, donor and recipient, form a diploid nucleus and may further divide by meiosis.

Yeast cells reproduce by forming buds called blastoconidia on the parent cell, which then break off and form a new yeast cell. Some yeasts, for example *Candida albicans*, can also form pseudohyphae or germ tubes when incubated in serum. *Figure 2.14* shows the main features of mould and yeast growth.

In vitro *diagnostic methods*

Selective media can be used to culture any pathogenic fungi from clinical specimens. As in other areas of microbiology there is an increasingly sophisticated range of media,

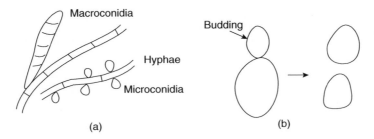

(a)　　　　　　　　　　　　　(b)

Figure 2.14
Principal microscopic features of mould and yeast growth. (a) This is characteristic of the dermatophyte mould *Trichophyton rubrum*, and represents a microscopic sample taken from a 21-day culture. (b) These yeast cells reproduce by budding, with the daughter cell breaking off and forming a new yeast cell.

including chromogenic agar containing chromophores, and selective agents that will distinguish between different genera of fungi and yeasts. Yeasts grow overnight on culture media, whereas filamentous moulds can take up to 21 days to show visible growth. Clinical samples from hair, skin and nails are first examined microscopically, as the presence of fungal elements, if any, can be reported before the culture is complete. Any growth of filamentous mould is first of all described by the colour and nature of the growth when viewed from the top and bottom of the Petri dish. A sample of the growth is then examined microscopically for the presence of characteristic hyphae, macroconidia and microconidia. This procedure is further described in *Chapter 13*.

Yeasts can be distinguished from bacteria on a culture plate by performing a Gram stain; yeasts are larger than bacteria, and do not fully take up the Gram stain. They appear as large ovoid cells, and often the long tubes of pseudohyphae are also visible. In severely immuno-compromised patients yeasts can spread into the bloodstream and also into the cerebrospinal fluid (CSF). Bloodstream infections, fungaemia, can be diagnosed by blood culture techniques or examination and culture of a specimen of CSF.

In common with bacteria, fungi can use different carbon sources and undergo different biochemical reactions. Biochemical tests, either singly or incorporated into an identification system, have been developed. Molecular methods have also been developed and are used to identify pathogens that would be dangerous to grow in the laboratory, including *Histoplasma capsulatum* and *Coccidioides immitis*.

Selective toxicity

Selective toxicity against fungal pathogens is more difficult to achieve than with prokaryotic bacteria, as there are fewer targets. Fungal pathogens are often slow growing and so treatment has to be more prolonged. The principal targets of antifungal treatments are the ergosterol in the cell membrane, RNA synthesis and interference with nutrient uptake.

Protozoa

Protozoa are microscopic single-celled eukaryotes ranging in size from 1 to 200 μm. They are chemoheterotrophs, absorbing nutrients primarily by ingestion. Many protozoa are free-living organisms that pose no clinical threat to human health; nevertheless, the parasitic members of this group are responsible for a significant burden of human disease worldwide. The protozoan parasite *Plasmodium* is the cause of malaria, and trypanosomes are responsible for sleeping sickness and Chagas' disease, all causing high levels of morbidity and mortality in susceptible areas of the world. More than 500 million people worldwide are infected with malaria and over 2 million, the majority of whom are children, die each year. While these diseases are not endemic to the UK, other protozoan parasites are implicated in disease and diagnosed from clinical specimens in microbiology laboratories across the UK.

Classification

Protozoa can be classified into groups by their method of reproduction and movement.

- ■ Rhizopods are free-living protozoans; some form commensal or parasitic relationships in human intestines. Rhizopods are amoebae with pseudopodic movement and include the Entamoebae, obligate intracellular parasites of the human intestinal tract. *E. histolytica* is the cause of amoebiasis, amoebic dysentery, found in either the trophozoite (amoebic) form or as characteristic cysts excreted in the faeces (the diagnosis is described in *Chapter 9*).

- Ciliates move with the use of cilia, are free-living and rarely parasitic.
- Flagellates move by means of flagellae and include the human pathogens trypanosomes, *Giardia*, *Trichomonas* and *Leishmania*.
- Sporozoa have no means of movement and include malaria, toxoplasmosis and *Cryptosporidia*.

Life cycles and transmission

It is important to understand the life cycle of any protozoan human pathogen in order to understand the diseases it causes and to develop treatment and prevention strategies. Some protozoans complete their life cycle in a single host and are then transmitted to another similar host. *Entamoeba histolytica* is passed from person to person via the faecal–oral route in the environmentally protected cyst form. Once in the small intestine of the human host the cysts disintegrate and release a parasite with four nuclei, which then divides to form four individual trophozoites, the active motile feeding stage of the sporozoan parasite. The trophozoites travel to the colon where they attack the epithelial cells and cause small ulcerations in the mucosa, leading to the symptoms of amoebiasis. They are excreted from the body as cysts, ready to infect a new host. *Giardia lamblia* (also referred to as *G. intestinalis* or *G. duodenalis*) is ingested in the cyst form; the cysts change into trophozoites and attach to the intestine where they cause diarrhoeal symptoms. Cysts are then excreted and transmitted to a new host.

The flagellate *Trichomonas vaginalis* is passed by sexual contact as a trophozoite, causing infection of the epithelial cells of the genitourinary tract. Trophozoites have five flagellae and an axostyle, a microtubule thought to be used for attachment to cells. Reproduction is by binary fission. There are four free flagella; the fifth is curved back on the body to form an undulating membrane. The trophozoites have no mitochondria and energy is generated in hydrogenosomes, membrane-bound organelles that produce hydrogen gas as they lack a TCA cycle and electron transport chains.

Some protozoans require more than one host to complete their life cycle:

- the definitive host is where sexual reproduction occurs
- the intermediate host is where asexual development takes place
- reservoir hosts are alternative hosts, passive carriers of the parasites.

Toxoplasma gondii is an obligate intracellular sporozoan parasite causing toxoplasmosis. The definitive host is the domestic cat. Studies have shown that 75% of cats have antibodies to toxoplasma, which means that they have been infected and formed an immune response. A quarter of humans also have antibodies and it is estimated that between 7 and 34% of the population of the UK have been infected, the majority of them showing no symptoms. Sexual reproduction takes place in the feline ileum, where trophozoite forms become merozoites. These merozoites differentiate into male and female gametocytes and are excreted in the cat faeces as oocysts. These mature in the external environment and remain stable in the soil for months. They can then be ingested by grazing animals and also by humans when they are gardening or cleaning cat litter. The infection can also be transmitted by consuming the oocysts in the meat of grazing animals, particularly if undercooked or raw. Human infection is caused when the oocysts change into sporozoites which invade tissues and form pseudocysts. The disease is usually controlled by the immune system and is therefore a problem for immuno-compromised patients whose immune system is unable to cope and the disease is reactivated. Infection in pregnancy can also be a problem as the sporozoites can cross the placenta to infect the fetus.

Cryptosporidium parvum is a small coccidian protozoan parasite which infects the human small intestine, where it undergoes sexual and asexual reproduction. Mature oocysts are shed in the faeces and passed from person to person by the faecal–oral route. Most vertebrates, particularly the young and immature, can be infected by various species of *Cryptosporidia* and act as a reservoir for the infection. *Figure 2.15* shows some representative structures of the protozoa described.

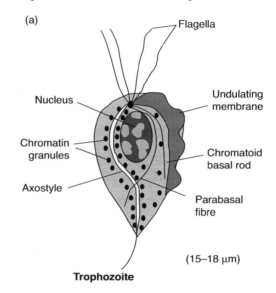

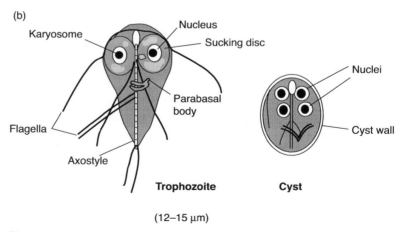

Figure 2.15
Structure of *Trichomonas vaginalis* (a) and *Giardia lamblia* (b). The trophozoite of *G. lamblia* is the motile, replicating form present during intestinal infection. The cyst is environmentally stable and is transmitted from host to host by the faecal–oral route.

In vitro *diagnosis of protozoan infection*

Designing appropriate diagnostic tests is dependent upon knowledge of the infection cycle of the specific disease. For example, *Cryptosporidia* infections can be diagnosed by staining a smear taken from a faecal specimen and examining the preparation microscopically for the characteristic cysts (see *Chapter 5*). Similarly, cysts of *Giardia lamblia* and *Entamoeba histolytica* can be seen in unstained faecal preparations (see *Chapter 9*). *Trichomonas vaginalis* is diagnosed either by staining of a smear taken from a vaginal swab, or by direct unstained microscopic examination of a sample from the swab (see *Chapters 5* and *9*).

It is known that *Toxoplasma gondii* provokes a specific immune response and appropriate antibodies can be demonstrated by latex agglutination tests. Molecular methods for protozoan infections have also been developed.

Treatment and prevention strategies

Protozoan pathogens cause a wide range of infections worldwide and the treatment is directed at specific points of the life cycle. Prevention is also a major consideration, especially in the case of malaria and trypanosome infections, where interrupting the life cycle of the parasites can vastly reduce the incidence of disease. An effective and safe vaccine for malaria would prevent millions of deaths; however, the complexity of the life cycle makes ensuring its efficacy in all populations difficult to achieve. *Giardia* and *Trichomonas* infections will respond to the antibiotic metronidazole, which is used for the treatment of anaerobic infections. Metronidazole is taken in to the cells by diffusion and then is non-enzymatically reduced by ferredoxin to create products that are toxic to anaerobic cells. Until 2002 there was no effective treatment for *Cryptosporidia* infections, leading to severe morbidity in immuno-compromised patients. Nitazoxanide, an anti-protozoal agent, and the aminoglycoside antibiotics paromomycin and azithromycin, have been shown to be partially effective in HIV infected patients. The infection is self-limiting in immunocompetent patients. Many cases of toxoplasmosis do not require treatment, but if required, the drugs pyrimethamine and sulphadiazine can be used. Pyrimethamine inhibits dihydrofolate reductase and nucleic acid synthesis, and sulphadiazine acts on the same pathway. Spiramycin, a macrolide antibiotic targeting protein synthesis, is used if treatment for toxoplasmosis is required in pregnancy.

Helminths

These parasites are the worms known to infect humans. Because they are multicellular eukaryotes, they are not microorganisms, but are often diagnosed by their microscopic forms, the eggs or larvae. With the exception of threadworms (pinworms) they are unlikely to be acquired in the UK and usually occur in patients with a history of travel to endemic countries. It is therefore important for requesting clinicians to provide travel history on the request forms accompanying faecal samples. The samples will then be examined more closely for the presence of helminth ova. Occasionally entire worms are passed and will be submitted to the laboratory for identification. The intestinal tract is not the only body system affected by parasitic worms; flukes can infect and live in human tissue and blood vessels for many years. Helminths are the largest parasites to infect humans and are multicellular eukaryotes, ranging in size from barely visible pinworms to tapeworms of up to 15 metres in length.

In some clinical microbiology laboratories the diagnosis of helminth infections is a rare occurrence and most experience of identification is gained from external quality control samples containing helminth ova rather than whole worms.

Classification

Helminths can be grouped into three classes, the nematodes (roundworms) and platyhelminthes (flat worms), the cestodes and the trematodes.

Nematodes are helminth roundworms inhabiting the intestine, or infecting the blood and tissues. The adults have a tapered cylindrical body containing an alimentary canal that goes all the way from the mouth to the anus. The infectious form may be eggs that are excreted in the faeces and ingested with food before they become larvae and penetrate the intestines (ascaris). Alternatively it may be the eggs passed out in the faeces which survive in the moist warm soil where they mature into larvae that penetrate the skin. Nematodes exist as separate sexes, and although there is no intermediate host for those infecting the intestine, the eggs need to remain in the external environment to rest and develop. Nematode infections are common in many developing countries where conditions are ideal, providing the preferred composition of warm moist soil and then ingestion with food or water or penetration into a new host. The most common intestinal infections are caused by *Ascaris lumbricoides*, *Trichuris trichuria*, *Necator americanus*, *Ancylostoma duodenale*, and *Strongyloides stercoralis*. The only example common in the UK is *Enterobius vermicularis*.

The tissue and blood nematodes such as *Onchocerca volvulus* and *Wuchereria bancrofti* are widespread in tropical regions where the infective larvae are spread by blackflies and mosquitoes, respectively. The adult forms are microfilariae, microscopic worm-like forms visible in the infected blood.

The cestodes are tapeworms which can live for 25 years in the human intestine, growing up to 15 metres in length. These worms are segmented, with each segment being called a proglottid. The terminal proglottids are shed from the body and each may contain up to 10 000 eggs. The head region, the scolex, is used to anchor the worm by disc-like suckers to the intestinal wall. Cestodes are hermaphrodites. Their eggs can remain in the soil for months before ingestion by cattle, followed by migration of the larvae into their tissue, which is then consumed by humans. Human infections can be caused by the pork tapeworm, *Taenia solium*, beef tapeworm, *Taenia saginata*, fish tapeworm, *Diphyllobothrium latum*, and by *Hymenolepis nana* and *Hymenolepis diminuta* (dwarf tapeworms found in humans, mice and rats). *Echinococcus granulosus* are canine tapeworms. Dog tapeworms do not develop in humans, but if the eggs are ingested by herbivores or humans, the onchospheres form hydatid cysts in the tissues. In this instance, humans act as a dead end or incidental host, because there is no further transmission to the definitive host.

The trematodes are flukes infecting human tissues and blood vessels, where they cause progressive damage. They are flat and leaf-like, varying in size from about 12 mm to about 7.5 cm in length, depending on the species. The schistosomes are sexual in their reproduction whereas others are hermaphrodites. Trematodes use snails as their intermediate hosts. Eggs released from humans hatch and release larvae which penetrate the snail, in which they develop into cercariae and from which they are excreted into the water. Schistosomes, such as *Schistosoma mansoni*, *S. japonicum* and *S. haematobium* invade the skin of humans and make their way via the portal veins to the intestine or bladder. *S. haematobium* causes calcification of ureters and increases the risk of developing cancer. Hermaphrodite species form cysts on animals or plants and produce metacercariae. Humans become infected when they eat the infected fish or plant. *Clonorchis sinensis*, the liver fluke, if untreated, can lead to fibrosis of the bile ducts, stones and even cancer. *Paragonimus westermani*, transmitted by infected crabs, infects the lung; consuming plants infected with *Fasciola hepatica* leads to disease in the bile ducts. Trematode eggs are distinctive and can be identified from faecal specimens and from urine samples. In common with other helminths, trematode infections are found most commonly in countries where raw sewage is discharged into lakes and rivers. Once again, travel history to an endemic area needs to be included on the request form to ensure that the specimen is examined for the presence of ova, cysts and parasites.

In vitro *diagnosis*
Many of the helminth infections described can be diagnosed from identifying ova and cysts from faecal samples (see *Chapter 9*). Reference laboratories provide courses in this specialist area and also distribute the external quality control samples to maintain expertise. Most laboratories will have reference material readily available and also a method for measuring the size of the egg under the microscope, as both size and appearance are important diagnostic tools. Schistosome ova can also be identified from urine specimens (see *Chapter 8*). Tissue and blood helminths will not generally be diagnosed in microbiology laboratories. Biopsies of tissues, lung, muscle, liver, brain and eye can be examined; blood smears will reveal the presence of filariasis. Specific antibodies to *Schistosoma*, *Strongyloides* and *Trichuris* species can be measured in serum samples. Molecular techniques involving PCR are used to detect the DNA of *Echinococcus*, *Onchocerca*, *Taenia* and *Wuchereria* species.

Treatment and prevention strategies
Selective toxicity against a multicellular organism can be difficult to achieve. There are now several effective drugs in routine use. Praziquantel is effective and safe in the treatment of schistosomes and for cestode infections. Niclosamide may also be prescribed for cestode infections. Intestinal nematodes can be treated with piperazine, benzimidazole, mebendazole and albendazole. Diethylcarbamazine and ivermectin are both effective drugs for filarial infections; diethylcarbamazine inhibits arachadonic acid metabolism in the microfilaria. Piperazine, praziquantel, ivermectin, levamisole and pyrantel all achieve their effect by paralysing the worms, whereas the benzimidazoles interfere with the polymerization of tubulin in the formation of microtubules in the helminth cytoskeleton. The development of drug resistance is also a problem – several countries have reported resistance to some of the principal drugs, yet measuring drug resistance is not as straightforward as it is with antibacterial drugs. Travellers to endemic countries can take sensible precautions to avoid contact with parasitic larvae and ova, but for the endemic population, who often have chronic infections with several parasites, treatment is less readily available, if at all. Prevention and control involves education, lifestyle changes, treatment and eradication programmes that are often beyond the country's financial means.

SUGGESTED FURTHER READING

This chapter has provided an introduction to the structure and function of the major prokaryotic and eukaryotic pathogens which are discussed in further chapters outlining their clinical diagnosis from microbiological specimens. Further background information on structure and function can be found in any good microbiology textbook.

SELF-ASSESSMENT QUESTIONS

1. Outline the principal components of the Gram-positive, Gram-negative and acid-fast cell walls. Suggest two ways in which structure influences bacterial behaviour.
2. What is meant by the term 'motile' in relation to bacteria? How is bacterial motility effected and why can this provide an advantage to the bacterium?
3. Which two major genera of bacteria produce endospores? Why are spores a problem in terms of disease transmission and infection control?
4. Outline the ways in which bacteria are classified in terms of their ability to survive in the presence of oxygen. How does this affect their ability to infect different body sites?
5. What is meant by the term 'selective toxicity'? Why is this more difficult to achieve in the treatment of fungal and protozoal infections than when treating bacterial infections?
6. Describe the principal stages of the bacterial growth curve and explain what is happening at each stage. How can the growth curve be manipulated for the purpose of food preservation?
7. Fungal infections are often opportunistic in nature. Explain what is meant by this term and give two examples of fungi acting in this way.
8. Outline the infection cycle of *Toxoplasma gondii*. Why is this protozoan infection a particular problem for pregnant women and patients suffering from AIDS?
9. Briefly describe the three classes of helminths.
10. With the exception of *Enterobius vermicularis*, helminth infections are uncommon in the UK unless the patient has a history of travel to endemic areas. Suggest some reasons for this.

Answers to self-assessment questions provided at:
www.scionpublishing.com/medmicro

Virology

Learning objectives
After studying this chapter you should confidently be able to:

■ **Describe the nature, characteristics and structure of viruses**
Viruses are simple cells composed of genetic material with a protein capsid, with or without an envelope. They are extremely small, 20–300 nm, beyond the resolution of the light microscope, and they rely on host cells for replication. They are intricately constructed, their nucleocapsids being in either a helical or icosahedral form. Their genetic material is in the form of either DNA or RNA, never both, and they are classified according to the Baltimore classification. They are transmitted between humans by respiratory, skin, faecal and oral routes, sexually, via blood and body fluid, by animals and insect vectors and by inanimate objects.

■ **Describe the principal steps in viral replication**
Viruses first attach to their target host cells by specific receptors before penetrating the cell and uncoating to release the nuclear material. DNA viruses replicate in the nucleus and RNA viruses in the cytoplasm. mRNA is transcribed and early proteins produced on the host ribosomes, followed by structural proteins. Replication of the DNA or RNA takes place and the genetic material is packed into the capsids prior to release from the host cell. An envelope is added from the lipid bilayer of the host cell on release.

■ **Explain the laboratory methods available for the diagnosis of viral infection**
Viral infections can be diagnosed by electron microscopy, cell culture, PCR-based molecular methods and by enzyme immunoassays, performed either manually or by an automated technique.

■ **Outline the diagnosis of several clinically important viral infections**
Many viral infections, such as the common cold, are self-limiting and do not require laboratory diagnosis. This is true of routine cold sores, chickenpox, shingles and many cases of viral gastroenteritis. It is, however, important to diagnose infections such as HIV, epidemic influenza, viral hepatitis and rubella. The following are diagnosed and confirmed by laboratory investigations: complications of other viruses, HSV encephalitis, varicella-zoster infection in pregnant women, outbreaks of mumps and measles, children hospitalized with respiratory syncytial virus or suffering from rotavirus or adenovirus diarrhoea, viral infections in immuno-compromised patients, and cases of glandular fever.

■ **Discuss the options available for the treatment of viral infections**
Treatment options for viral infections are not as varied as for bacterial infections because it is more difficult to achieve selective toxicity for virally infected host cells. The range of therapeutic options available are based on knowledge of viral structure and pathogenesis. HIV combination therapy targets several different aspects of the viral replication cycle. Treatment for HSV, VZV and CMV is with aciclovir and analogues of the drug, which target DNA replication. Hepatitis B is treated with interferon and a drug that targets the reverse transcriptase activity, adefovir dipivoxil. Influenza treatment targets the neuraminidase on the surface of the virus. For most other viruses, there are no effective treatments.

Viruses (see *Box 3.1* for a list of useful definitions) are obligate intracellular parasites, passed successfully between hosts yet unable to replicate and multiply outside host cells. This is because they are very simple cells consisting of their genetic material and protein, which may or may not be surrounded by a lipid envelope. They rely on host cells for raw materials, nucleotides, amino acids, lipid envelopes and replication machinery, enzymes and ribosomes. They are also extremely small, beyond the resolution of the light microscope and visible only by electron microscopy. Viruses are intricately constructed and yet able to dismantle into their component parts after entry to a host cell, where, after replication, they repackage their genetic material once more into complex structures prior to leaving the cell. They are strong enough to survive in the external environment, some for extended periods, while others require close contact and little exposure between hosts.

Box 3.1 Definitions

Viruses consist of a genetic component containing either RNA or DNA, but never both. The RNA or DNA can be either single- or double-stranded.
Capsid is the protein coat, the shell that surrounds the nucleic acid. The majority of viruses have either a helical or icosahedral capsid.
Capsomeres are the protein molecules that form the capsid structure.
Complex viruses do not have a simple helical or icosahedral capsid but, as the name suggests, involve a more complex structure, e.g. pox viruses have a rectangular shape surrounded by an envelope.
Envelope is the phospholipid bilayer containing glycoproteins that surrounds the capsid in enveloped viruses, and is also known as the viral membrane.
Virion denotes the complete infectious viral structure: nucleic acid plus capsid in a non-enveloped virus; nucleic acid plus capsid plus envelope in enveloped viruses.
A **retrovirus** is a virus whose RNA genome has a DNA intermediate as part of its replication cycle.

Viruses have been responsible for significant pandemics and high death rates over time. Viruses are believed to have spread within human populations from the time that man progressed from hunter-gatherers and lived in agricultural communities; viruses could then spread more easily among the increased population. Egyptian carvings depict men with dropped feet, a classic sign of polio. Measles was recognized as early as 4000 BC, showing similar symptoms to the cattle disease rinderpest and canine distemper; this was perhaps an early transmission of viruses between species.

Until a successful vaccination was developed for smallpox, the virus was responsible for over 300 million deaths worldwide in the twentieth century, with millions more survivors scarred for life. Emperors of Japan and Burma along with kings and queens of Europe became victims of smallpox. Viral infections sweeping through one of the opposing armies influenced the outcome of significant battles. The Spanish invaders Cortés and Pizarro defeated the armies of the Mexican Aztecs and Peruvian Incas when they introduced the smallpox and measles viruses to the susceptible populations. Yellow fever played a role in the import of African slaves to Mexico and the southern states of America; Caucasian and Native Americans were susceptible to the mosquito-borne virus, whereas the black Africans had natural resistance and were brought in to boost the falling numbers of workers. Smallpox, measles, yellow fever and polio (which caused epidemics in the nineteenth century and first half of the twentieth century) are now vaccine-preventable diseases. Influenza viruses have produced pandemics in recent history and genetic changes within avian influenza viruses still pose a threat. New viruses continue to emerge, notably HIV, Ebola virus, hantavirus and Lassa fever. The UK vaccination schedule includes measles, mumps and rubella, and vaccinations are available to travellers (e.g. hepatitis A and yellow fever) and to other groups of susceptible individuals (e.g. for hepatitis B).

3.1   VIRAL STRUCTURE AND CLASSIFICATION

Virus structure was impossible to study until the advent of electron microscopy and, more recently, data from the analysis of computerized images, three-dimensional construction methods and X-ray crystallography. Brenner and Horne were among the early researchers in the 1950s who, using electron-dense dyes, negative staining and electron microscopy, investigated the detailed structure of viruses. Watson and Crick in 1956 first suggested that virus capsids had numerous protein subunits arranged in either helical or icosahedral shapes.

Size

One of the principal differences between viruses and bacteria and the eukaryotic pathogens is size. Viruses range in size from 20 to 300 nm (nanometres; $1\,nm = 10^{-3}\,\mu m$). They pass through filters designed to retain bacteria and are invisible by light microscopy. This is a pity because viruses are intricate and attractive structures. Viruses are impossible to grow on culture media, as they have to infect cells in order to replicate; they can, however, be cultured in cell lines and in the membranes of eggs.

Figure 3.1 shows some size relationships between an average bacterium and viruses.

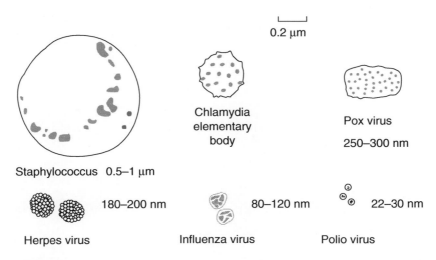

Figure 3.1
The relative sizes of bacteria and viruses. Viruses range in size from 20–300 nm (1 nm = $10^{-3}\,\mu m$). Shown here are representative staphylococci cells, a chlamydia elementary body (the infective form of chlamydia), a small obligate intracellular bacterium, and a range of viruses from the large pox virus to the small polio virus.

Genetic material

Viruses have a simple structure, carrying their genetic material in the form of either RNA or DNA, but never both. RNA viruses are the only organisms to have their nucleic acid in this form; the RNA is present either as a single genome or in several segments (influenza viruses have a segmented RNA genome). Both RNA and DNA genomes can consist of double-stranded or single-stranded nucleic acid. The production of viral messenger RNA (mRNA) is necessary for the replication of viral proteins on host ribosomes. All viral mRNA is designated positive and so viral

Table 3.1 Examples of common viruses and their Baltimore classification

Baltimore class	Nucleic acid	Family	Examples	Enveloped or naked	Capsid symmetry
I	dsDNA	Herpes Adenovirus Papovavirus	HSV1, 2. CMV, EBV VZV Adenovirus Papillomavirus	Enveloped Naked Naked	Icosahedral Icosahedral Icosahedral
II	ssDNA	Parvovirus	Parvovirus	Naked	Icosahedral
III	dsRNA	Reovirus	Rotavirus	Naked	Icosahedral
IV	(+) ssRNA	Togaviruses Picornavirus Calicivirus	Rubivirus: rubella Flavivirus: yellow fever, dengue, hepatitis C Polio Rhinovirus (common cold) Hepatitis A Norovirus Hepatitis E	Enveloped Naked Naked	Icosahedral Icosahedral Icosahedral
V	(-) ssRNA	Orthomyxovirus Arenavirus Paramyxovirus	Influenza Lassa fever Mumps Morbillivirus: measles	Enveloped	Helical
VI	(reverse)RNA (+) ssRNA with DNA intermediate in replication cycle	Retrovirus	Lentivirus: HIV	Enveloped	Icosahedral
VII	(reverse)DNA dsDNA with RNA intermediate	Hepadnavirus	Hepatitis B virus	Enveloped	Icosahedral

RNA is classified as positive if it has the same sequence as the mRNA, or negative if it contains the complementary base sequence. The Baltimore classification divides viruses into seven classes based on their genetic structure, as shown in *Table 3.1*.

Because they have no intracellular structures, viruses depend on host ribosomes to translate their proteins and on host nucleotides for raw materials to replicate their nucleic acids. Not all types of host cells would be suitable and this means that host specificity is important. Some viruses only infect animals or plants, whereas others are capable of successfully infecting humans. The ability to infect animals, birds and humans or to adapt to new species by combining significant genes can lead to the emergence of new infections and diseases. Avian influenza is a good example.

Capsids

A protein coat, the capsid, made up of individual protein molecules, called capsomeres, surrounds the nucleic acid. The capsid protects the more fragile nucleic acid from physical damage, from chemical damage such as UV radiation in sunlight, and from enzymic damage from nucleases (from dead cells or as part of the host defence). In relation to viral function, the capsid is responsible for host cell recognition, where it operates as a specific attachment protein to a recognized cellular receptor molecule. Depending on the type of virus, the capsomeres are arranged in symmetry to form either a helical or an icosahedral coat around the nucleic acid molecules.

The capsid of helical viruses forms a cylindrical shape around the nucleic acid, and is either a straight and relatively rigid rod shape, or a more curved or coiled helix that is more flexible and can be curled into an envelope. The proteins are assembled using repeating components that have a constant special relationship with each other. If the virus has multiple segments of genome, each one is enclosed in an individual helical capsid. If the helical virus is enveloped, the capsid coils inside the lipid envelope and the resulting virus can appear roughly spherical (see *Figure 3.2*).

Icosahedral capsids consist of a rigid 20-faced box composed of equilateral triangles and 12 vertices (corners). The simplest icosahedron has 20 faces made up of three identical capsomere subunits, i.e. 60 subunits in total. The overall shape appears almost spherical. An example of this simple structure is poliovirus, a naked single-stranded RNA of the picornavirus family. The structure is very stable and enables the virus to withstand the harsh environmental conditions encountered in the digestive tract as well as survival in the external environment. Others, for example the double-stranded DNA viruses of the herpes family, contain the proteins of the icosahedral capsid, a protein layer between the capsule and the envelope called the tegument, and glycoproteins forming spikes within the lipid envelope. DNA viruses are not as hardy in the environment and this is reflected in their method of transmission, where they are passed from person to person in saliva, blood and respiratory droplets (see *Figure 3.3*).

Envelopes

The envelope comprises a lipid bilayer into which proteins are inserted to enhance recognition and attachment to receptors on host cells. The lipid bilayer is often of host cell origin and is added to the virions as they leave the host cell. The proteins are either matrix proteins linking the nucleocapsid to the envelope, or glycoproteins, which are transmembrane proteins. External glycoproteins are anchored in the envelope

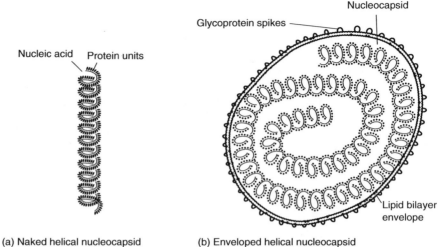

(a) Naked helical nucleocapsid   (b) Enveloped helical nucleocapsid

Figure 3.2
This diagram shows a naked (a) and an enveloped (b) helical virus. The capsid forms a cylindrical shape around the nuclear material. The structure is flexible enough to be coiled inside the lipid envelope (comprising a lipid bilayer with glycoprotein spikes on the outside) if necessary.

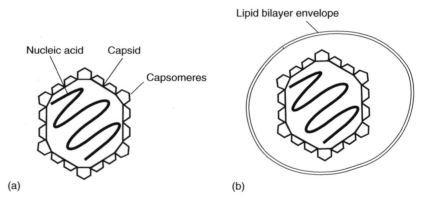

(a)   (b)

Figure 3.3
This structure represents a naked (a) and an enveloped (b) icosahedral virus. The icosahedral capsid consists of 20 protein capsomeres arranged as equilateral triangles and pentons. The virus appears spherical when viewed under the electron microscope. Many icosahedral viruses also have glycoprotein spikes protruding from the surface of the lipid envelope.

but most of the protein structure is on the outside of the virion, often appearing as 'spikes' on the virion surface. These spikes can then act as binding molecules to host receptors. The other proteins in the envelope act as transport channels, as shown in *Figure 3.4*. A good example of the role of envelope glycoproteins can be seen in the influenza viruses. There are two types of glycoproteins appearing as spikes, the haemagglutinin H and the neuraminidase N, and each virus has 500 molecules of

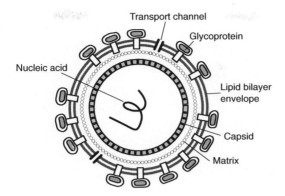

Figure 3.4
Viruses have envelopes modified from the host cell lipid membrane, into which they insert their own proteins. Matrix proteins link the nucleocapsid to the envelope; glycoproteins comprise the major antigens of enveloped viruses. The envelope also contains transport proteins.

haemagglutinin and 100 neuraminidase. They are antigenic in nature and give the influenza virus its characteristic H and N classification, e.g. swine flu is H1N1.The haemagglutinin has the ability to agglutinate red blood cells but also to bind to the sialic acid present on host cells. The neuraminidase removes the *N*-acetyl neuraminic acid from host glycoproteins and allows the passage of virion out of epithelial cells and into new cells, disrupting the mucous fluid of the respiratory tract and easing the viral spread through cells. Both helical and icosahedral viruses can be enveloped.

Some viruses have a complex structure that does not fall easily into the definition of either helical, icosahedral, enveloped or non-enveloped. Poxviruses, of which smallpox is an example, are large, oval or brick-shaped enveloped viruses, between 200 and 400 nm in length. The complex structure contains more than 100 different proteins, ten of which function as enzymes.

Nomenclature

Viruses are classified by family and genus. The family name always ends in -viridae and the genus in -*virus*. For example, the family Picornaviridae contains the genera *Enterovirus*, *Rhinovirus* and Hepatovirus, causing polio, common colds and hepatitis A, respectively. The family Herpesviridae includes herpes simplex virus (cold sores and genital infections), varicella-zoster (chickenpox and shingles) and Epstein–Barr virus, EBV (infectious mononucleosis). Viruses are also described by the type of DNA or RNA they contain, whether single-stranded or double-stranded, positive or negative stranded, the type of capsid and whether they are enveloped or not. The Baltimore classification is based on the nucleic acid present in different viruses. Baltimore classifications, with examples of specific viruses, are shown in *Table 3.1*.

3.2 VIRAL PATHOGENESIS

The way in which viruses cause symptomatic disease is the result of their infection and replication process within the specific cells they infect and damage. A virus targeting intestinal epithelial cells damages the normal cell function as it takes over the cells and replicates, leading to symptoms of sickness and diarrhoea; a virus preferentially replicating in the liver leads to symptoms of hepatitis and jaundice; similarly, a virus targeting the mucous membranes of the respiratory tract produces a variety of respiratory symptoms. Complications arise when the virus is not readily cleared by the immune system, the viral infection has produced irreversible damage to cells or nerves, or viral damage to the cells has been superseded by a secondary bacterial infection. The method and ease of transmission between hosts also determines whether large numbers of people are infected at one time (influenza, chickenpox, norovirus) or whether the viral disease is sporadic and affects only specific groups of people who are exposed to infection with the virus through lifestyle (for example intravenous drug abusers), by their profession (medical staff, police, etc.) or through travel to endemic countries. Examples include hepatitis A, B and C, HIV and yellow fever. Vaccination programmes for mumps, measles, rubella, hepatitis B and smallpox now control a considerable number of previously potentially severe viral diseases.

Viral infection and replication follow a series of steps from transmission until new viruses are replicated, released and transmitted again. The principal stages are:

- adsorption (attachment)
- penetration into the host cell
- uncoating
- transcription of mRNA
- translation of the mRNA into structural and non-structural proteins on host ribosomes
- replication of the nucleic acid
- assembly of new virions
- release to infect more cells.

Transmission

The ways in which microorganisms are transmitted from person to person are described in *Chapter 4*. All of the routes described are applicable to viral infection and examples are given for each of them.

- **Respiratory**, via droplet infection transferred by coughs, sneezes and saliva – respiratory viruses include influenza, adenoviruses and infectious mononucleosis (glandular fever), chickenpox, rubella, mumps, measles, respiratory syncytial virus.
- **Skin**, via shedding of skin cells or direct contact with infected skin lesions – wart viruses.
- **Faecal–oral**, transmission via food, water and poor hygiene – norovirus, rotavirus, hepatitis A.
- **Sexual** transmission, via mucosal contact with infected individuals – HIV, genital warts, genital herpes, hepatitis B.
- **Blood-borne**, via contact with the blood of an infected person – hepatitis B and C, HIV, CMV, congenital rubella.
- **Animals,** zoonotic transmission from vertebrates and vector-borne disease from invertebrate, arthropod vectors – orf virus, rotavirus. The following would need

exposure during travels – yellow fever, West Nile fever, dengue, Ebola virus, Marburg disease, Lassa fever, Japanese encephalitis.

■ **Inanimate objects**, fomites, where the pathogen survives before infecting the next host. This includes clothing, bed linen, clinical instruments, door knobs, surfaces of kitchen or furniture – influenza, norovirus.

Attachment

Viral attachment is, like bacterial attachment, a specific interaction between the virion and the host cell receptor. The infectious dose is important because the greater the number of viruses present, the greater the possibility of them coming into contact with susceptible cells. Not all viruses can attach to all types of host cell, giving the virus a host cell, species and tissue specificity. Different viruses recognize different receptors on human host cells and these receptors fulfil a cellular function of their own as well as providing attachment points for viruses to be adsorbed onto the cell surface. In some cases a co-receptor is also necessary for viral attachment. Knowledge of the specific receptor and virus interactions increases understanding of viral pathogenesis and can lead to the development of new treatment strategies.

Viral penetration and uncoating

Receptor virus binding initiates the internalization and uncoating of the virus prior to replication of the genome and the transcription and translation of structural proteins on the host ribosomes in the cytoplasm. In DNA viruses, the genome is replicated in the nucleus of the host cell, whereas RNA replication takes place in the cytoplasm. *Figure 3.5* shows two methods used by viruses to penetrate and uncoat after initial receptor binding to the host cell. Uncoating, the shedding of the envelope and capsid to release the nucleic acid, is an essential step in viral replication. The viral envelope, if present, is derived from the host cell membrane and, mediated by fusion proteins, fuses with the new host membrane and delivers the nucleocapsid into the cytoplasm. Some viruses uncoat at the cell membrane and the nucleic acid is then released into the cytoplasm. Other viruses shed their capsids in the cytoplasm. Receptor-mediated endocytosis is also used by viruses to enter cells. After attachment, the virus is taken into an early endosome and transported to the cytoplasm. The early endosome changes into a late endosome, which is more acidic and helps with the uncoating of the virus. Uncoating is completed when the endosome fuses with a lysosome and the nuclear material is released.

Transcription of mRNA

DNA viruses replicate and transcribe mRNA within the host cell nucleus. Larger DNA viruses encode their own DNA polymerase enzyme and other proteins to enhance their transcription and replication, including enzymes to scavenge for the deoxynucleotides they need for replication. Here again, tissue specificity is important because the DNA binding proteins have to be compatible. The smaller DNA viruses are more dependent on the host cell; parvoviruses can only replicate in growing cells such as very early blood cells and fetal cells. The first mRNA transcribed is for the early proteins required for replication and may include polymerases. Viral proteins are translated as one large protein, one portion of which acts as a protease to cleave

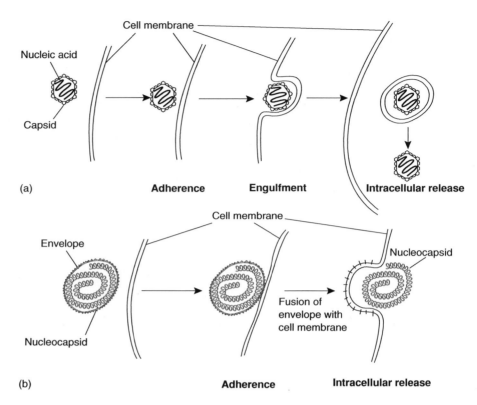

Figure 3.5
Entry of a naked virus (a) by receptor-mediated endocytosis, where the nucleocapsid is engulfed and transported to the cytoplasm in an endosome, which fuses with a lysosome prior to release. (b) shows an enveloped virus uncoating at the cell membrane and releasing the nucleocapsid into the cytoplasm.

the polyprotein into smaller functional units. Protease inhibitors are used as part of the combination therapy in the treatment of HIV.

Replication of the viral DNA commences in the nucleus. The late proteins for the capsids are produced in the cytoplasm using host cell ribosomes and raw materials, and then transported into the nucleus for assembly.

Replication and transcription of RNA viruses takes place in the cytoplasm and the production of the mRNA by RNA polymerase is dependent on whether the genomic RNA is double-stranded or single-stranded, positive or negative, as described in the Baltimore classification classes III, IV and V. Double-stranded RNA viruses synthesize mRNA from the positive strand. If a single-stranded RNA virus is positive, then the mRNA is the same as the genome and immediately begins to transcribe proteins; a negative strand is synthesized to enable the RNA to replicate. Negative strand RNA viruses must first replicate to produce a positive strand for use as the mRNA. In both situations, RNA polymerase has to be produced as quickly as possible to generate mRNA because the human cell does not normally replicate RNA, only DNA, and RNA is degraded easily. As the viral RNA replicates it provides more templates for the production of mRNA and viral replication is accelerated. *Figure 3.6* shows the

(a) Double-stranded RNA genome

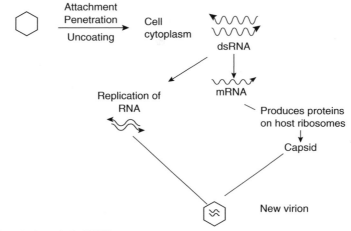

(b) Positive single-stranded RNA genome

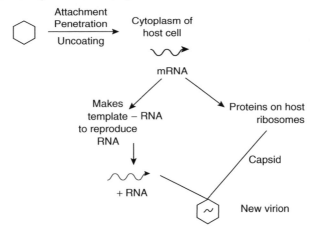

(c) Negative single-stranded RNA genome

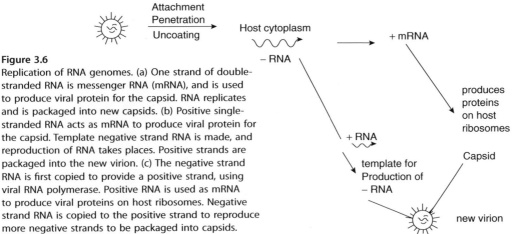

Figure 3.6
Replication of RNA genomes. (a) One strand of double-stranded RNA is messenger RNA (mRNA), and is used to produce viral protein for the capsid. RNA replicates and is packaged into new capsids. (b) Positive single-stranded RNA acts as mRNA to produce viral protein for the capsid. Template negative strand RNA is made, and reproduction of RNA takes places. Positive strands are packaged into the new virion. (c) The negative strand RNA is first copied to provide a positive strand, using viral RNA polymerase. Positive RNA is used as mRNA to produce viral proteins on host ribosomes. Negative strand RNA is copied to the positive strand to reproduce more negative strands to be packaged into capsids.

principal steps in the replication of DNA viruses, while *Figure 3.7* shows those for RNA viruses.

Viruses in classes VI and VII of the Baltimore classification are more complex in their replication. HIV, a single-stranded positive RNA virus, produces the enzyme reverse transcriptase to produce a DNA intermediate that integrates into the genome of the host cell from where it is transcribed. Hepatitis B virus is unusual, and unique for a DNA virus, in that it has a double-stranded DNA genome and uses a reverse transcriptase to produce an RNA intermediate during replication.

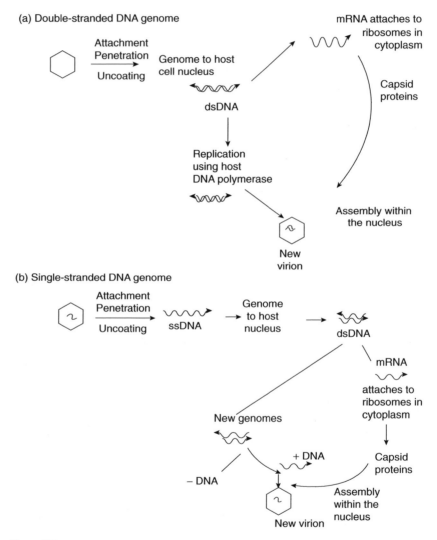

Figure 3.7
Replication of DNA genomes. (a) One strand of the double-stranded DNA is used to transcribe messenger RNA (mRNA). mRNA attaches to ribosomes in the host cytoplasm and transcribes proteins. Double-stranded DNA is replicated in the nucleus using host DNA polymerase. (b) shows the single-stranded DNA genome. The transcription of single-stranded DNA viruses involves an extra step to produce double-stranded DNA templates.

Assembly and release of new virions

Once the genome has replicated, packaging within the capsids takes place. The location for this, either in the nucleus or cytoplasm, is dependent on the type of virus. The whole process is remarkable for its precision and intricacy, bearing in mind the size of the complete virus and the complexity of the capsid structure. Individual capsomeres join together precisely to form either a helical or an icosahedral shape after being sorted in the Golgi apparatus. They have to be moved around the cell in the microtubules or vesicles to locate other protein molecules and then the nuclear material has to be packaged inside them. For some viruses the assembly takes place at the same time as the genome is produced; for others the genome is packaged into the already formed capsids. This can only be achieved with accuracy because the nuclear material has a packaging signal composed of a specific base sequence, and there are still empty capsids released. Non-enveloped viruses assemble in the host cell nucleus; enveloped viruses assemble close to the area where they will acquire their envelope, be it the nuclear membrane, organelle membrane or outer cell membrane.

Enveloped viruses acquire their envelopes from host membranes, often the outer cell membrane, as they bud out of the cell. Budding from the cell has the advantage that the host cell does not necessarily die. Viral glycoproteins, transport proteins and matrix proteins, all of viral origin, are inserted into the lipid membrane to form the complete enveloped virion. *Figure 3.8* shows the budding of influenza virus through the host membrane.

Naked viruses accumulate within the cell, and when the numbers are sufficiently high, the cell bursts, or lyses, and the new virions are released. This is called the viral lytic infection cycle. The viruses then infect neighbouring cells, by either attacking their outer membranes or spreading intracellularly. The latter has the advantage that the immune system is less likely to be alerted.

If the virus is, for example, a rhinovirus causing cold symptoms, damage to the epithelial cells causes an increase in the amount of virus-rich fluid produced, fluid that can be spread to other hosts by sneezing and nasal secretions on hands and inanimate objects.

Lytic, latent and chronic infection

Many acute viral infections are the result of lytic infection of the target cells. The host immune system is alerted by the damage to the cells and produces natural killer cells, cytotoxic T cells, interferon and both a cellular and antibody response to contain and control the infection and also to give immunity. Herpesviruses are good examples of latent infection. After the initial acute infection, the viruses are not cleared but 'hide' either within specific cells or in the nerve ganglions, where they exist with minimal gene expression, controlled by immune cells. If conditions in the host change and the immune system is less vigilant they can reactivate. Herpes simplex virus is a good example: the initial lytic infection causes cold sores and the release of virus-rich fluid from the blisters on the mucous membranes. The viruses then travel along the nerve fibres to the dorsal root ganglion where they remain latent. Re-emergence can be triggered by stress, sunlight or menstruation, depending on the individual, at which point the viruses travel back along the nerve fibres and produce a lytic infection on the mucous membranes.

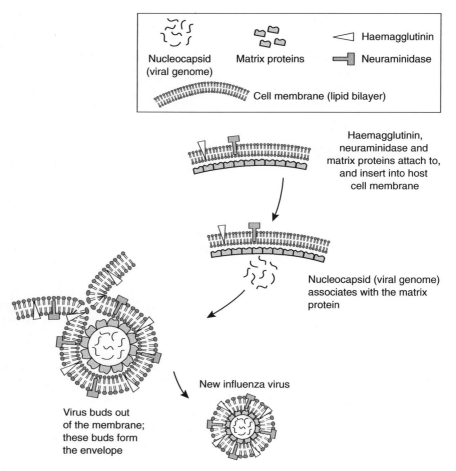

Nucleocapsid
(viral genome)

Matrix proteins

◁ Haemagglutinin

Neuraminidase

Cell membrane (lipid bilayer)

Haemagglutinin,
neuraminidase and
matrix proteins attach to,
and insert into host
cell membrane

Nucleocapsid (viral genome)
associates with the matrix
protein

New influenza virus

Virus buds out
of the membrane;
these buds form
the envelope

Figure 3.8
Budding of an influenza virus through the host cell cytoplasmic membrane.

In chronic infections the patients recover from the initial acute infection but continue to carry the virus and so become carriers. Unlike in latent infections, the virus can be detected continuously. Hepatitis B is a good example.

Finally, some viruses have the potential to be oncogenic, i.e. leading to the formation of cancer. The herpesvirus EBV is associated with both Burkitt's lymphoma and nasopharyngeal carcinoma in specific geographical areas of the world; chronic infection with hepatitis B can increase the chances of a patient developing liver cancer. However, the mechanisms for the development of malignancy are different for both viruses. Human papilloma viruses, types 16 and 18, are associated with the development of cervical cancer in susceptible patients.

Viral infection of cells results in either cell death or sufficient alteration in the cells to trigger an immune response and the appearance of distinctive symptoms in the patient. The combination of symptoms and the presence of viral antigen or antibodies in the patient's blood serum provide sufficient evidence for an accurate diagnosis to be made.

3.3 LABORATORY DIAGNOSIS OF VIRAL INFECTIONS

Traditionally, virus infections were diagnosed by cell culture techniques, by visualizing viral particles using electron microscopy (EM) and by haemagglutination methods. Cell culture and EM methods are still in routine use, but haemagglutination techniques have been replaced by more sensitive and specific monoclonal antibody based methods (enzyme-linked immunosorbent assay, ELISA, sometimes known as EIA), fluorescent antibody techniques (immunofluorescence, IF) and by molecular based techniques (PCR amplification using specific nucleic acid sequence primers). The principles of the methods in current use are explained in *Chapter 5* (EM, IF) and *Chapter 6* (molecular methods and ELISA). Some laboratories still use the complement fixation test (described in *Chapter 6*) to diagnose rising viral antibody titres in acute and convalescent serum.

Diagnosis of virus particles in faecal specimens using immune electron microscopy

Grids for the electron microscope are prepared by coating them with protein A, and IgG and IgM derived from human convalescent serum as the capturing antibody. The grid is then floated on to a drop of the faecal specimen and left at room temperature for 2 hours. After incubation the grid is stained for a few seconds with a negative stain, phosphotungstic acid, and then viewed at a screen magnification of at least 50 000. For optimum recovery of virus particles, the test is performed on faecal specimens 48 hours after the onset of symptoms and one gram of the sample is used. At this stage the maximum number of viruses are excreted; the high number is important as the method requires at least 1 million virus particles per 1 ml of solution. The cost of an electron microscope is beyond the budget of routine laboratories and so specimens usually have to be referred to a regional laboratory.

Cell culture

Herpesviruses, varicella-zoster and CMV can be diagnosed from clinical samples such as vesicle fluid using human diploid fibroblasts MRC-5 line or Vero cells. The specimen is added to two cell culture tubes, each containing 0.2 ml of VTM (viral transport medium) which are then incubated for a minimum of 7 days at 35–37°C. They are examined daily for cytopathic changes indicating the presence of the viruses. Molecular methods are gradually replacing cell culture in many laboratories.

Molecular methods

Real-time PCR methods (see *Chapter 6* for more details), giving a quantitative result of the level of virus present in the sample, use specific viral primers for RNA or DNA, and have the advantage of a rapid turn-around time of less than 24 hours. This makes them an attractive replacement for culture and ELISA for the diagnosis of some viral pathogens. Influenza A, H1–15 and B can be detected in naso-pharyngeal aspirates, broncho-alveolar lavage, endotracheal aspirates, nose and throat swabs and sputum after extraction of the nucleic acid. The precision of the method not only enhances accurate diagnosis of outbreak strains but also provides reliable epidemiological data for monitoring the levels of, for example, H1N1 swine flu in the population.

Molecular methods are also used for adenovirus and norovirus and for measuring the viral load of HIV in blood plasma when the infection is diagnosed, and during the monitoring of the effectiveness of specific anti-retroviral treatment.

Enzyme-linked immunosorbent assays

Enzyme-linked immunosorbent assays (ELISAs, sometimes referred to as EIAs or enzyme immune assays) are easy to use and enable large numbers of clinical specimens to be screened at a time. The tests can be in either 96 well plates or single strips, and can be manual or automated. Single-use kits are also available, where the specimen is added to a strip into which are embedded the antigen antibody and substrate. As the specimen travels along the strip, a coloured product is visualized if the antigen–antibody complexes are present. This is a form of immunochromatography that is used commercially in home-use pregnancy test kits. A wide variety of virus infections can be tested using ELISA on serum samples or, as in norovirus and rotavirus, from faecal samples. The solid phase (coated wells), can either be a specific antigen or antibody; specific ELISAs will also detect IgM or IgG antibodies, useful in differentiating acute infection or past immunity. The scope of the method is broad in terms of the antigens and antibodies detected and the ability to ascertain a serological profile, and thus, information about the disease stage and progression. This is important in hepatitis B and Epstein–Barr infections and in determining whether varicella-zoster infection or rubella infection is acute or representative of past immunity in susceptible pregnant women.

3.4 THE DIAGNOSIS AND TREATMENT OF CLINICALLY IMPORTANT VIRAL INFECTIONS

Viral infections that are self-limiting and have predictable symptoms, such as the common cold, mild respiratory infections and episodes of viral gastroenteritis, do not need confirmation by laboratory tests. This is true of some childhood diseases, such as chickenpox, where the symptoms can be diagnosed with some accuracy, and with common cold sores and shingles. However, if symptoms persist and complications occur, laboratory diagnosis can confirm the causative organism and guide treatment if available.

It is important to diagnose infections such as HIV, epidemic influenza, viral hepatitis and rubella, and to check the immune status of a pregnant woman exposed to chickenpox. Symptoms of a persistent throat infection that does not respond to antibiotic treatment could be caused by Epstein–Barr virus. Unexpectedly high levels of vaccine-preventable diseases need to be confirmed to provide epidemiological data.

Human immunodeficiency virus

The diagnosis, treatment and prevention of human immunodeficiency virus (HIV) is a global challenge. Throughout the world the number of infections is estimated at 33 million. In the UK over 80 000 people (2009 HPA figures) are thought to be infected with HIV. Unlinked anonymous data from pregnant women, intravenous drug users and sexual health clinics, covering the 15–59 years age range, suggest that up to a quarter of infections remain undiagnosed. In developed countries treatment regimes allow patients to live with the virus, whereas in endemic countries, where treatment is unavailable or too expensive, the mortality rates are much higher, and globally, 2 million adults and children have died from the infection.

HIV is a member of the *Lentivirus* genus of the Retroviridae family, Baltimore classification VI, as shown in *Table 3.1*. The virus is a complex icosahedral structure with 72 external spikes of the major envelope glycoproteins gp120 and gp41 and contains host cell proteins in the lipid bilayer. The dense cone-shaped nucleocapsid is composed of the core protein p24 and two copies of the singe-stranded RNA genome associated with the enzymes viral reverse transcriptase, RNase H, integrase and protease. Two major types of the virus have been identified, HIV1 and HIV2. HIV1 is more commonly diagnosed in the UK, with HIV2 infections more often found in western Africa and in India. The infection is primarily transmitted in blood and body fluids, sexually, from mother to child and by intravenous drug use. The virus infects the heart of the immune system, the CD4 lymphocytes and macrophages as well as dendritic cells, by attaching to specific receptors, CD4 and CXCR4 on T lymphocytes and CD4 and CCR5 on macrophages, via the viral envelope proteins gp120 and gp41.

The incubation from exposure to clinical onset is between 1 and 4 weeks. The primary infection may go unnoticed as it takes the form of a self-limiting flu-like or mononucleosis infection and may involve a skin rash. After this initial illness the infection may remain clinically latent for up to 10 years, after which time the classic signs of immunodeficiency disease appear, such as opportunistic infections, skin cancer lesions of Kaposi's sarcoma, neurological symptoms, night sweats, chronic tiredness and malaise. The CD4 lymphocyte count drops to levels where effective immune responses and memory are no longer possible. Kaposi's sarcoma is also caused by a herpesvirus, HHV8, controlled in immuno-competent individuals by the immune system. During the clinically latent phase the virus is not latent but is controlled by the continual turnover of CD4 cells. The virus continually makes errors as it multiplies, giving rise to extensive mutations during the course of an infection.

It is important to diagnose the disease and start treatment as soon as possible; however, there are large numbers of infected individuals who are not aware that they are carrying the virus. Specific antibodies to the virus are formed between 2–4 weeks and 3 months after infection. In the early stages the p24 antigen is also detectable and so the laboratory tests should include detection of both antigen and antibody to maximize the detection of early infection. There are strict protocols in HIV testing to ensure that the laboratory diagnosis is correctly made. It is also important to provide a rapid test result, preferably while the patient is still in the clinic. Counselling and confirmatory testing are then possible in as short a time as possible, reducing the stress of the patient waiting for the result, and also enabling an accurate diagnosis to be made.

Rapid automated single-use ELISAs detecting both antigen and antibody provide accurate, sensitive and specific results. If the result is positive, the serum is re-tested directly from the clotted blood sample and then an EDTA sample is requested. The plasma is separated from the cells within 6 hours and subsequently tested for HIV viral load using a reverse transcriptase PCR technique. The result gives an indication of the number of RNA copies per ml of blood and provides the baseline count for treatment.

HIV is a good example of how knowledge and understanding of the structure and replication of a virus can lead to the development of effective drug therapy. The high mutation rate of HIV means that the virus will quickly develop resistance to a single antiviral agent, and so in highly active anti-retroviral therapy (HAART), a combination of drugs is used. Reverse transcriptase copies the viral RNA into double-stranded DNA which is then incorporated into the host genome. Nucleosides are the building blocks of DNA; nucleoside analogues are used in nucleoside reverse transcriptase inhibitors (NRTIs) to compete with reverse transcriptase activity by incorporation into the DNA chain and halting chain elongation. Non-nucleoside reverse transcriptase inhibitors (NNRTIs) block reverse transcriptase at a different site and are not incorporated into the DNA. The drug regime incorporates anti-reverse transcriptase inhibitors, for example, efavirenz (NNRTI) plus tenofir or abacavir (both NRTIs) plus lamivudine or emtricitabine. Treatment is highly successful and recent data in the UK showed that 90% of patients treated within 3 months of diagnosis had undetectable viral loads (<50 copies/ml) after one year. There will, however, always be reservoirs of the virus latent in metabolically inert cells or in areas with limited drug penetration and so drug therapy has to be continuous. A summary of the classes of drug available is shown in *Table 3.2*. Transmission from mother to child is reduced by treating the mother either with zidovudine monotherapy or a combination of zidovudine and lamivudine. Combination therapy is monitored by viral load measurement – a rise in the viral load can indicate development of resistance to one or more of the drugs and the need to change the therapy.

Table 3.2 Examples of the classes of drugs used in the treatment of HIV

Class of drug	Activity	Examples
Nucleoside reverse transcriptase inhibitors (NRTI)	Competitive inhibition of reverse transcriptase	Zidovudine, abacavir, lamivudine, tenofir, emtricitabine
Non-nucleoside reverse transcriptase inhibitors (NNRTI)	Non-competitive inhibition of RT	Efavirenz
Protease inhibitors	Inhibit the enzyme necessary to produce cleaved functional proteins	Atazavir, darunavir, fosamprenavir, indinavir
Fusion and envelope inhibitors	Inhibit fusion of virus to host cells	Enfuvirtide
Integrase inhibitors	Inhibit integration of HIV genome into nucleus	Raltegravir
CCR5 receptor antagonists	Inhibit receptor binding	Maraviroc

Influenza

There are three genera of influenzavirus, A B and C, belonging to the family Orthomyxoviridae, enveloped single-stranded RNA viruses, Baltimore classification V. Genera B and C only infect humans, whereas influenza A (avian) infects birds, swine, horses and humans. The viruses have two different spikes protruding from their surface, the haemagglutinin H and the neuraminidase N, which act as surface antigens. Viral attachment to host cells is via the haemagglutinin and antibodies produced against it are protective. This is not true of the neuraminidase which splits off neuramic acid from the host cell virus receptor and is also believed to play a role in the release of new virus particles from the cell. There are 15 different subtypes of haemagglutinin and nine of neuraminidase, responsible for the strains causing either sporadic or epidemic disease, for example H1N1 and H3N2. Influenza A also has matrix protein surrounding the nucleocapsid and nucleoprotein associated with the segmented genome. The two surface antigens are renowned for undergoing subtle changes (known as antigenic <u>drift</u>), and provided the change is not too significant, protective antibodies will remain effective. However, if the antigens, H and N, change significantly, there is an antigenic <u>shift</u> and previous immunity is not protective. Because the genome is segmented, re-assortment or recombination can take place. If a host is infected with two different types of the virus, a new strain can emerge, particularly if human and bird or swine viruses mix in a host (see *Box 3.2*).

Box 3.2 Influenza shift and drift

The two glycoprotein spikes, haemagglutinin and neuraminidase on the surface of the influenza virus are able to change subtly (antigenic <u>drift</u>) or more significantly (antigenic <u>shift</u>). Antigenic drift is a continuous event and, providing the changes are small, antibodies raised against the original virus will continue to be protective. The shift occurs because, apart from HIV, influenza is one of the fastest mutating viruses. RNA viruses mutate faster than DNA viruses because the enzymes that produce the RNA are less accurate than those reproducing DNA. Therefore, small changes in the viral genome lead to small changes in the envelope proteins and antigenic drift. New, epidemic strains of influenza arise when there are large changes in the RNA genome that are not recognized by the immune system. These emergent strains of influenza A often occur in countries where animals and birds live in closer proximity to humans and the viruses are able to infect several species. The influenza genome is composed of 7–8 segments of single-stranded RNA which makes it easier for mixing to occur. If an animal or bird becomes co-infected with two strains of influenza, genetic re-assortment and recombination can take place. This could be poultry infected with an avian and human strain, or a pig infected with two strains, in which case the pig acts as a mixing vessel for the virus.

One of the largest flu pandemics was the Spanish flu epidemic that occurred at the end of the First World War in 1917 and 1918, so called because it was the Spanish press which published details of the disease. The strain is believed to have originated in large army camps in France, where great numbers of chickens were kept and killed for food. The 1918 strain was a not a recombination of poultry and human viruses but an adaptation of an avian virus able to reproduce in humans. After the war, the men dispersed across Europe, taking with them the new virus that swept through populations, killing more than 50 million. This was more than the number killed in the war and more than in the Black Death. Modern cloning techniques have shown that the H5N1 virus is very similar, except for a few amino acids in the polymerase proteins, to the 1918 strain. Further changes in the H5N1 virus, enabling human-to-human infection, are closely monitored by global surveillance schemes. The aim of this concerted effort is to reduce exposure, contain the virus and monitor the genome structure in readiness for vaccine development, activities that were not possible in 1918.

The 1957 Asian flu and 1968 Hong Kong flu epidemic strains were examples of genetic re-assortment of H2N2 and H3N2 viruses respectively. Asian flu originated from a recombination of wild duck and human strains in China and spread to the west through Hong Kong, killing between 1 and 4 million people. In 1968–69 the H3N2 virus was the result of antigenic shift and re-assortment of the H2N2 virus, resulting in 1 million deaths. The latest pandemic of H1N1 swine flu in 2009 originated in Mexico as a result of re-assortment of two swine viruses and caused 6000 deaths worldwide.

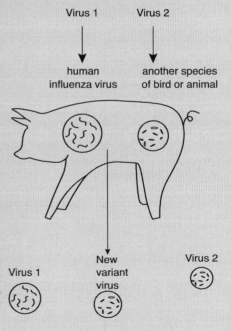

Influenza is spread by aerosols, from person to person and, after an incubation period of one to four days, the typical symptoms of fever, chills and muscle pain appear, often quite suddenly. Additional symptoms of a dry cough, chest pain, other respiratory symptoms and pharyngitis are also common. Most patients will recover within a few days, whereas complications can occur in elderly patients and those who have underlying disease or respiratory problems. The annual death toll from influenza in the UK is often in the thousands, with some strains affecting particular age groups more than others. Fortunately, influenza is a vaccine-preventable disease if the sequence of the infecting strain is known; the annual vaccine is based on the circulating epidemic strains. When a new strain of the virus emerges and causes disease, a vaccine is developed as soon as possible. This was demonstrated in 2009–10 with the development of the H1N1 swine flu vaccine, which is now incorporated into the annual flu vaccine. However, the WHO has developed a global surveillance scheme to monitor the emergence of new strains and their transmission, amid concerns that the avian H5N1 virus is evolving into a strain that can be transmitted easily from person to person, with the potential to cause serious disease.

Particularly when there is an epidemic strain circulating, and for an accurate diagnosis, specific and sensitive laboratory testing is required. In the past influenza A and B were diagnosed retrospectively by the complement fixation test, using paired acute and convalescent serum from the patient and looking for a rising titre of antibodies. Molecular techniques now offer rapid and accurate results using probes for A H1–H15 and B, and real-time PCR methodology.

Influenza can be treated with either oseltamivir (tamiflu) or zanamivir. Both of these drugs are neuraminidase inhibitors.

The herpesviruses: HSV, EBV, varicella-zoster, CMV

The herpesviruses are a family of double-stranded DNA viruses, Baltimore classification I. A summary of the characteristics of these viruses is shown in *Table 3.3*. They all have the potential to cause acute, latent and recurrent disease. EBV also

Table 3.3 The herpesvirus family, Herpesviridae

	Virus name	Target cell	Latency	Spread
Alpha	HHV1 HSV1 HHV2 HSV2 HHV3 VZV	Muco-epithelial cells	Neurons	Close contact, droplet, saliva
Beta	HHV5 CMV HHV6* Herpes lymphotropic virus HHV7*	Monocytes, lymphocytes, epithelial cells	Monocytes and lymphocytes	Close contact, saliva transfusion, placenta, tissue transplant
Gamma	HHV4 EBV HHV8 Kaposi's sarcoma related virus	B lymphocytes, epithelial cells	B lymphocytes	Saliva

*HHV6 is the cause of roseola or sixth disease, a largely asymptomatic illness in young children; if symptomatic, a rash is present. HHV7 is also associated with roseola in children.

has the potential to be oncogenic and is associated with the development of Burkitt's lymphoma and nasopharyngeal carcinoma in specific geographical areas of the world, whereas in the UK it is associated with infectious mononucleosis in young adults.

Herpes simplex virus 1 and 2

HSV 1 and 2 have a worldwide distribution and are the cause of vesicles on the face and mouth, cold sores, and genital herpes. After the primary infection, which also involves systemic symptoms of fever and malaise, the viruses remain latent in the neurons of the sensory ganglia for life, a persistent infection that can be reactivated. When reactivated, the viruses travel along the ganglia and erupt on the skin surface with the symptoms of acute disease. Generally, HSV1 is associated with mouth and facial infection and HSV2 with genital infections; the differences between the two viruses are demonstrated by restriction enzyme analysis. Both are strictly human pathogens spread by droplets or close contact. They attach to human target cell receptors via their envelope glycoproteins and once inside the cell are transported to the nucleus where they undergo replication.

Herpetic whitlows, also called digital herpes simplex, are a further local form of the infection where the blisters form on the finger or around a fingernail. In addition to local infections, HSV is associated with more serious complications of encephalitis, and generalized disease in immuno-compromised patients. HSV is also associated with some cases of Bell's palsy, a condition where viral infection of the seventh cranial nerve results in loss of sensation on one side of the face, causing weakness in the facial muscles, as if one side of the face has dropped. Accurate diagnosis is therefore essential and is achieved either by using molecular PCR-based techniques or by tissue culture. A differential diagnosis of HSV can eliminate syphilis vesicles, and differentiate between HSV and varicella-zoster.

The symptoms of HSV can be treated with aciclovir, but this does not eliminate the latent virus. Aciclovir is an analogue of guanosine triphosphate; aciclovir triphosphate is incorporated into the extending DNA and terminates the chain. The drug is inactive until it is phosphorylated by the viral enzyme thymidine kinase of HSV and varicella-zoster viruses.

Varicella-zoster (VZV)

Varicella is the Latin word for vesicles, and primary infection with the virus causes chickenpox. This is primarily a childhood disease spread by direct contact or droplets. After an incubation period of 2–3 weeks the symptoms of malaise and fever occur, followed by the appearance of a characteristic rash with vesicular spots all over the body, which last for about a week. In some cases there may be few or no lesions and the disease is subclinical. Protective antibodies are raised against further primary infection but do not protect from reactivation. The virus, a strictly human pathogen, becomes latent in the dorsal route ganglia. In common with other herpesviruses, reactivation of the virus can be triggered by stress and a weakened immune system. The virus travels back along the nerve to the skin and causes the localized painful vesicles and symptoms of shingles. The most common sites for the infection are along the path of the thoracic nerve and the trigeminal nerves in the face, but can occur along any nerve route.

Complications can occur with both primary and secondary infection. Chickenpox is a more serious disease for adults and particularly so if it is contracted by women in

Box 3.3 Viral haemorrhagic fever

The viruses causing viral haemorrhagic fevers (VHF) are all RNA viruses with a lipid envelope. They have animal or insect hosts, such as ticks and mosquitoes, and are restricted to areas of the world where these hosts are found. They cause sporadic zoonotic infections and small outbreaks in susceptible areas. Humans are not natural reservoirs but human-to-human transmission can take place through body fluids in cases of Ebola virus, Marburg disease, Lassa fever and Crimean Congo haemorrhagic fever (CCHF). The four families of viruses involved are:

- Arenaviruses – Lassa fever
- Bunyaviruses – hantavirus causing Rift Valley fever; *Nairovirus* – Crimean Congo haemorrhagic fever
- Filoviruses – Ebola virus and Marburg disease
- Flaviviruses – dengue and yellow fever.

Typical symptoms include fever, oedema, hypotension, shock, flushing of the face and chest, petechiae (small bruise-like rash), malaise, myalgia, diarrhoea and vomiting. Because of the risk of spreading the infections in hospitals, patients are treated in bio-containment facilities and any laboratory diagnosis is carried out in specialist laboratories with containment level 4 facilities. The full VHF syndrome, involving liver damage, disseminated intravascular coagulation (DIC) and bone marrow dysfunction, is dependent on the virulence of the virus. VHF syndrome is a feature of the filovirus infections, Ebola virus, Marburg disease and CCHF but is less likely in dengue, Lassa fever and Rift Valley fever, although DIC is a complication in the latter. Interestingly, the second attack of dengue with a different strain is more serious than the first because antibodies formed against the first strain enhance the symptoms of the second.

the perinatal stage just before or immediately following delivery. Because the mother cannot pass on protective antibodies, there is a risk that the baby may develop serious varicella which could be fatal if untreated. Immuno-compromised patients are also at high risk from the infection from serious systemic disease. Smokers, sufferers of chronic lung disease and pregnant women are also at greater risk of developing potentially fatal varicella pneumonia. Meningoencephalitis is a rare but serious complication of primary VZV infection, where the viruses gain access directly to the central nervous system.

Chickenpox and shingles are diagnosed clinically, but laboratory diagnosis of past or present infection is useful if there is a risk of exposure in a susceptible adult. Serum samples are tested for the presence of IgM antibodies, suggesting current infection and IgG antibodies formed in response to past infection. If the infection is acute in pregnant women, protective immunoglobulin from pooled and appropriately screened donations from immune individuals can be administered. The presence of antibodies formed to an earlier infection provides reassurance. ELISA methods, often single-use automated tests, enable rapid, sensitive and specific results. Molecular-based methods can also be useful to detect specific DNA from vesicle fluid and from CSF, differentiating VZV from HSV.

Varicella-zoster infection can be treated with aciclovir and famciclovir, a structural analogue of aciclovir.

Epstein–Barr virus (EBV)

The complexity and variety of disease caused by EBV makes it one of the most interesting to study. It is a typical herpesvirus in that it causes acute, chronic, persistent and reactivated infection. Furthermore, it is also associated with a diverse range of malignant disease in susceptible patients and in different regions of the world. It is most prevalent in adolescents and young adults. The virus is transmitted in saliva, often from asymptomatic carriers, and the infection is often called 'kissing disease'. Childhood infection with EBV is usually asymptomatic and 50% of children have antibodies to the virus by the age of 5 years. Symptomatic infection, infectious mononucleosis (IM, also known as glandular fever) is seen predominantly in adolescents and young adults in the UK, particularly those in the higher socio-economic groups who have not encountered the virus earlier in their lives. 90–95% of adults have antibodies to EBV. EBV targets the epithelial cells in the oropharynx and is the site of acute lytic infection. Immediate latency is established in the B lymphocytes where the virus enters the cell via the complement receptor CD21. B lymphocytes containing the EBV genome become immortalized or transformed.

After infection, the incubation period before symptoms are observed is between 30 and 50 days. Typical symptoms include enlargement of the lymph nodes and tonsillitis, sometimes accompanied by a rash. Liver enzyme levels are usually raised and in some cases the spleen becomes enlarged. The condition is frequently diagnosed as tonsillitis, and treated with amoxacillin, which can cause the further complication of a rash. The majority of patients recover from IM without complications but a proportion have a prolonged convalescence with chronic tiredness and a low grade fever. Haemolytic anaemia is a recognized complication of IM. EBV is associated with chronic fatigue syndrome, where sufferers experience the symptoms of EBV infection accompanied by muscle fatigue, memory and concentration problems, which may last for months or years. HIV-infected patients can develop wart-like lesions on their tongues. These oral hairy leukoplakia lesions are characterized by a hairy surface. There is also evidence of EBV involvement in Kawasaki disease, a childhood syndrome associated with coronary artery involvement.

EBV is also associated with tumours in which the EBV genome is found in the malignant cells and EBV nuclear antigen is expressed or antibody levels to EBV antigens are raised. The first tumour found to be associated with EBV was Burkitt's lymphoma, a facial lymphoma occurring in children of 5–10 years of age in malarial areas of eastern Africa. Nasopharyngeal carcinoma is a poorly differentiated cancer occurring in southern China, Taiwan, Hong Kong and Singapore but rare in other countries. In Malaysia it is the most common tumour in men. The incidence of specific disease is often the result of several co-factors, and it is thought that a combination of genetic and environmental factors are responsible. The EBV genome is also associated with Hodgkin's lymphoma and X-linked lymphoproliferative syndrome. HIV-infected patients and patients on immunosuppressive treatment also have a higher incidence of EBV-associated lymphomas.

The clinical diagnosis of IM is not always straightforward because the symptoms can be mistaken for bacterial tonsillitis or a different viral infection. The laboratory diagnosis is based on both haematology and serology results. Infectious mononucleosis refers to the abnormal differential blood picture, where there is a raised white cell count of predominantly atypical monocytic cells with an enlarged irregular cytoplasm, often called 'angry cells'. They are in fact enlarged activated T lymphocytes attacking EBV-infected B lymphocytes.

During the course of the primary infection heterophile antibodies are formed that react against red blood cells from sheep, horses and goats. A commercial slide test using latex particles coated with pig kidney extracts is used to detect these heterophile antibodies. In the microbiology laboratory serological diagnosis helps in the diagnosis of acute and past infection. EBV produces different antigens during replication and it is these antibodies to the various antigens that enable an accurate diagnosis, and the distinction between current and past infection. During the acute illness IgM antibodies to the virus capsid antigen, VCA, are present. The VCA antibodies switch to IgG as the infection becomes convalescent and antibodies are formed to the nuclear antigen, EBNA. The antibodies can be simultaneously detected by ELISA in 96 well plates, individually by automated ELISA and also by immunoblot methods. The presence of EBV antigen in tumour samples can be detected in the histopathology department either by a molecular *in situ* hybridization method, where the presence of Epstein–Barr encoded RNA is recognized by immunofluorescently labelled oligonucleotides, or by an immunohistochemical stain using labelled antibodies to the EBV latent membrane protein.

Unlike other herpesviruses there is no effective antiviral treatment for EBV. However, aciclovir is effective in the treatment of oral hairy leukoplakia.

Cytomegalovirus (CMV)

CMV is the largest virus in the herpes family and generally causes asymptomatic infection, transmitted in saliva, blood transfusions and organ donations. The virus is readily inactivated and so requires close contact for transmission. Up to 90% of adults are seropositive. In tissue culture the infected cells become characteristically large, their nuclei filled with inclusion bodies, hence the name cytomegalovirus, referring to the large cells. The virus can cause serious congenital disease, and severe interstitial pneumonia in immuno-compromised and transplant patients. The virus becomes latent in lymphocytes and endothelial cells and can be reactivated if the host becomes immuno-deficient. Because the infection can be transmitted via transfusion and transplantation, it is imperative that blood and donated organs are screened for CMV if they are to be given to susceptible patients, i.e. those who are seronegative.

CMV can be transmitted across the placenta, at the time of birth and post-natally. If the mother contracts a primary CMV infection during pregnancy and the fetus is infected, there is a 5–10% chance of the neonate having symptoms at birth. Even if the symptoms are not serious at birth there is still a risk of deafness or brain dysfunction. Infections acquired at birth or later are more likely to be asymptomatic or cause an IM-like infection.

It is important to diagnose the infection in cases of congenital disease and to distinguish the infection from toxoplasmosis, as the clinical outcome and treatment strategies are different. Infants with symptoms of congenital disease can be screened using a group of serological tests, together called the ToRCH screen (toxoplasma, rubella, CMV and herpes). CMV IgM and IgG antibodies can be detected in serum to distinguish between acute and past infection. IgG levels rise significantly in reactivated disease. The virus can be detected in cell culture in MRC-5 cells and CMV-specific DNA detected by molecular methods.

CMV infection is treated with ganciclovir, a derivative of aciclovir that is phosphorylated by a CMV-specific phosphotransferase enzyme.

Viral hepatitis, hepatitis A, B and C

Viral hepatitis is caused by different viruses with similar initial clinical manifestations. However, laboratory diagnosis is necessary to distinguish between them, as the clinical outcomes are significantly different.

Hepatitis A (HAV)

HAV is a single-stranded positive sense, naked RNA virus of the picornavirus family. It is able to survive in the environment and is resistant to heat, freezing and solvents. Transmission is through the faecal–oral route and following ingestion the virus multiplies in the cells of the Peyer's patches before travelling to the liver where it multiplies in the hepatocytes and Kupffer cells. The incubation period is between 2 and 6 weeks, after which symptoms of fever, abdominal pain, headache, muscle pains, anorexia, nausea and vomiting appear, followed by jaundice. Liver function tests are abnormal, with raised levels of liver enzymes. The symptoms are caused by host T cells attacking the infected liver cells, and by the viral damage to these cells, resulting in the release of liver enzymes and increased levels of bilirubin, leading to jaundice. Hepatitis A is endemic in many countries, although only sporadic in the UK, and so vaccination is advised for travellers to these areas. Seropositivity is again a useful indication of exposure, and is above 90% in endemic areas. Levels in Europe and the USA have fallen significantly; the disease was much more common in people born before the middle of the twentieth century.

After the infection anti-HAV antibodies are formed and the host has lifelong immunity. The virus is cleared from the body and there are no long-term effects.

There is no specific drug treatment for hepatitis A.

Hepatitis B

Hepatitis B is a hepadnavirus, enveloped, with a partially double-stranded circular DNA genome, Baltimore classification VII. The virion is called the Dane particle. It is unusual in that it uses a reverse transcriptase enzyme during replication to produce an RNA intermediate. Unlike hepatitis A, hepatitis B is transmitted through blood contact, intravenous drug use, semen, milk and other secretions. It does not survive well outside the human body but is highly infectious. For this reason, vaccination is essential for anyone who is at risk from contact with blood and body fluids. The virus targets the liver where it infects the hepatocytes and provokes an immune response, both of which damage the liver cells and result in the symptoms of fever, malaise, nausea, rash and aching joints, dark urine and pale stools. The liver becomes enlarged and the patient becomes jaundiced. Viral replication takes place within 3 days of infection but the symptoms may not be observed for 45 days or more.

The outcome of the infection can be acute, chronic, symptomatic or asymptomatic, with the possibility of long-term illness and malignant liver disease. The majority of patients with acute disease will mount an effective cell-mediated immune response and clear the virus completely. If the immune response does not eliminate the virus, the symptoms are milder and the disease becomes chronic, with up to 20% of these patients developing cirrhosis of the liver, which may progress to liver failure. Co-infection with hepatitis D contributes to chronic disease. The other significant problem with chronic infection is the possibility of developing hepatocellular carcinoma. In countries where levels of hepatitis B are high, levels of hepatocellular cancer are also high. The virus can be passed from mother to child; 90% of children infected at birth will become chronic carriers and a source of infection to others. Over a third of the world's population has been infected with hepatitis B and there are estimated to be 350 million chronic carriers of the disease.

Because of the high infectivity of the virus it is often important to know a patient's hepatitis B status, particularly before they are admitted to a dialysis unit, for example.

Hepatitis B has three antigens to which detectable antibodies are formed, providing the basis for laboratory serological tests and the patient's hepatitis B status. The virus produces large quantities of its glycoprotein surface antigen found on the cell envelope, HbsAg. The presence of this indicates either current infection or carrier status. Antibodies to this antigen (HbsAbs) are found in everyone who has been successfully vaccinated. If an individual has been exposed to the whole virus, rather than the manufactured vaccine form, they will have antigens or antibodies to the core antigen, HbcAg and the e antigen HbeAg, which have much of their protein sequence in common. The serological profiles are complex and a profile of the presence or absence of the antibodies and antigens helps to determine the stage of the disease. In a past infection the HbsAg is negative, and the anti Hbc and antiHbs are both positive, whereas in early acute infection the patient will be positive for HbsAg and HbeAg. The results are achieved using ELISA techniques, either manual or automated, and the presence of hepatitis B DNA can also be tested for using quantitative PCR methods. Positive results should be repeated from the initial specimen.

The recommended treatment for chronic hepatitis B is peginterferon alfa (interferon with the addition of polyethylene glycol) and adefovir dipivoxil, a nucleoside analogue reverse transcriptase inhibitor. Other NRTIs are also effective.

Hepatitis C

Hepatitis C is an icosahedral enveloped positive RNA virus of the flavivirus family transmitted sexually and by intravenous drug abuse, and, prior to routine testing for the virus, by blood and blood product transfusion and organ donation. Hepatitis C accounts for 90% of viral hepatitis previously called non-A non-B hepatitis. Unlike hepatitis B there is no vaccine and large numbers of drug users are infected. Nine thousand new cases were reported to the HPA in 2009. However, hepatitis C infection has similarities to hepatitis B in that it causes acute and chronic infection, which can lead to cirrhosis. Up to 35% of cases resolve after initial infection and the percentage who develop chronic hepatitis is between 55 and 80%. The disease progresses slowly over 20–30 years and so patients may not know that they were infected during blood transfusions before routine screening was introduced. Hepatitis C is tested by measuring the number of copies of the virus in a patient's serum by a molecular amplification method using real-time PCR.

Chronic infections can be treated with a combination of ribavirin and peginterferon alfa. Ribavirin, a nucleoside analogue, inhibits a wide range of DNA and RNA viruses.

Mumps, measles and rubella

Vaccination against these three childhood diseases is incorporated in the MMR vaccine, and if sufficient people are protected to provide herd immunity, the incidence of disease should be low. The MMR vaccine was introduced in 1988 and since then the incidence of the three viral infections has dropped significantly. The levels in the

UK for measles now average around 1000 cases per year, 7–8000 for mumps and less than 20 for rubella. When the uptake of MMR temporarily declined, the mumps virus was able to circulate, resulting in an outbreak in 2005 affecting over 43 000 susceptible young people who were born before the introduction of MMR. Rises in the level of measles is also seen when herd immunity drops. Mumps and measles are both members of the paramyxovirus family, measles in the genus of *Morbillivirus* and mumps in the *Rubulavirus* genus. They can be tested by detection of antibodies in blood and oral secretions. Both are spread by saliva and aerosols and have the potential to cause serious complications in some patients. For this reason they and rubella were ideal candidates to include in a vaccination programme. Screening for rubella antibodies continues to be an important aspect of pre-pregnancy planning and antenatal care.

Rubella is a mild disease, but can have serious consequences for the unborn child if a non-immune mother contracts the virus during the first 4 months of pregnancy. The virus can pass across the placenta and affect the developing fetus, leading to spontaneous miscarriage or congenital defects including deafness, eye and heart problems, known as congenital rubella syndrome (CRS). Rubella is in the genus *Rubivirus* and family of Togaviridae, Baltimore classification IV, and is a positive sense single-stranded RNA virus. It is so called because members of the family have an outer lipoprotein membrane, the 'toga'. The damage to the developing fetus is because the virus retards cell division at the point where the organs are developing and so causes malformations.

In common with many virus infections, the laboratory diagnosis is achieved by measuring antibody levels by an ELISA technique. For routine antenatal specimens the tests can be performed in batches, either manually or automated on a machine. However, single-use tests are available if an urgent result is required to determine either the presence of IgG if a susceptible patient has been exposed to the infection, or IgM if acute infection is suspected.

Adenoviruses

Adenoviruses are double-stranded DNA viruses, Baltimore classification I. They are interesting because the 47 serotypes can cause gastrointestinal disease by faecal–oral spread, respiratory disease (nose and throat infections) by aerosol transmission and conjunctivitis of the eye. They are a common cause of childhood viral infections and also infect adults. Many viral infections are not diagnosed but if the illness requires accurate diagnosis this is achieved by EM examination of stool samples and diagnosis of respiratory infection by ELISA or molecular methods. There is no effective anti-viral treatment.

Rotavirus, norovirus and respiratory syncytial virus

These are included in *Chapter 9* (rotavirus and norovirus) and *Chapter 10* (respiratory syncytial virus, RSV).

SUGGESTED FURTHER READING

Asaria, P. & MacMahon, E. (2006) Measles in the United Kingdom: can we eradicate it by 2010? *BMJ*, **333**: 890–895.

Clementi, M. (2000) Quantitative molecular analysis of virus expression and replication. *J. Clin. Microbiol.* **38**: 2030–2036.

Dalgleish, A.G. & Weiss, R.A. (1999) *HIV and the New Viruses*, 2nd edn. Academic Press.

Espy, M.J., Uhl, R. *et al.* (2006) Real-time PCR in clinical microbiology: applications for routine laboratory testing. *Clin. Microbiol. Rev.* **19**: 165–256.

Gulley, M.L. & Tang, W. (2008) Laboratory assays for Epstein–Barr virus-related disease. *J. Mol. Diagnost.* **10**: 279–292.

Gupta, R.K., Best, J. *et al.* (2005) Mumps and the UK epidemic 2005. *BMJ,* **330**: 1132–1135.

Henrickson, K.J. (2003) Parainfluenza viruses. *Clin. Microbiol. Rev.* **16**: 242–264.

Knipe, D.M., Howley, P.M., Griffin, D.E. *et al.* (2007) *Field's Virology*, 5th edn. Lippincott Williams & Wilkins.

Leland, D.S. & Ginocchio, C.C. (2007) Role of cell culture for virus detection in the age of technology. *Clin. Microbiol. Rev.* **20**: 49–78.

Mahony, J.B. (2008) Detection of respiratory viruses by molecular methods. *Clin. Microbiol. Rev.* **21**: 716–747.

Richmond, J.K. & Baglole, D.J. (2003) Lassa fever: epidemiology, clinical features, and social consequences. *BMJ,* **327**: 1271–1275.

Tuaillon, E., Mondain, A.-M., Meroueh, F. *et al.* (2010) Dried blood spot for hepatitis C virus serology and molecular testing. *Hepatology,* **51**: 752–758.

Williams, H. & Crawford, D.H. (2006) Epstein–Barr virus: the impact of scientific advances on clinical practice. *Blood,* **107**: 862–869.

SELF-ASSESSMENT QUESTIONS

1. Explain the different types of viral genomic structures that form the basis of the Baltimore classification system.
2. Outline the various routes of viral transmission.
3. Describe the nature and function of viral envelopes.
4. Explain the methods currently used to diagnose viral infections in the laboratory. Give an example of viral infections diagnosed by each of them.
5. HIV is treated with a combination of drugs. Explain the reasons for this and outline the principal classes of drugs used.
6. The 1918 H5N1 influenza virus is described as an adaptation of an avian flu virus to infect humans, whereas the H2N2 epidemic strain of 1957 is a re-assortment virus. Explain the difference.
7. Herpesviruses cause acute, chronic and recurrent infections. Illustrate this fact using one example of a herpesvirus.
8. Why is it important to ensure a laboratory diagnosis of a patient with clinical signs of infectious hepatitis?
9. Haemorrhagic fever viruses (VHF) cause serious disease in endemic countries and to travellers in these areas. They are not endemic in the UK. Why is this? Give two examples of viral haemorrhagic fevers.
10. Why is it important to maintain high levels of immunity to mumps, measles rubella and other vaccine preventable diseases?

Answers to self-assessment questions provided at:
www.scionpublishing.com/medmicro

Host–pathogen interactions in health and disease

Learning objectives
After studying this chapter you should confidently be able to:

■ **Define the terms used to describe the interactions between hosts and microbes in health and disease**
A pathogen is a microbe (bacteria, viruses, fungi and protozoa) capable of causing host damage in the course of infection. Pathogenicity is defined as the capability of a microbe to cause damage to the host. Bacteria are described as pathogenic, depending on their ability to cause damage by the expression of virulence factors. Opportunistic pathogens are able to cause disease if the host is in some way immuno-compromised or they are given the opportunity to leave their normal niche and invade tissue beyond the epithelial layer. The term infection is sometimes used to describe infectious disease but can also mean that bacteria are present at a site but not causing disease. Disease suggests that the infectious process has caused damage to the host.

■ **Discuss the importance of the presence of normal flora in the host**
The normal flora is a collection of microorganisms found on the bodies of normal healthy individuals, consisting of bacteria and some fungi. It is present on all parts of the body that communicate with the outside world. By occupying receptor sites on the cell surfaces, the normal flora discourage the attachment of other microorganisms and also carry out several important functions for the host, including the stimulation of the immune system and production of vitamins. Conversely, they also provide a source of opportunistic pathogens.

■ **Describe how knowledge of the presence or absence of normal flora at a given site, in conjunction with knowledge of the most likely pathogens, guides the interpretation of the significance of cultures from clinical specimens in the microbiology laboratory**
Knowledge of, and familiarity with the appearance and composition of normal healthy flora enables the presence of potential pathogens from a specific body site or type of specimen to be recognized and subsequently identified.

■ **Describe the role of the innate and adaptive host defence mechanisms and the ways in which pathogenic microorganisms circumvent and challenge them**
The components of the innate immune system include natural defences, antibiotic substances, acute phase proteins, the complement cascade and phagocytic cells. Together they provide the first defence and inflammatory response to infection and provide foreign antigen for the components of the adaptive immune response. The adaptive immune response provides specific effector cells and antibodies to control the infection and memory cells to recognize subsequent challenges by the same microorganism.

■ **Describe the stages of infection and the ways in which infectious disease is expressed in the host**

Infectious disease is characterized by the stages of encounter, entry, adhesion and colonization, invasion from the site of infection and spread to other areas of the body (does not occur in all infectious disease), multiplication and damage, outcome of the disease and transmission to a new host and a new encounter. Some infectious encounters will always have the same aetiology, i.e. signs, symptoms and disease process. Some bacteria, *Staphylococcus aureus* for example, can infect a wide variety of tissues, leading to differing symptoms and severity of disease. The yeast *Candida albicans* may be carried harmlessly by a healthy individual but cause serious infection in an immuno-compromised person. Infection with Group A streptococci can cause an unpleasant and painful sore throat, whereas invasion by the bacteria could lead to life-threatening septicaemia in another individual. Different pathogens may cause similar symptoms in patients, such as chest infections, skin and wound infections, urinary tract infections, meningitis and sexually transmitted infections, but may be the result of bacterial, viral or fungal infections. Accurate diagnosis is therefore of prime importance.

■ **Describe the ways in which virulence factors are genetically controlled and transferred between bacteria**

Some virulence factors form part of the structure of the pathogen; bacterial LPS is a good example. Other virulence factors are genetically controlled by sensing and regulating mechanisms influenced by the changing conditions within a human host. Genes controlling virulence may be clustered together on a pathogenicity island or situated on separate sections of the genome. Transposons are discrete sequences of DNA originating from the chromosome or a plasmid, inserted into other positions on the genome, leading to mutations and increased virulence. Genetic material encoding virulence factors can be transferred by plasmids during conjugation, by bacteriophages in the process of transduction and by transformation, where DNA from dead bacteria is absorbed by living bacteria.

4.1 INTRODUCTION TO HOST–PATHOGEN RELATIONSHIPS

Humans are constantly challenged by microorganisms and the outcome can depend as much upon the host reaction to this encounter as the power of the microorganism. This host–pathogen relationship can be of mutual benefit – a symbiotic relationship, as in the case of the normal flora resident on all mucosal surfaces – or it can be parasitic, where the balance of the relationship shifts in favour of a pathogenic microorganism, resulting in disease. Some infectious diseases are caused by 'professional pathogens' which always cause disease in susceptible hosts, whereas others, known as 'opportunistic pathogens', are normally harmless but take advantage when host defences are breached or the host is compromised in some way. Usually the host is well protected by the innate and adaptive immune system, a challenge successfully overcome and circumvented in various ways by successful pathogens, either as the result of sheer force of numbers or the expression of genetic factors that enhance their ability to cause disease. Bacteria, in particular, spontaneously adapt and mutate as they reproduce, in response to selective pressures from the hostile environment that they encounter within the human host. These pressures include the activity of the immune system and the presence of antimicrobial drugs. This chapter describes the ways in which the host protects itself from infection and the ways in which successful pathogens overcome these defences and establish disease, which can be mild or life-threatening.

The early parts of this chapter describe the complex relationship between human hosts and their resident microbial population, the normal flora. This relationship is commensal, where host and microbes live in harmony. It is also symbiotic, the host providing a niche and nutrients for the largely bacterial flora, in return for which the bacteria provide resistance to outside, exogenous infection, through occupation of the receptor sites, expression of defensive chemical mediators and the production of essential nutrients, e.g. vitamin K.

Box 4.1 Definitions

A **pathogen** is a microbe (bacteria, viruses, fungi and protozoa) capable of causing host damage in the course of infection.

Pathogenicity is the capability of a microbe to cause damage to the host.

Bacteria are described as pathogenic depending on their ability to cause damage by the expression of **virulence factors.**

Microorganisms are described as **opportunistic pathogens** if the host is in some way immuno-compromised or they are given the opportunity to leave their normal niche and invade tissue beyond the epithelial layer.

Infection can be used to describe infectious disease but can also mean that bacteria are present at a site but not causing disease.

Disease is an abnormal condition that impairs bodily function. It is associated with specific signs and symptoms, discomfort and dysfunction, suggesting that infectious disease involves some damage to the host.

Terms used to describe interactions between hosts and microorganisms

A pathogen is a microbe (bacteria, viruses, fungi and protozoa) capable of causing host damage in the course of infection. Some microbes are classic or professional pathogens, causing infectious disease whenever they infect a susceptible host. *Neisseria gonorrhoeae* (gonorrhoea), *Corynebacteria diphtheria* (diphtheria), measles, dengue fever viruses and malarial parasites are good examples. Other pathogens, such as *Streptococcus pyogenes* and *S. pneumoniae*, and *Neisseria meningitidis*, cause serious disease but can also be carried harmlessly in small numbers in healthy people. *Mycobacterium tuberculosis,* the bacteria causing human tuberculosis (TB), infect many people but do not always lead to active TB because the host immune system attacks and isolates the bacteria in calcified nodules, rendering the host susceptible during their lifetime to reactivation of the disease if their immune system weakens.

Pathogenicity is defined as the capability of a microbe to cause damage to the host. Bacteria are described as pathogenic depending on their ability to cause damage by the expression of virulence factors. Some virulence factors are part of the bacterial structure, such as lipopolysaccharide; others are proteins expressed on the cell surface, while some are genetically controlled, such as capsules and toxins. Constituents of the normal flora, bacteria and yeasts are normally considered to be of low pathogenicity and possess few virulence factors. They can, however, act as opportunistic pathogens if the host is in some way immuno-compromised or they are given the opportunity to leave their normal niche and invade tissue beyond the epithelial layer. With greater numbers of patients receiving chemotherapy and undergoing life-saving invasive procedures or suffering from HIV, the importance of opportunistic infections has escalated. Fungal infections, previously considered insignificant, can be life-threatening to immuno-compromised patients. In a similar way, *Pseudomonas aeruginosa*, an environmental bacterium, poses little threat to a healthy person, yet causes serious infections in burns patients (where protection mechanisms associated with the skin are destroyed) and people suffering from cystic fibrosis, for whom it causes a chronic destructive lung infection.

These paradigms illustrate the complexity of human–pathogen relationships.

The definition of disease as an abnormal condition that impairs bodily function, associated with specific signs and symptoms, discomfort and dysfunction, suggests that infectious disease involves some damage to the host. Infection, however, is sometimes used to describe infectious disease but can also mean that bacteria are present at a site but not causing disease. An example of this could be that a significant number of hosts may be infected with *Staphylococcus aureus* on their skin in small numbers, but in the majority of cases it will not be causing damage and disease. As another example, most people are infected with *Streptococcus sanguinis* as part of their oral flora; however, the bacteria only travel in the bloodstream to the heart valves and cause bacterial endocarditis in a minority who are susceptible to the disease.

4.2   NORMAL FLORA

The normal flora is a collection of microorganisms found on the bodies of normal healthy individuals, consisting of bacteria and some fungi, such as the yeast *Candida albicans*. Normal flora is present on all parts of the body that communicate with the outside world and is therefore found in conjunction with the skin and mucous membranes, where the constituents have a commensal and often beneficial co-existence with the host. Mucous membranes are characterized by a layer of epithelial cells and resident bacteria surrounded by mucus which serves to trap foreign particles, including bacteria, and expel them. The level of normal bacteria associated with different parts of the body varies, but overall humans have 10^{13} cells and 10^{14} bacteria associated with them. Considering that there are significant areas of the body that are normally sterile, without normal flora, the numbers in other areas, for example the oral cavity and the intestine, are extremely high. *Figure 4.1* shows the concentrations of normal flora in different areas of the human body.

The composition of the normal flora varies with age, diet and the environment. It is affected by the individual's hormonal state, their general health, sanitary conditions and personal hygiene.

Acquisition of normal flora

Conditions in the uterus are sterile and the fetus first comes into contact with microorganisms as it passes through the birth canal containing normal vaginal flora. If the mother has any infection in the vagina, the neonate may also be infected. The next encounter with microorganisms comes from the mother's skin. Fortunately,

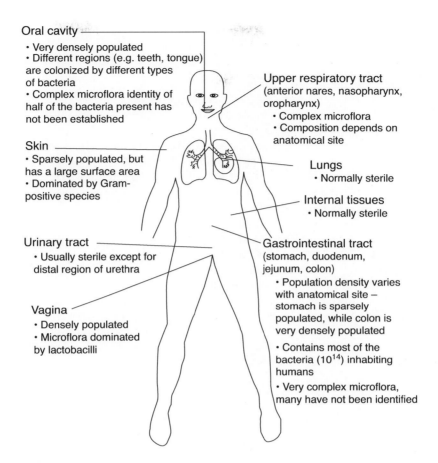

Oral cavity
• Very densely populated
• Different regions (e.g. teeth, tongue) are colonized by different types of bacteria
• Complex microflora identity of half of the bacteria present has not been established

Skin
• Sparsely populated, but has a large surface area
• Dominated by Gram-positive species

Urinary tract
• Usually sterile except for distal region of urethra

Vagina
• Densely populated
• Microflora dominated by lactobacilli

Upper respiratory tract (anterior nares, nasopharynx, oropharynx)
• Complex microflora
• Composition depends on anatomical site

Lungs
• Normally sterile

Internal tissues
• Normally sterile

Gastrointestinal tract (stomach, duodenum, jejunum, colon)
• Population density varies with anatomical site – stomach is sparsely populated, while colon is very densely populated
• Contains most of the bacteria (10^{14}) inhabiting humans
• Very complex microflora, many have not been identified

Figure 4.1
Distribution of the normal flora within the human host.

protective antibodies are able to cross the placenta and so the neonate is protected by maternal antibodies during the first weeks of life. Protective antibodies are also passed via breast milk. The newborn then gradually acquires its own microbial flora through human contact, contact with the environment and via food. Studies of the composition of gastrointestinal (GI) tract flora in babies has demonstrated that breast-fed babies have large numbers of lactic acid streptococci and lactobacilli, whereas bottle-fed babies have a greater variety of bacteria. As the baby's diet becomes more varied, so does the normal flora of the GI tract.

The skin is colonized first, followed by the oropharynx, the gastrointestinal tract and other mucosal surfaces. If adults are treated to make them free of normal flora, they will re-establish their normal levels within six weeks.

Distribution of the normal flora

Normal flora is found on the skin, respiratory tract, digestive tract, urinary tract and genital areas, with varying concentrations at different sites. Some areas of the body are always sterile: blood, cerebrospinal fluid and the deep tissues and organs such as heart, kidneys, lungs and liver.

Several factors influence the type of microorganisms found as part of the normal flora at a particular body site:

- Oxygen availability. Strict aerobes would not be able to survive in the restricted oxygen levels of the GI tract, but would thrive on the skin.
- pH levels. Few bacteria can survive the harsh acid environment of the stomach.
- Osmolality. This is a measure of osmotically active particles in solution and salt levels; both affect bacterial survival. Skin bacteria, *Staphylococci*, *Corynebacteria* and *Micrococci* can survive in the higher levels of salt. High levels of osmolality are found in the kidney, a normally sterile area. However, *Staphylococci*, uropathogenic *Escherichia coli* and *Proteus* species are able to cause infection in the area if they gain access.
- Moisture. Gram-positive bacteria survive better on the dry areas of the skin.
- Temperature. Some bacteria grow better at the core temperature of the body, rather than the cooler areas of the skin.
- Nutrient availability. This affects the distribution; some skin bacteria can break down the fatty acids secreted on to the surface, others cannot.
- Antimicrobial secretions. These are inhibitory at some body sites.
- Physical removal. Resident bacteria have to use effective attachment mechanisms to live on surfaces such as the urethral epithelium where they are constantly flushed by the passing of urine.

As shown in *Figure 4.1*, the density of normal flora varies between sites. In highly protected areas such as the gingival crevice between the gum and the teeth, and within the microvilli of the large intestine, the bacteria are densely packed. The average bacterium has a volume of 1 μm^3 and where they are packed most densely, this results in 1 x 10^{12} bacteria per ml. In less hospitable areas of the body, levels of 1–10 million bacteria per ml are found.

Skin

Skin provides a variety of niches for bacteria and yeast to become resident flora. The areas under the arms (axillae) and the groin area provide a moister and warmer environment than the more exposed areas of skin. There are more sebaceous glands, and sweat and sebum provide the principal sources of nutrients. The fatty acids and low pH produced after lipids have been metabolized are toxic to many species of bacteria and the skin also has higher levels of salt, which again can be inhibitory to some bacteria. Skin residents must therefore be aerobic or facultatively anaerobic; they must be able to adhere to skin cells, tolerate salt and use lipids. Common constituents of skin flora include *Staphylococci*, *Micrococci*, *Corynebacteria* and *Propionibacteria*. The yeast *Candida albicans* and the coliform bacteria also occupy the moister areas. Skin flora is present on all clinical samples taken from skin swabs and has a characteristic appearance and odour.

Oropharynx

The oral cavity is one of the richest areas for normal flora, providing a variety of habitats for bacteria to grow, each with different oxygen contents, redox potential, pH and nutrient sources. Because of the flow of saliva and the action of chewing, resident bacteria must have good methods of adhesion and resist flushing mechanisms. It has been shown that after brushing the teeth or using mouthwash, the bacteria re-adhere to the various surfaces in a particular order of attachment, allowing a multiple layer or pellicle to form on the surface. The teeth provide a non-shedding surface for bacteria, allowing biofilms to develop on them. Biofilms are formed when bacteria exist in a multiple layer held together with extracellular polymeric substance. If the biofilms are allowed to form over a period of time, hard plaque is formed. Tooth surfaces are colonized by aerobic streptococci and *Neisseria* species. Interestingly, the oral cavity supports the growth of very anaerobic bacteria as well as aerobes in the gingival pockets. Gingival pockets or crevices are the areas between the gum and the tooth, filled with gingival crevicular fluid, creating an anaerobic environment where bacteria such as *Fusobacterium* species, *Veillonella* species and spirochaetes can live. There are also many more bacteria, known to be present by the use of molecular probes, forming part of the oral flora. As yet, they have not been fully characterized. The complex interactions of the oral flora as they compete for nutrients maintains the balance of the total population.

Upper respiratory tract

The normal flora of the nose is very similar to that of the skin, containing *Staphylococci* and *Corynebacteria*. Nose swabs can be important in the identification of carriers of MRSA and *Staphylococcus aureus,* either because the patient is being admitted to hospital or because they have had frequent staphylococcal infections and they could be harbouring the bacteria in their nasal passages. In addition, the flora of the nasopharynx contains Gram-negative bacteria such as *Haemophilus influenzae*, *Moraxella catarrhalis* and *Neisseria* species. Throat flora is more diverse as it is influenced by the oral cavity and food intake. Alpha haemolytic streptococci are the dominant bacteria. Up to 10% of the population also carry small numbers of the pathogenic bacteria *Streptococcus pyogenes* and *Streptococcus pneumoniae*, which, although present in a culture from a throat swab, are very much in the minority and are being carried asymptomatically rather than causing an infection. Resident bacteria of the upper respiratory tract are associated with mucous membranes and must therefore be able to survive in the presence of the normal innate mucosal defence system including lysozyme, lactoferrin and the secretory antibody IgA.

The lower respiratory tract is a sterile area, protecting the gaseous exchange in the lungs.

Gastrointestinal (GI) tract

The GI tract covers a large surface area of approximately 200 m^2 and contains the highest levels of normal flora. There are several discrete areas providing distinct niches: the stomach, duodenum, jejunum, ileum and colon. Many of the bacteria form anaerobic ecosystems with nutrients readily available from endogenous sources. Distinct niches are created by the folding of the intestinal surface to create large surface areas for the absorption of nutrients, and these provide numerous fluid-filled cavities in which the bacteria live. Depending on their position in the GI tract, bacteria are exposed to differing pH levels and the presence of proteolytic enzymes and bile salts.

The stomach, with a pH of less than 2, is a hostile area for bacteria, with levels as low as 10^3 per ml. The principal bacteria in this area are *Helicobacter pylori*, many strains of which are harmless commensals. There are, however, some pathogenic strains of *Helicobacter pylori* associated with the development of ulcers and chronic infection, which may in a minority of cases lead to gastric cancer and lymphoma.

Levels in the duodenum and jejunum are also relatively low, 10^5 per ml, but consist of a greater variety of bacteria, including Gram-negative anaerobic rods, *Bacteroides* species, and Gram-positive anaerobic rods, *Bifidobacteria*. Bacteria in these areas have to be able to survive in the presence of the secreted bile salts. The ileum supports a greater diversity of flora at a concentration of 10^9 per ml and includes enterococci, *Clostridium* species and *Escherichia coli*.

By far the most densely populated area of the GI tract is the colon, where approximately 500 different species are represented and form 55% of the solid weight of the faeces. Ninety per cent of the bacteria are obligate anaerobes including *Clostridium* species, around 10% are *Bacteroides* species and there are lower levels of *Escherichia* and *Enterobacter* species, *Proteus* species and lactobacilli. Routine faecal specimens are cultured in an aerobic environment and so the flora observed on the culture plate represents the aerobic and facultative anaerobes only, as the majority of bacteria are strictly anaerobic.

Urogenital tract

The urinary tract is sterile apart from the distal portion of the urethra, where the mucosal surfaces are colonized by skin, anal and vaginal flora. Bacteria are shed on the surfaces of the epithelial cells whenever urine passes through the urethra.

In females, the composition of the vaginal flora is age- and hormone-dependent. Before puberty and after the menopause, vaginal secretions are alkaline and the flora consists mainly of staphylococci, streptococci and coliforms. From the menarche to the menopause, the presence of oestrogen influences the presence of glycogen producing bacteria (the lactobacilli), and the pH is lowered to around 5. The presence of the lactobacilli and the lower pH help to protect the area from pathogens.

The benefits of normal flora

One of the prerequisites of the infectious process is adhesion to host cells by attaching to specific receptor sites on the epithelial cell surface. One of the important benefits of having the epithelial cells of mucous membranes covered with normal flora is that receptor sites are already occupied, thus providing colonization resistance to potential pathogens. They also produce antimicrobial substances, bacteriocins, to deter potential invaders. This is not always effective as pathogens have developed strategies to overcome the resident bacteria. The presence of bacteria also acts as a stimulant for the immune system, and protective IgA antibodies are secreted into the mucous layer.

The importance of the gastrointestinal flora has been extensively studied. Evidence from research using gnotobiotic (germ-free) mice has demonstrated important differences in the structure and activity of the gut tissue with and without gut flora. There are several important functions of the gut floras that demonstrate their symbiotic relationship with their human hosts:

- Colonization resistance – large numbers occupy the surface area of the GI tract. The resident flora also discourages other bacteria from colonizing the area by the production of fatty acids, peroxides and bacteriocins. The passage of antibiotics through the GI tract destroys the normal flora and can lead to diarrhoea as a side-effect of the antibiotic treatment in otherwise healthy individuals. Susceptible patients may also become infected with *Clostridium difficile*, and risk developing more serious antibiotic-associated diarrhoea.

■ Stimulation and 'training' of the immune system. The presence of the gut flora provides a stimulus for the production of protective IgA antibodies in the mucous membrane. Bacteria in the intestinal flora behave as antigens and stimulate the immune system to produce antibodies. An example is the formation of naturally occurring antibodies to antigens of the ABO blood group system. Antibodies are only produced to red cell antigens that are not present in the individual; hence a blood group O will have antibodies to A and B. Germ-free mice have poorly developed gut lymphatic tissue.

■ Healthy gut development is assisted by the presence of the bacteria. The presence of the bacteria stimulates growth and development, whereas germ-free mice have enlarged thin-walled, fluid-filled intestines.

■ Resident bacteria are involved in the production of vitamins; *Escherichia coli* produces vitamins B and K, and evidence of vitamin K deficiency has been demonstrated in germ-free mice. Bacterial enzymes also play a part in breaking down substrates; glucuronides are deconjugated by bacterial glucuronidases.

Potential hazards of normal flora

The most important disadvantage of a large resident microbial population is the risk of opportunistic endogenous infection. This can happen in several ways, as shown in *Table 4.1*.

Table 4.1 Potential for endogenous, opportunistic infection by members of the resident flora

Opportunity	Infection sites	Causative organisms
Access to sub-epithelial tissue as a result of damage	Burns	*Pseudomonas aeruginosa*
	Lacerations/trauma	*Staphylococcus aureus* from skin
	Rupture of bowel or appendix	Gut flora released into peritoneal cavity
Entry by, or attachment to foreign body	Urinary catheter	Urethral flora
	Cannulae, prosthetic heart valves, respirators	Staphylococci and yeast from skin, oral bacteria attaching to heart valve
Bacterial flora transferred to another body site	Gut and vaginal flora causing urinary tract infection	*Escherichia coli* and other coliforms, staphylococci, enterococci
	Oral flora attaching to prosthetic heart valve	Oral streptococci
	Intestinal perforation by trauma or pelvic surgery	GI flora
Immunosuppression of the host by chemotherapy, immune deficiency and disease processes	Multiple, depending on type of infection	Yeasts and fungi
		Staphylococci
		Protozoa, viruses
Overgrowth or imbalance of resident flora	Oral flora imbalance leading to gingivitis and dental caries	Anaerobic oral flora
		Overgrowth of *Streptococcus mutans*

Host tolerance

The presence of bacteria on the surface of epithelial cells normally triggers an inflammatory response in the host. However, a healthy person is constantly supporting a large number of bacteria on their skin and mucosal membranes without any sign of inflammation. This suggests that the commensal nature of this relationship must incorporate mechansims of tolerance, but inflammation and stimulation of the immune response will still be triggered by the presence of 'foreign' bacteria from an outside (exogenous) source. Studies on mice in which certain cytokines (interleukins, chemical messengers) IL2 and IL10 had been genetically 'knocked out' demonstrated that if they had normal flora in their GI tract, they developed colitis. Germ-free knockout mice did not develop the disease, suggesting a role for cytokines in the tolerance mechanisms. The interaction between the epithelial cells and the bacteria living on them is thought to be complex, involving down-regulation of inflammatory mediators and up-regulation of inhibitory mediators in both the bacteria and the epithelial cells.

For their part, resident bacteria do not express their virulence genes or bacterial hormones controlling their virulence, but do express their own chemical messengers called bacteriokines, to interact with host cytokine networks. The epithelial cells express antibiotic peptides to control bacterial growth, and inhibitory factors including cytokines that down-regulate bacterial virulence factors including lipopolysaccharide (LPS) present in the cell walls of Gram-negative bacteria. The immune system is very sensitive to the pro-inflammatory effect of LPS. A state of peaceful co-existence is achieved through these complex chemical interactions, with the bacteria forming micro-ecosystems, occupying receptor sites and providing a defence mechanism for the host. If, as described earlier, conditions change and the bacteria are given the opportunity to penetrate the epithelial layer, they find themselves in the more hostile environment of the sub-epithelium. If they possess the appropriate virulence factors, these will be expressed, provoke an inflammatory response and infection and disease will result. Conversely, small numbers of potentially pathogenic bacteria can exist harmlessly within the normal flora, without expressing their virulence factors. The immune system also forms specific antibodies to the carrier strain. However, if the host is infected with large numbers of a virulent strain to which they have no pre-existing antibodies, infectious disease may well result, as shown in *Figure 4.2*.

In further chapters the diagnosis of infectious disease from specific body sites is discussed. Specimens taken from the patient are cultured on to suitable media and examined after appropriate incubation for the presence of bacteria. It is therefore very important to know the site from which the specimen was taken and whether that site normally supports the presence of normal flora. Familiarization with the appearance and composition of normal healthy flora enables the presence of potential pathogens to be recognized and then identified as the most likely cause of the infectious disease. *Table 4.2* gives examples of the specimen types received in the microbiology laboratory, the presence or absence of normal flora and some examples of potential pathogens. It is by no means exhaustive, but gives an illustration of the factors to consider when reading clinical cultures. Appreciation of the extent of normal flora and knowledge of the most likely pathogens guides the development of standard operating procedures and range of culture media to be inoculated, as discussed in *Chapters 6* and *7*.

Table 4.2 Potential pathogens and the presence of normal flora in bacterial cultures from a range of different specimen types

Specimen type	Presence of normal flora	Potential pathogens
Skin swabs taken from lacerations, bites, folliculitis Infected eczema, ulcer swabs Skin scrapings	Staphylococci including coagulase-negative species and *Staphylococcus aureus*. *Micrococcus* species, *Propionibacterium* species, *Corynebacterium* species. Coliforms.	*Staphylococcus aureus.* Coagulase-negative staphylococci Group A streptococcus, other beta-haemolytic streptococci, *Pseudomonas aeruginosa,* anaerobes (see *Chapter 10*) Dermatophyte and non-dermatophyte fungi (see *Chapter 13*)
Throat swabs Pernasal swabs	A mixture of *Haemophilus* species, streptococci, *Moraxella* species, streptococci, *Candida* species	Group A streptococcus (*Streptococcus pyogenes*) *Corynebacterium diphtheriae, Fusobacteria* (see *Chapter 10*) *Bordetella pertussis*
Ear swabs	Skin flora including coliforms	Group A streptococcus, *Staphylococcus aureus, Streptococcus pneumoniae, Haemophilus influenzae, Moraxella catarrhalis, Pseudomonas aeruginosa,* mixed anaerobes (see *Chapter 10*)
Sputum	Similar to oropharynx	*Haemophilus influenzae, Streptococcus pneumoniae,* TB, *Mycoplasma pneumoniae, Chlamydia pneumoniae, Pseudomonas aeruginosa* viruses (see *Chapter 11*)
Blood	Sterile. Possible contamination by skin flora during venepuncture	Any clinically significant isolate (see *Chapter 12*)
Cerebrospinal fluid (CSF)	Sterile	*Neisseria meningitidis, Streptococcus pneumoniae,* Group B streptococci, *Escherichia coli,* TB, viruses such as herpes simplex virus, *Cryptococcus neoformans* (in immuno-compromised (patients) (see *Chapter 12*)
Fluids – joint, ascitic, pleural	Sterile	Growth of clinically significant isolate e.g. *Staphylococcus aureus*
Urine	Small numbers of skin flora. Dependent on specimen type, midstream or catheter urine	Significant numbers of *Escherichia coli* and other coliforms. *Staphylococcus aureus,* coagulase-negative staphylococci, Group B streptococci, *Candida albicans, Pseudomonas aeruginosa* (see *Chapter 8*)
Genital swabs	Vaginal flora in females, age dependent, skin flora in men	Group B streptococci, *Candida albicans, Staphylococcus aureus, Proteus* species. Mixed anaerobes, *Trichomonas vaginalis,* gonorrhoea, *Chlamydia trachomatis,* syphilis (detected by serology), genital herpes (see *Chapter 10*)

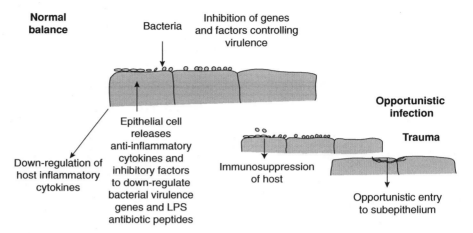

Figure 4.2
Benefits of normal flora occupation of skin and mucous membranes. Opportunistic infection from the normal flora can occur if the host is immunosuppressed or if trauma facilitates entry.

4.3 THE INNATE AND ADAPTIVE IMMUNE SYSTEMS

Interactions between the host and potential pathogens determine whether the host will develop infectious disease or remain healthy. The human body is constantly challenged by microorganisms yet most people, most of the time, do not succumb to infection. This is because of the efficiency of the innate (non-specific, constitutive) and the adaptive (inducible) immune systems. If these responses are compromised the host becomes more susceptible to opportunistic infectious disease.

The innate system plays an important role in the overall immune response by initiating the attack on potential pathogens and presenting foreign antigen to the cells of the adaptive arm of the immune response. The effector cells of the adaptive response take several days to produce specific antibodies and effector cells and during this time the innate system produces an inflammatory response to the infecting microorganisms. The folowing sections describe the principal barriers to infection and outline the host immune responses.

Innate defences

The body is protected by a number of non-specific defence mechanisms that react in the same way every time they are challenged. These include physical barriers, antimicrobial chemicals, mechanical removal, pathogen recognition receptors, the presence of the normal flora, phagocytic cells and the complement system.

Physical barriers

The skin forms a protective barrier and is composed of squamous epithelial cells. The top layer, the stratum corneum, comprises dead cells filled with keratin. As well as providing a hostile environment for pathogens, the top layer is constantly being shed. Some specialized fungi, the dermatophytes, can infect this area and cause skin lesions, yet cannot penetrate beyond the epithelium to deeper layers. Ear wax provides a physical barrier because it is relatively impenetrable for pathogens, while nasal hair provides the first filter for air entering the respiratory system, followed by trapping of pathogens in the mucous surface of the nose.

Mechanical removal

Potential pathogens can be removed from surfaces by the flow of fluid; tears prevent the colonization of the eye surface, saliva washes bacteria away from the mucosal surfaces in the mouth and fluid flow through the intestines aids in the removal of bacteria. Bacteria are actively trapped and removed by the activity of the mucosal surfaces in the upper respiratory tract by the action of the muco-ciliary escalator: bacteria are trapped in the mucus and then actively wafted upwards by the activity of the ciliated epithelial cells. In the nasal area they are directed to the back of the throat where they are subsequently swallowed. In the urogenital tract bacteria are continually flushed away with the passing of urine and the sloughing of the top layer of epithelial cells.

Changes in the pH value

Changes in the relative acidity and alkalinity at mucosal surfaces can limit the number of microorganisms, particularly bacteria, able to survive there. This was shown earlier in this chapter in relation to normal flora on mucosal surfaces, and is effective as a deterrent for the colonization of exogenous pathogens. The pH of the stomach is extremely low, while that of the skin and vaginal areas is around 5.0. The skin is acidic because of the end products of the resident bacteria and lactic acid produced from sweat and the antibacterial presence of lipids, whereas the acidity of the vaginal area in adult females is the result of the acid-producing lactobacilli. The action of bile salts helps to keep the lower intestine relatively alkaline, which again is inhibitory to exogenous pathogens.

Antibacterial substances

A variety of substances produced at mucosal surfaces provide protection from potential invaders. They can be up-regulated significantly in the presence of foreign bacteria, and are particularly responsive to the presence of LPS. The complex interactions between the normal flora and the epithelial cells allow them to survive in the presence of an impressive array of antibacterial molecules. Mucin is one of the principal components of mucus which acts as a lubricant and protector for the epithelial cells, in addition to trapping non-resident bacteria and acting as a medium in which a variety of antibacterial molecules are present, such as:

- Secretory IgA, an immunoglobulin (antibody) which is produced by plasma cells in the sub-epithelial layers in response to foreign antigen and transported to the surface where it binds to specific epitopes (a region on the antigen surface).
- Lactoferrin, a glycoprotein produced by neutrophils and epithelial cells, which binds iron very effectively, thus denying bacteria the free iron they need for growth. Lactoferrin also attaches to LPS and components of the Gram-positive cell wall.
- Collectins, which are the serum protein mannose-binding lectins (MBL) and the lung surfactant proteins A and D (SP-A and D). They are produced by most mucosal surfaces where they act as lectins that recognize and bind to carbohydrate on bacterial surfaces. They act as opsonins, either coating bacteria to make them more obvious to the complement proteins or as pattern recognition receptors, alerting the immune system to foreign antigen.

■ Lactoperoxidase, a glycoprotein enzyme present in mucus, saliva and tears. Together with thiocyanate (SCN) ions and hydrogen peroxide also found in these biological fluids, it forms the lactoperoxidase system. Oxidation of the thiocyanate ions by the hydrogen peroxide forms intermediary oxidation products that have both bactericidal and bacteriostatic activity, providing a natural defence system. Lysozyme, an enzyme present in tears and mucosal membranes, attacks the β 1–4 linkages of Gram-positive peptidoglycan and has activity against LPS.

Pattern recognition receptors and cells of the innate immune system
Cells of the innate immune system, the neutrophils (polymorphological neutrophils, polymorphs) and the macrophages and dendritic cells, are alerted to the presence of foreign antigen by pattern recognition receptors that recognize bacterial molecules. Bacteria have developed multiple ways in which to evade the immune system, but throughout their evolution, the essential molecules recognized cannot be changed. They are known as pathogen-associated molecular patterns (PAMPs) and include aspects of the bacterial cell such as LPS, peptidoglycan and lipoarabinomannan (a component of the cell wall of mycobacteria) and other cellular components. PAMPs are also recognised on eukaryotic pathogens, for example glycans on the surface of schistosomes.

Macrophages have CD14 receptors recognizing LPS on Gram-negative bacteria, and are activated by LPS bound to LPS binding protein. Macrophages have an important role in the immune system; they are long-lived cells found in the blood circulation and in the tissues. Along with dendritic cells, they phagocytose bacteria and present fragments of them to the cells of the adaptive immune system. Neutrophils are short-lived, circulating cells attracted to sites of infection where they phagocytose bacteria and kill them with a burst of noxious chemicals. Dead neutrophils form the pus often associated with localized infections.

It is no surprise that pathogenic bacteria have developed strategies for avoiding and killing macrophages and neutrophils or achieving intracellular survival.

Complement
The complement cascade is one of several effective protein cascades in the protection of the host and is believed to be a very ancient defence mechanism. The complement cascade involves the activation of a single protein which triggers a coordinated reaction to produce an active end product, the membrane attack complex, which punctures the membrane of the bacterial cell. Initiation of complement activity is via the attachment of the protein C3b, derived from the continuous low level cleavage of C3 to C3a and C3b, to bacterial cells (the alternative pathway), by the binding of bacterial mannose to mannose-binding lectins (MBL pathway), or by the classical pathway where a complement protein attaches to pre-formed antibody on the surface of the bacterium. Complement activity is controlled by regulatory proteins to ensure a measured, appropriate response. Because of the destructive activity of complement, bacteria have developed ways of avoiding the attachment of complement proteins to their surfaces (see Box 4.2).

Inflammation
The combined activity of an influx of neutrophils to the site of infection, the presence of complement and subsequent damage to the host cells, results in an inflammatory

Box 4.2 Complement activity

Complement is a protein cascade system, where the initiation of the cascade proceeds to the formation of a membrane attack complex (MAC) that damages bacterial cell walls. In bacterial infection the complement cascade is often initiated by the deposition of C3b onto bacterial cell surfaces (the alternative pathway). The recognition of mannose on bacterial cell surfaces by mannose-binding lectins initiates the mannose-binding lectin pathway. The classical pathway of complement activation is via antibodies attaching to antigens on the bacterial cell surface.

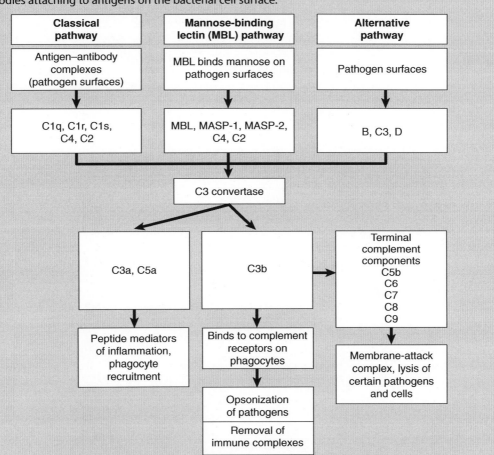

response. For the host, this is characterized by heat, swelling and pain at the infection site. There is a significant increase in the levels of circulating acute phase proteins, including cytokines, produced by the liver and epithelial cells, giving symptoms of a raised temperature and aching muscles.

Acquired immune system

Foreign antigen is presented to the effector cells of the immune system by antigen-presenting cells, the macrophages and the tissue dendritic cells, whereas neutrophils effectively phagocytose and kill bacteria, but do not process the antigen. The antigen fragments are presented to T and B lymphocytes in a controlled manner, so that the immune system is not over-stimulated, causing immunopathological damage to the host. The cells present their antigen associated with specialized molecules on their cell surface, called the major histocompatibility complex (MHC). Lymphocytes are programmed to recognize a specific antigen when it is presented to them in this way and respond via their T cell receptors. Depending on the source of the antigen, whether viral, bacterial, intracellular or from a parasite, an appropriate response is generated. This may involve the differentiation of B cells into plasma cells producing antibodies, or the activation of T cells or macrophages to attack and kill the pathogen. Once again, the outcome of a successful host response is detrimental for the pathogen, especially as memory cells are formed ensuring that the response is accelerated if the same antigen is encountered in the future. Successful pathogens have evolved ways of circumventing the activities and products of the adaptive immune system.

Evasion strategies

For a pathogen to cause infectious disease and damage to the host it must have the ability to switch on virulence genes to produce virulence factors, enabling it to spread throughout the infected area and beyond, and for simultaneous survival in the presence of the defences described above. Needless to say, the most successful pathogens have an impressive array of virulence factors. They are not all expressed at every stage of the infectious process, only as required. *Table 4.3* gives examples of pathogen evasion strategies of the innate system and *Table 4.4* details those for the adaptive immune system.

The production of excreted toxins (exotoxins) is also an effective way to overcome the immune response and cause significant damage to host cells. In some bacterial disease the damage is primarily caused by these toxins. This is especially true of the the genus *Clostridia*, anaerobic Gram-positive rods which are able to survive as

Table 4.3 Pathogenic evasion of the innate immune defence system

Innate defence target	Virulence factor	Mode of action	Examples
Secretory IgA	Inactivation of IgA by enzymes	Enzyme activity of IgA proteases. Glycosidases and sialidases	*Neisseria meningitidis, Neisseria gonorrhoeae*, streptococci, *Haemophilus influenzae*
Lactoferrin	Siderophores (iron-binding chemicals) proteases, receptors for iron-binding proteins	Free iron is released from iron-binding proteins	Used by a wide range of bacteria, including *Escherichia coli, Streptococcus pneumoniae, Neisseria meningitidis, Neisseria gonorrhoeae*
Ciliary beat in upper respiratory tract	Pyocyanin toxin of *Pseudomonas aeruginosa* Effect demonstrated in *Haemophilus influenzae*, but virulence factor not yet fully characterized, ?protein D	Ciliary beat of host cells slowed sufficiently to allow bacterial access to respiratory epithelial cells	*Pseudomonas aeruginosa* *Haemophilus influenzae*

Innate defence target	Virulence factor	Mode of action	Examples
pH – low pH of stomach	Urease Acid tolerance genes	Raises pH around bacteria in acidic environment of stomach Survival in stomach acid	*Helicobacter pylori* *Salmonellae, Shigellae, Campylobacter, Vibrio cholerae, Escherichia coli O157, Listeria monocytogenes*
Complement	Capsules	Opsonization resistance	*Streptococcus pyogenes, Streptococcus agalactiae, Neisseria meningitidis, Neisseria gonorrhoeae, Staphylococcus aureus, Escherichia coli* and other capsulated bacteria
	Protease	Inactivation of C3b	Elastase produced by *Pseudomonas aeruginosa*
	M proteins	Bind regulatory proteins and thus prevent opsonization by C3b	*Streptococcus pyogenes*
	Side chains of LPS	C3b binding, but distance too great for complement membrane attack complex to be effective	Gram-negative bacteria
Antibacterial peptides	*PagP* gene product	Alters LPS to reduce susceptibility	*Salmonella typhimurium*
Phagocytes (neutrophils and macrophages)	Production of proteins and enzymes	Prevents intracellular killing and enhances survival within phagocytes	*Mycobacterium tuberculosis, Salmonella typhimurium, Legionella pneumophila, Listeria monocytogenes, Coxiella burnetii*
Cytokines and cell signalling	Interfere with host cytokine networks Produce cytokine homologues	Interferes with level of TNF produced by natural killer cells	Epstein–Barr virus, cytomegalovirus, adenoviruses
Inhibition of apoptosis (cell suicide)	Interfere with specific signals in infected cells	Keeps cell alive for parasite to occupy	Toxoplasma
Intact, non-phagocytic intestinal epithelial cells	Type IV secretion systems	Injection of chemicals into cell by secretion system to alter cytoskeletal structure and induce phagocytosis, thereby evading mucosal defence	*Shigella* species and *Salmonella* species. Induced uptake into intestinal epithelial cells
	Cytolytic toxins	Kill phagocytic cells	*Staphylococcus aureus* leucocidin
Recognition of PAMPs	C type lectins	Modification or shielding of PAMPs reduces recognition by phagocytes and complement	Schistosomes
Complement proteins	Viral products	Block complement activity by producing homologue regulatory proteins	Herpes viruses Pox viruses

Table 4.4 Evasion of the adaptive immune response

Target	Virulence factor	Mode of action	Examples
Pre-formed antibodies	Protein A	Binds antibodies by Fc receptor (the wrong way round)	*Staphylococcus aureus*
		Coat with host antibodies – appears as host protein rather than pathogens	Parasites –schistosomes, hydatid disease
Presentation of foreign antigen to immune system in conjunction with MHC	Superantigen toxins Viral immunoevasins	Bypass MHC restriction on T cell activation, leading to over- or under-stimulation of immune response	Toxic shock syndrome toxin of *Staphylococcus aureus*, toxin involved in necrotizing fasciitis
		Interfere with MHC/peptide presentation	Cytomegalovirus, adenovirus
Antibody recognition	Antigenic variation Variation in pilin protein expression Antigenic shift and drift	Changed target for pre-formed antibodies Changed target for neutralizing antibodies	*Trypanosoma brucei* *Neisseria gonorrhoeae* Influenza viruses
Host effector cells	Latency in host, minimal gene expression	Latent in nerves after initial infection	Herpes zoster, Herpes simplex
		Latency in B lymphocytes	Epstein–Barr virus
T cells	Virus binds to CD4 on cell surface	Destroys effective immune response	HIV

spores in the environment for extremely long periods of time. When the spores are inhaled, inoculated or injected (often by trauma) into a human host they vegetate back into viable cells and also produce powerful toxins.

■ Some of the toxins target cells of the nervous system (neurotoxins), for example botulinum toxin (*Clostridium botulinum*) binds to acetyl choline receptors at neuromuscular junctions, inhibits the flow of acetyl choline and therefore muscle contraction, resulting in a floppy paralysis. The neurotoxin of tetanus, (*Clostridium tetanus*) binds to the γ-aminobutyric acid receptors (GABA) resulting in a rigid muscular paralysis.

■ *Clostridium difficile* toxins are excreted when these toxin-producing bacteria infect the gastrointestinal tract, often as a result of the removal of the normal flora by antibiotic treatment. The infection can develop into a serious condition called pseudomembranous colitis (see *Chapter 9*) whereas the toxin of *Clostridium perfringens* destroys tissue and creates a necrotic area and gas gangrene (see *Chapter 10*).

■ Toxins of the aerobic Gram-positive rods *Bacillus anthracis* and *Bacillus cereus* are the causative agents of anthrax and food poisoning respectively.

■ The cause of some of the world's largest pandemics, *Vibrio cholerae* is the result of bacteria attaching to the intestinal epithelial cells and the production of a powerful enterotoxin.

■ *Staphylococcus aureus*, *Streptococcus pyogenes* and *Escherichia coli* O157 also produce powerful toxins affecting a variety of cells during their infection processes.

■ Toxin production is a feature of the pathogenesis of fungi: aflatoxin produced by *Aspergillus fumigatus* affects liver function and is a co-factor for the development of cancer in patients already infected with hepatitis B virus.

4.4   ESTABLISHMENT OF INFECTIOUS DISEASE IN THE HOST

There are several prerequisites to the establishment of infectious disease when a pathogen infects a human host. These can be summarized as:

■ encounter
■ entry
■ adhesion and colonization
■ invasion from the site of infection and spread to other areas of the body
■ multiplication and damage
■ outcome of the disease
■ transmission to a new host and a new encounter.

Some infectious encounters will always follow a set pattern and aetiology (signs, symptoms and disease process), such as sleeping sickness caused by trypanosomes, a common cold virus, or whooping cough in a non-immune individual. Others take a less predictable course, for example *Staphylococcus aureus* can infect a wide variety of tissues with differing symptoms and severity of disease, while *Candida albicans* may lead to serious infection in an immuno-compromised person, yet be carried harmlessly by a healthy individual. Group A streptococci in the throat can cause an unpleasant and painful sore throat, whereas invasion by the bacteria could lead to life-threatening septicaemia in another. Different pathogens may cause similar symptoms in patients; for example, a chest infection, skin and wound infections, urinary tract infections, meningitis and sexually transmitted infections may have several bacterial causes or may be viral or fungal in origin. This highlights the importance of the diagnostic clinical microbiology laboratory in differential diagnosis.

Transmission of infectious disease

The transmission of disease is an important factor in controlling the spread of infection among susceptible populations (the study of patterns of health and disease in the population is called epidemiology) and guides the development of national vaccination programmes and infection control strategies. It is essential that information on the occurrence and distribution of disease is collated centrally to inform public health agencies of higher than usual levels of, for example, healthcare-acquired infection or community cases of a specific influenza strain; swine flu is an excellent example. For this reason there is a requirement to inform the appropriate agencies of cases of specific communicable diseases. From the microbial viewpoint, transmission to new hosts is essential to provide new niches and to preserve the species.

Transmission of microorganisms from one host to another can be effected by horizontal or vertical transmission. Horizontal transmission can be achieved in a variety of ways from person to person, whereas vertical transmission is from parent to child, either before birth across the placenta or ascending via the cervix causing congenital infection, or at birth causing perinatal or neonatal infection. Vertical transmission can also be via sperm, ovum, milk or blood. Examples of vertical infection include toxoplasmosis, viral infections such as cytomegalovirus, parvovirus or rubella, hepatitis B, HIV, syphilis, gonorrhoea, chlamydia and listeriosis (*Listeria monocytogenes*).

Successful transmission depends on the number of microorganisms shed from the host, their stability in the environment and resistance to drying, and the minimum number required to cause infectious disease in a new host. For several infectious processes described in later chapters, particularly *Chapter 9*, the infectious dose is stated in relation to different bacteria infecting the GI tract. If the infectious dose is very low, for example in *Escherichia coli* O157 (this may be only 10 organisms), the relative likelihood of transmission via food or from person to person is high. Stability in the environment dictates to some extent the route of transmission. A bacterium well equipped to survive in dry environments, of which *Staphylococcus aureus* is a good example, is able to survive in dust or on doorknobs until it comes into contact with a new host, whereas *Neisseria gonorrhoeae* is very fragile and must be kept warm and moist. Viruses with a lipid envelope do not survive long outside a human host, whereas those without can infect inanimate surfaces and wait for transport to a new host via food or water.

The principal routes of infection include:

- respiratory, via droplet infection transferred by coughs, sneezes and saliva
- skin, via shedding of skin cells or direct contact with an infected skin lesion
- faecal–oral transmission via food, water and poor hygiene
- sexual transmission via mucosal contact with infected individuals
- blood-borne via contact with the blood of an infected person
- transmission from animals; zoonotic transmission from vertebrates and vector-borne disease from invertebrate, arthropod vectors
- inanimate objects, fomites, where the pathogen survives before infecting the next host; this includes clothing, bed linen, clinical instruments, door knobs, surfaces of kitchen or furniture.

Adhesion and colonization

Attachment to host cells is not a random event and is the result of specific structures on the pathogens, adhesins, attaching to specific molecular structures on host cells. Attachment can be to mucosal surfaces found in the oral, respiratory, gastrointestinal and genitourinary tracts, skin cells and the non-shedding surface of the teeth. Invasive bacteria will also have mechanisms to attach to a variety of different cells at different stages of the disease process as they move from their entry site to deeper tissues. Some receptors may be available at a range of body sites, whereas some are restricted to specific areas. This combination of adhesins and receptors is described as tissue tropism. If the receptor is only present in one area of the body, the pathogen can only cause infectious disease at that site, and this explains why *Campylobacter* species cause gastrointestinal symptoms but not respiratory disease, and *Bordetella pertussis* (whooping cough) does not lead to diarrhoea.

Several parts of the cell structure can act as adhesins: bacterial capsules, fimbriae, lipoteichoic acid, slime layers, flagellae, viral surface structures such as haemagglutinins, and envelope proteins. Specific receptors on host epithelial cells include glycolipids, proteins, collagen, fibrinogen, fibronectin, existing receptors for cytokines, complement or hormones. Some bacteria also switch on genes to produce structures called secretion systems to inject the host cell with proteins which act as the receptor for the pili on the bacterial cell surface, or the proteins induce the host cell to phagocytose the bacteria.

For some pathogens, the site of adhesion is also the site of infection, where they remain, and do not progress any further into the host. The common cold viruses produce predictable symptoms after infecting the nasal mucosa. Benign wart viruses produce skin lesions at the site of attachment and infection. Dermatophyte fungi cause lesions only on the keratinized outer layer of skin; *Corynebacterium diphtheriae* secretes a powerful toxin at the site of attachment, producing the characteristic symptoms of the disease. Similarly, *Vibrio cholerae* attaches to intestinal epithelial cells and causes the symptoms of cholera via a powerful toxin. Pathogens such as *Streptococcus pyogenes,* which cause pharyngitis or skin infection, will, in the majority of cases, remain a local infection, but have the capacity to switch on virulence factors enabling them to spread into the blood and deeper tissues.

Invasion

Dissemination of, in particular, bacteria to deeper tissues and the bloodstream necessitates breaching the epithelial layer and crossing the endothelial layer, surviving in the blood, or within phagocytes after switching on different virulence factors, called invasins. Some bacteria are injected into the host by arthropods, examples being *Borrelia burgdorferi* (tick bite) and *Yersinia pestis* (flea bite). Damage to the epithelial layer also offers access to bacteria such as *Pseudomonas aeruginosa* into burns and ulcers, and *Pasteurella multicida* following a dog or cat bite. Others are capable of breaching the epithelial and endothelial layers: *Salmonella typhi* (typhoid fever), *Neisseria meningitidis* (meningitis*), Haemophilus influenzae, Streptococcus pneumoniae* and *Escherichia coli. Chlamydia trachomatis* (genital infections), *Mycobacterium tuberculosis, Listeria monocytogenes* and *Legionella pneumophila* survive in phagocytic cells. Salmonella and shigella bacteria induce intestinal epithelial cells to phagocytose them (see *Chapter 9*). Their spread through tissues is aided by specific enzymes and toxins capable of breaking down collagen or hyaluronic acid. Bacteria capable of surviving in the blood are able to resist the effect of complement via expression of capsules.

Damage to the host

Damage to host cells is the result of a combination of pathogenic virulence and host reaction to the infectious process. The inflammatory response invoked to attack the invading pathogen causes pain, swelling, redness and heat, which are the cardinal signs of inflammation. The influx of neutrophils leads in many instances to the formation of pus in the infected area. If the infected area is the central nervous system and the inflammation is taking place between the brain and the skull, with no room for expansion outwards, the symptoms of the disease are severe headaches, pressure on the brain and loss of consciousness. Given that the invading organism may be *Neisseria meningitidis*, which possesses a wide range of virulence factors and is able to survive in the blood, septicaemia may also be a symptom and a characteristic rash is evident (see *Chapter 12*). Septicaemia and septic shock are exacerbated by the immune response to the infection, resulting in loss of circulation to vital organs, hypovolaemic shock and possible multi-organ failure. Excessive macrophage reaction to the presence of *Mycobacterium tuberculosis* and the formation of calcified nodules is another example of immunopathological damage (see *Chapter 11*). Viral infections cause damage to the cells they attack; diarrhoea is the result of damage to the microvilli epithelial cells and the subsequent loss of dead cells in rotavirus infection.

Bacterial toxins are either endotoxins (LPS, a component of the Gram-negative cell wall) or protein exotoxins secreted from growing cells. Exotoxins act in three different ways to damage host cells:

■ Membrane-acting toxins damage host cell walls. Examples are the pore-forming alpha toxin of *Staphylococcus aureus*, Panton–Valentine leukocidin of *Staphylococcus aureus*, *Streptococcus pneumoniae* pneumolysin, lecithinase of *Clostridium perfringens* and streptolysin O of *Streptococcus pyogenes*.
■ A-B toxins, a large family of toxins comprising a biologically active A subunit and the B binding domain. The A subunit is inserted into the host cell and disrupts cell functions in various ways. Examples are the clostridial toxins, *Corynebacterium diphtheriae* toxin, *Pseudomonas aeruginosa*, cholera toxin and Shiga toxin (shigella).
■ Superantigen toxins bypass the usual antigen processing and presentation system and directly bring T cells and antigen-presenting cells into contact, the result being either over- or under-stimulation of the immune system. The former can lead to toxic shock (*Staphylococcus aureus*) or necrotizing fasciitis (*Streptococcus pyogenes*).

Exotoxins produced by some bacteria cause symptoms and damage to the host often at a distance from the initial infection. Powerful toxins from clostridial bacteria cause potentially fatal botulism and tetanus, anthrax, pseudomembranous colitis, gas gangrene and necrotizing fasciitis.

Outcome of infection and disease

The outcome of an infectious disease is multifactorial, dependent on the ability of the host to overcome the pathogenic process and recover from the ensuing damage and the relative pathogenicity of the causative organisms. The initial infectious dose, nature of the infection and the ability of the host immune system are important host factors. An immuno-competent individual will follow a predictable path when infected with a cold, influenza, chickenpox or *Cryptosporidia* infection. For an immuno-compromised patient, a cold may linger and the other infections may prove fatal. A healthy susceptible individual, however, would become seriously ill if infected with a large dose of *Clostridium botulinum* or bitten by a mosquito carrying malaria.

Recovery from disease often involves complete elimination of the infectious agent from the body and a strong immune response, ensuring that re-infection would be promptly dealt with by memory cells able to produce either antibodies or effector cells. Some pathogens, however, persist in the body in a latent form, kept under control by the immune system but able to cause recurrent infection if host defences weaken. Recurrrent cold sores (*Herpes simplex*), shingles (*Herpes zoster*), recurrence of mononucleosis symptoms (EBV) and reactivated tuberculosis are good examples.

Dissemination

Transmission to a new host completes the infection cycle; this transmission occurs by the same routes as the initial infection, giving bacteria, viruses, fungi and parasites the opportunity to transfer to new hosts. This can happen either directly or, in the case of some parasites, via an intermediate host.

4.5 GENETIC CONTROL OF VIRULENCE

Earlier sections have described how a virulence factor can be a constituent of the cell structure that is permanent, such as peptidoglycan or LPS, or expressed as necessary during the course of infection, for example capsules. Other virulence factors such as toxins, iron-binding proteins, proteases, adhesins, invasins and immune response modulators are only expressed in response to signals from the host environment because the bacterium is stressed by the lack of nutrients or by components of the immune response.

Two component regulatory systems

Bacteria constantly 'sense' their environment and the genes for specific virulence factor expression can be switched on by changes in temperature and essential ions such as phosphorus, magnesium and iron. A sensor protein in the bacterial cytoplasmic membrane monitors the appropriate environmental parameter and signals the response regulator via a signalling process involving phosphorylation. The response regulator has DNA binding activity which then switches on the relevant gene or genes. The virulence factor is then produced. When conditions change again the sensor protein no longer sends the signal to the regulator and the relevant genes are switched off. *Bordetella pertussis*, the bacteria causing whooping cough, respond to raised temperature and lowered magnesium, sulphate and nicotinic acid levels by the expression of toxins, a characteristic of the disease process. From the bacterial point of view such regulation ensures that virulence factors are only employed inside a human host and not in the environment. These two component regulatory systems are also used to regulate genes involved in the uptake and metabolism of specific compounds; *Escherichia coli* regulates uptake of glutamine, arginine, histidine and nitrate in this way. Genes for virulence factors are often located in a similar area of the genome and one signal may be enough to trigger the production of several virulence factors in a coordinated way (see *Figure 4.3*).

Quorum sensing

Quorum sensing is a process employed by bacteria to sense the cell density around them and coordinate their gene expression. The bacteria secrete a chemical called an auto-inducer into the surrounding environment. If there is a significant density of bacteria, the concentration of auto-inducer rises which triggers a sensor protein and signal transduction system linked to a DNA binding protein, as described earlier. *Pseudomonas aeruginosa* are known to regulate several virulence enzymes, biofilm formation, toxins and invasion systems by quorum sensing. *Streptococcus pneumoniae* regulate competence, the ability to take in naked DNA from dead bacteria, either to acquire genes or as supply of nucleotides for generating new DNA. *Staphylococcus*

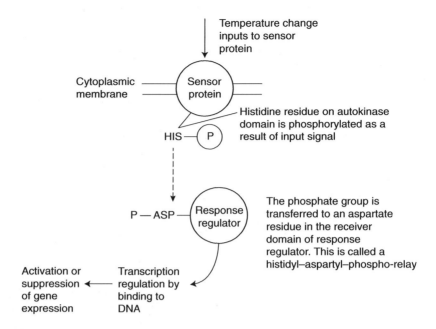

Figure 4.3
Two component regulatory systems. The example shown is a temperature change, but it could also be the binding of a ligand to a receptor.

aureus use the system for expression of exotoxins, enzymes, coagulase and protein A and *Enterococcus faecalis* for plasmid transfer (see *Figure 4.4*). Gram-positive cells secrete oligopeptides while Gram-negative cells secrete *N*-acyl homoserine lactone (AHL). Both Gram-positive and -negative cells secrete AI2, a furanosyl borate diester, the product of the *LuxS* gene. This is an auto-inducer that can be received by a wide range of bacteria. Communication between different genera of bacteria also occurs, known as quorum sensing 'cross talk': *Escherichia coli* and *Salmonella enterica* react to auto-inducers from other bacteria and change their expression to fit in with these populations. A further form of cooperation between bacteria of the same species has been observed: when challenged with the antibiotic norfloxacin, resistant members of the bacterial population produce indole, although they do not require it themselves. The indole enables sensitive bacteria to activate reflux pumps to pump out the antibiotic.

Transfer of genetic material

Genetic material is passed between bacteria in several ways. Major DNA acquisitions have taken place during the evolution of bacteria, creating pathogens with enhanced virulence, for example the transfer of toxin genes and other virulence factors. Horizontal mutations leading to antibiotic resistance occur as a result of selective pressure to survive. An ever-increasing range of novel enzymes (extended spectrum β-lactamases), capable of hydrolysing B lactam drugs, are being recognized.

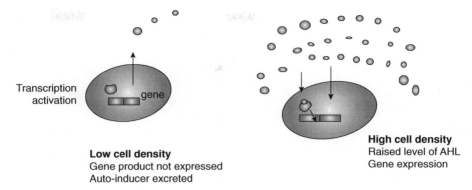

Figure 4.4
An example of quorum sensing controlling the transcription of the hypothetical product of gene A in a Gram-negative bacterium.

Transposons

Genes can also be recombined or inserted into the genome by a random process called transposition. The discrete sequences of DNA transposed can either be chromosomal or plasmid in origin. These genetic elements, called transposons (or sometimes jumping genes), cause mutations and often code for antibiotic resistance genes.

Transformation

This is a process by which naked DNA from dead organisms is taken up by other bacteria and is dependent on the ability (competence) of the new bacteria to accommodate the new DNA.

Pathogenicity islands

In some bacteria, such as enterococci, *Salmonellae* and *Escherichia coli*, there are distinct regions integrated into the chromosome with a different G–C content from the rest of the genome. These have been acquired by horizontal transfer and contain the genes for virulence factors. They are called pathogenicity islands and can code for toxins, iron uptake, fimbriae and invasion systems.

Plasmids, conjugation and recombination

Virulence and antibiotic resistance genes may also be carried on smaller, extrachromosomal genetic material called plasmids. Virulence genes carried within the chromosome are more stable, but the smaller plasmids are more easily transmitted between bacteria. This is a problem for infection control in hospital settings because plasmids coding for antibiotic resistance can be passed between bacteria with relative ease. Plasmids can be passed by conjugation between bacteria, as shown in *Figure 4.5*. The plasmid may also become incorporated into the recipient chromosome at recombination sites, giving the cell a larger chromosome. These cells, known as Hfr (high frequency of recombination) cells, can then pass on the genetic information to a negative cell. The new recipient does not generally become a donor cell and the DNA it receives replaces a segment of its DNA rather than enlarging the chromosome.

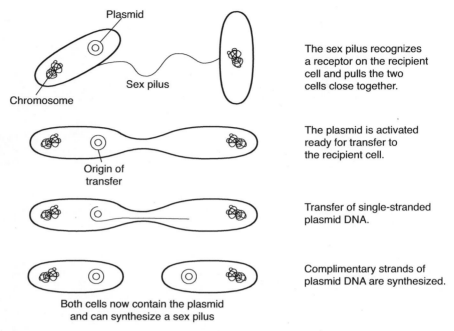

Figure 4.5
Transfer of genetic material between bacteria by conjugation.

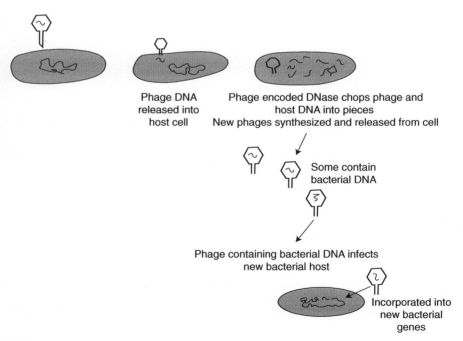

Figure 4.6
Transduction. Transfer of bacterial DNA between host cells by incorporation into phages.

Transduction

Bacterial DNA can also be passed by transduction, where the genetic material is transferred by bacteriophages (phages), viruses that infect bacteria. When a bacterium is lysogenized by a phage, the phage chromosome becomes incorporated into the bacterial genome and is passed on through thousands of generations. *Corynebacterium diphtheriae* toxin is a good example of lysogeny, as the toxin gene is coded for by a phage. During the course of a lytic bacteriophage infection, the host bacterial cell is lysed and new bacteriophages are released to infect other bacteria. In the process of packaging the new phages with DNA, some of the host DNA is incorporated and transferred via the phage to a new host where it is incorporated into the genome (see *Figure 4.6*).

SUGGESTED FURTHER READING

Favoreel, H.W., Van de Walle, G.R., Nauwynck, H.J. & Pensaert, M.B. (2003) Virus complement evasion strategies. *J. Gen. Virol.* **84:** 1–15.

Hannigan, B.M., Moore, C.B.T. & Quinn, D.G. (2009) *Immunology*, 2nd Edition. Scion Publishing.

O'Hara, A.M. & Shanahan, F. (2006) The gut flora as a forgotten organ. *EMBO reports*, **7:** 688–693.

Schmid-Hempel, P. (2009) Immune defence, parasite evasion strategies and their relevance for 'macroscopic phenomena' such as virulence. *Phil. Trans. R. Soc. B.* **364:** 85–98.

SELF-ASSESSMENT QUESTIONS

1. Explain what is meant by the term 'opportunistic infection'.
2. A hospital patient has been taking several antibiotics over a period of several weeks. He develops diarrhoea. Give two possible reasons for this and explain why it is important to send a faecal sample to investigate the possible presence of *Clostridium difficile* toxins.
3. Give two examples of how members of the normal flora can cause infection after being transferred to another body site.
4. Outline three components of the innate immune system.
5. Name the three pathways through which the membrane attack complex of complement can be activated.
6. Why is the MHC system important in regulating the adaptive immune response? How can the MHC restriction be overcome by superantigens?
7. Describe two strategies by which bacteria evade the activity of complement.
8. Exotoxins are powerful proteins used by pathogens to evade the immune response. Outline three diseases where the symptoms are produced by the production and activity of a toxin. Name the three principal classes of toxins.
9. What is meant by a two component regulatory system? How do these enable bacteria to regulate their virulence factors?
10. Give some examples of the ways in which infection can be transmitted from person to person by horizontal transmission.

Answers to self-assessment questions provided at:
www.scionpublishing.com/medmicro

The use of microscopy and staining in microbiology

Learning objectives
After studying this chapter you should confidently be able to:

■ **Explain the development of microscopy from the late sixteenth century to the present day**
Early microscopes were really versions of the telescope. A simple single lens microscope enabled van Leeuwenhoek to describe bacteria and protozoans. The development of the condenser and compound lenses increased the amount of light reaching a sample and reduced the distortion. Staining methods and improved lenses and objectives enabled the classification of bacteria. More sophisticated forms of microscopy were later developed.

■ **Describe the different types of microscopy used in microbiology**
Light microscopy is used extensively in routine laboratories along with immunofluorescence microscopy. The use of electron, scanning electron and confocal microscopy has enabled the ultrastructure of viruses as well as large and dense surface structures to be visualized. Images can be three-dimensional and transmitted via video technology to observe cellular behaviour.

■ **Describe the role of microscopy in the diagnostic laboratory**
Light microscopy is used to identify cells and casts in urine samples, and to identify parasites in faecal samples or stained preparations. It can be used for counting cells in CSF specimens. Immunofluorescence techniques have a role in identifying pathogens in clinical samples. Electron microscopes are used for virus identification and are mainly found in research and reference laboratories as they are usually beyond the budget of routine laboratories.

■ **Describe the various staining methods used for identification of a range of microorganisms**
Gram stains are used routinely for the initial identification of bacteria, Ziehl–Neelsen stains for *Mycobacteria* and *Cryptosporidia* species, acridine orange for *Trichomonas vaginalis*, phenyl auramine for *Mycobacteria* and for *Cryptosporidia* species, and calcofluor for initial identification of fungal elements in clinical samples.

The microscope is often regarded as a symbol for the practice of biomedical science, particularly in microbiology, histology and to a certain extent immunology. Of these disciplines it is probably microbiology that has contributed most to the early use of the microscope and its development from a curiosity to an analytical tool. A number of staining methods that were developed in tandem are still the mainstay of identification and diagnostic techniques in microbiology, for example the Gram and Ziehl–Neelsen (ZN) stains.

5.1   THE HISTORY AND DEVELOPMENT OF MICROSCOPY

Although the compound microscope had been developed by the late sixteenth century as a version of the telescope with a short focal length, the image quality was poor. Satisfactory illumination was a problem with increasing magnification and the thick object and eyepiece lenses suffered from both chromatic and spherical aberration. When light passes through glass some of the wavelengths are bent at different angles and there is a dispersion, which can give the effect of a rainbow. This can mean that there is a difference in focusing of the different colours, known as chromatic aberration, and the resulting image is blurred with strongly coloured edges. Spherical aberration occurs because the lens is curved and the images are again distorted. In 1674 when Anton von Leeuwenhoek first described bacteria and protozoans he was using a simple single lens microscope, which had superior optical properties at higher magnification. The major disadvantage was the need to build a dedicated microscope for each specimen, yet despite this the simple microscope remained in popular use throughout the seventeenth and eighteenth centuries.

Microscopy improved in the mid- to late nineteenth century as a result of two major innovations: the condenser and compound lenses. The condenser developed by Abbe was able to concentrate and focus light onto the sample, and the construction of compound eyepiece and objective lenses significantly reduced the distortion of the final image. The objective lens, placed nearest to the specimen, produces the initial magnification with the image being further magnified by the lens of the eyepiece. The use of higher quality flint glass meant that thinner lenses could be used, and this further reduced the effects of both spherical and chromatic aberration.

The ability to visualize the causative agents of disease was a major breakthrough in the history of microbiology, as described in *Chapter 1*. In 1859 the Austrian pathologist Rudolf Virchow initiated the concept of cellular pathology through the application of the more advanced compound microscope to the examination of tissue samples. The development of staining methods, notably by Christian Gram in 1884, and later the development of the Ziehl–Neelsen (ZN) stain, allowed bacteria to be classified by shape and staining characteristics – these are still the basis of initial identification today. The ZN stain was particularly important in research aimed at understanding the cause and transmission of tuberculosis.

The work of Coons in 1943 led to the development of antibodies for the selective identification of antigens in tissue samples. His initial work involved raising polyclonal antibodies to streptococci that were then used to demonstrate the association of the bacteria with rheumatic fever. The last 25 years have seen a rapid expansion of antibody techniques in a number of specialist areas of diagnostic pathology. Rapid development of microscopy in the second half of the twentieth century has enabled a range of sophisticated techniques to be developed, including ultraviolet, electron, epi-fluorescent and confocal microscopy.

The light microscope

All the early developments in microscopy described above rely on the use of the light microscope with standard Köhler illumination (see *Figure 5.1*). Modern student microscopes are set so that light from the condenser lens system is focused at the plane of the specimen being viewed; this is known as critical illumination. *Figure 5.1* shows a comparison of both critical and Köhler illumination. Köhler illumination

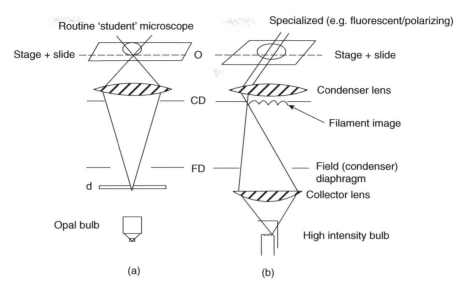

Figure 5.1
Light paths for critical (a) and Köhler (b) illumination. With critical illumination, conjugate planes are the illuminating bulb filament and sample plane (O). When adjusted correctly, the image of the filament is seen coincident with the sample image. A diffusing glass filter (d) is used to blur the filament image. With Köhler illumination, the image of the field diaphragm and the sample are coincident when adjusted correctly. The filament is out of the plane of focus. FD, field diaphragm; CD, condenser diaphragm.

is still used in specialized microscopy because the double lens condenser system is more efficient at collecting and focusing light. The limitations of their resolution relate to the illumination and the numerical aperture of the objective lens. Most light microscopes (see *Figure 5.2*) have a choice of objective lenses that give a magnification of 10×, 40× or 100×, giving a total magnification of 10 times this value when the eyepiece lens is included in the overall magnification. The resolution of the light microscope, i.e. the size of the smallest object that can be seen clearly, is determined by the nature of the light used; the shortest wavelength that the human eye can see is 400 nm (0.4 μm) and the resolution of the light microscope is half the wavelength of light used, i.e. 200 nm or 0.2 μm. For visualizing bacteria this is ideal, as most bacterial cells are around this size, but it is not possible to see detail within the bacteria, apart from the presence of spores indicated by a non-staining area within the cells. Most identification is performed using the 100× objective and the addition of a drop of immersion oil between the specimen and the lens. The oil improves the resolution by minimizing the refraction, or scattering, of light. A greater angle of light is trapped and the resulting image is clearer. Oil should never be used on any objective unless it has 'oil immersion' written on it.

The advantage of light microscopy is that it is possible to view living organisms and tissue directly from the patient specimen. In an unstained specimen, movement of the organism can also be observed, for example the tumbling activity of bacteria, or the twitching of protozoa such as *Trichomonas vaginalis* from a vaginal specimen.

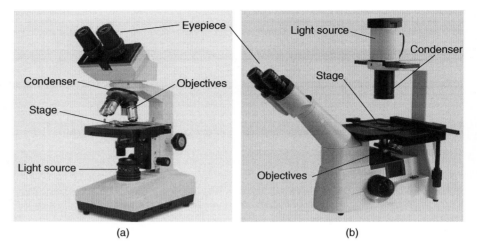

(a)   (b)

Figure 5.2
Photographs of standard light (a) and inverted light (b) microscopes.

The inverted light microscope

As the name suggests, the light source and the objective lens are in reverse positions. The light source is above the stage and the objective lens below the microscope stage, as shown in *Figure 5.2*. The advantage is that specimens can be observed directly in Petri dishes or in flat-bottomed wells; this allows the observer to view the contents of the specimen directly. Whole Petri dishes of living organisms can be observed in this way.

5.2   THE LIGHT MICROSCOPE IN ROUTINE DIAGNOSTIC MICROBIOLOGY

Light microscopy is a valuable tool in most areas of the clinical laboratory and for a variety of different specimen types, using both stained and unstained samples. Microscopic examination can be used to demonstrate the presence or absence of bacteria, with an indication of the staining reaction, morphology of the cells, and the presence of a capsule or spores. Blood cells, fungal elements, protozoan and helminth eggs are also important diagnostic indicators visualized by light microscopy. The examples outlined in the rest of this section demonstrate the importance of light microscopy, and are all explained more fully in the relevant chapters on sample types later in this book.

Urine microscopy

Microscopy is performed on all urine specimens received in the microbiology laboratory, and provides valuable information when interpreted in conjunction with clinical details and the results of the bacterial culture. Infected urine samples usually contain large numbers of white blood cells and may also contain red cells, epithelial cells, bacteria and protein casts from the kidney tubules. Flat-bottomed 96-well microtitre trays are used, into which a measured volume of urine is added.

The samples are left to settle and then viewed using the 40× objective of an inverted microscope. The presence of raised numbers of cells and the presence of casts can be evaluated and recorded after examining at least ten high-powered fields to give an estimated count (see *Chapter 8*).

Figure 5.3 shows a typical infected urine specimen, as seen on the inverted light microscope.

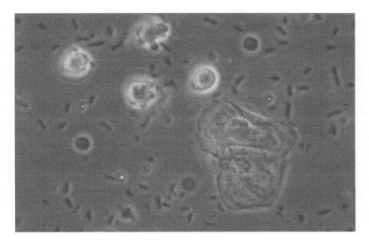

Figure 5.3
Microscopic image of infected urine at ×40 magnification. The small rod shapes are bacteria; the largest, irregular shape cell is an epithelial cell. The smallest cells are red blood cells and the medium sized cells are white blood cells.

Examination of faecal samples

Wet preparations and concentrations

One of the standard methods for viewing specimens under light microscopy is to add a small amount of the sample to a drop of diluent on a microscope slide, apply a coverslip and view at low and then high power. The microscopic appearance of a small amount of faeces is viewed in this way. The sample may contain large amounts of irrelevant material such as fat globules, meat and vegetable fibres, but with practice the presence of blood cells, both red and white, as well as yeasts and protozoan cysts can be distinguished. Ova and cysts from helminths, nematodes and cestodes are likely to be present in small numbers within a specimen and are identified more easily if the specimen is cleared of debris and concentrated before being thoroughly examined under the microscope. This identification is further helped by temporarily replacing one of the eyepieces with a special eyepiece called a graticule that contains a measurement grid. The graticule has to be calibrated for a specific microscope and magnification using a stage micrometer (see *Box 5.1*). Measurement is important in the identification of cysts and ova, as some of them have a similar morphology but can be distinguished by their relative size. Sizes range from the relatively small *Clonorchis sinensis* ova at 30 μm to the large ova of schistosomes, measuring 150 μm.

Box 5.1 Calibrating a microscope for measurement

The size of a specimen can be determined using an eyepiece micrometer. Calibration of the microscope is carried out using an eyepiece micrometer and a stage micrometer, as follows:

1. The eyepiece scale is broken down into 100 small divisions.

2. The stage micrometer scale extends over 1 mm. This millimetre is itself divided into 0.1 mm divisions, and each of these is again subdivided into 0.01 mm sections.

3. Insert the eyepiece graticule into the eyepiece, and replace in the microscope.

4. Place the stage micrometer on the microscope stage.

5. Focus the low-power objective onto the stage scale.

6. Adjust the eyepiece and stage scales as necessary, until they are parallel and overlapping.

7. Note the number of eyepiece divisions and their corresponding stage measurement. For example, 10 eyepiece divisions = 0.2 mm on the stage scale.

8. Calculate the value of one eyepiece division, as follows: If 10 eyepiece divisions = 0.2 mm, then 1 eyepiece division will be 0.2÷10 = 0.02 mm = 20 µm.

9. Repeat from step 5 for each objective, noting and recording the reading from each.

10. Calibration need only be done once for each microscope and its objectives and eyepieces.

Sellotape slides

The sticky side of Sellotape (adhesive tape) can be used to directly pick up specimens from either a patient or from a patient specimen. The sticky side is then pressed onto a microscope slide (*Figure 5.4*). As seen in *Figure 5.5*, the nematode *Enterobius*

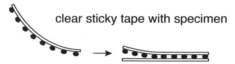

clear sticky tape with specimen

Figure 5.4
Sellotape slide preparation. Any eggs of *Enterobius vermicularis* can be seen using a low magnification.

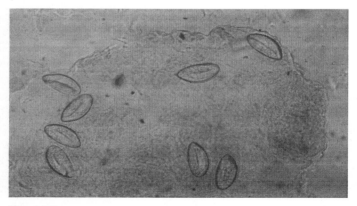

Figure 5.5
Ova of *Enterobius vermicularis*. These threadworm or pinworm eggs are shown on a Sellotape slide.

vermicularis can be diagnosed by taking a Sellotape sample from the skin around the anal area, pressing it onto a slide and examining it unstained for the presence of the pinworm eggs. The eggs are large and can easily be seen using a low power objective (see *Chapter 9* for further details).

Staining of faecal parasites

Staining of parasite samples helps in their morphological identification, especially in the identification of amoeba and *Giardia* trophozoites. Either Giemsa's stain or a rapid Field's stain is used for identifying *Dientamoeba fragilis* and *Blastocystis hominis.*

The Nomarski technique (see *Box 5.2*) can also be used to enhance the appearance of cysts.

Direct examination of genital swabs

The patient swab is pressed on to a microscope slide, a coverslip applied and the slide viewed at 40× magnification. Some laboratories use this method routinely for all genital swabs, whereas others use the method to confirm the presence of the protozoan parasite *Trichomonas vaginalis,* after it has been seen in a stained preparation. In an unstained swab specimen, the cells of *T. vaginalis* resemble large white cells and are often observed to be moving; if the swab has already been refrigerated, gently warming the slide can be sufficient to restore mobility. A Gram-stained specimen taken directly from a genital swab is often examined in the clinic as soon as the swab is taken, to show the presence of the characteristic Gram-negative diplococci, *Neisseria gonorrhoeae,* the causative agents of the sexually transmitted disease gonorrhoea. The bacteria are fragile outside the human body and need to be cultured as soon as possible. The confirmation of their presence by microscopy can help in the early diagnosis and management of the patient. *Chapter 10* describes the investigation of infections of the genital tract.

Microscopic examination of fungal samples and cultures

Examination before culture

Samples of hair, skin, nails or other tissue are sent to the laboratory to be examined for the presence of fungal pathogens. At the same time as they are inoculated into culture media, a small amount of the sample is examined microscopically. The specimen is placed onto a drop of potassium hydroxide and Indian ink on a microscope slide. A coverslip is applied and the slide is viewed at 10× and 40× magnification. If the sample is infected, fungal elements are visible as short strands of blue hyphae, more complex branching hyphae or discrete yeast-like structures. An interim report can then be sent out and a final diagnosis made after culture, which may take up to 3 weeks.

The fluorescent stain calcofluor has replaced Indian ink as the staining method of preference in many laboratories. Calcofluor is one of a group of chemicals added to washing powder and liquids. It binds to glycans in fibres and then fluoresces a blue colour, neutralizing the effect of white materials that have become yellow with age. Its ability to bind to glycans is useful in microbiology, because calcofluor will selectively bind to fungal wall structures.

Box 5.2 The Nomarski technique

The Nomarski technique, or differential interference contrast, is used to enhance the contrast in unstained samples. The principle of the technique is that when light passes through a sample made up of differing refractive indices, the phase of the wavefront is altered because light travels more slowly where the refractive index is higher. In simple terms this method relies upon the fact that different densities found within a specimen alter the path of polarized light by differing amounts (the more dense, the greater the effect). Before passing through the specimen the polarized light is split into a double beam that is slightly divergent. Before entering the upper (analyser) filter the divergent rays are combined by a second Wollaston prism. Any variation in path length induced by the specimen will generate interference, adding or subtracting from signal strength. This results in a pseudo-3D image that translates physical density into optical density. This is shown diagrammatically on the right. The microscope used has to be set up for brightfield illumination and have Nomarski prisms, which are then adjusted with the condenser rings to give the desired effect (an appropriate standard operating procedure will be provided if the microscope is equipped for Nomarski). The contrast results from the phase changes being converted to amplitude changes, which produces a three-dimensional image. The method is useful for viewing living cells, and the examples shown here are a *Giardia* cyst (left) and an *Entamoeba coli* cyst (right).

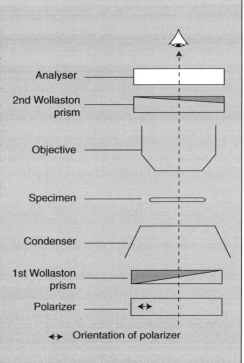

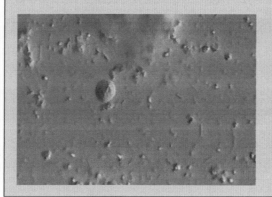

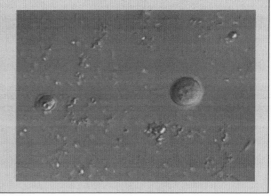

Examination of cultures

Light microscopy is used in conjunction with the appearance of the colonies to identify fungal pathogens. The Sellotape method is ideal (see *Figure 5.4*); the sticky side is pressed on to the downy surface of the colony and placed on to a drop of either lactophenol cotton blue or acid fuchsin on a microscope slide. When viewed at 40×, the size, arrangement and shape of the hyphae and conidia guide the identification.

If the presence of the capsulated yeast *Cryptococcus neoformans* is suspected, a preparation can be stained with Indian ink. The capsule does not take up the stain and the yeasts appear as spheres with a clear halo around them (see *Chapter 13* for more on examination of yeast cultures).

Cell counts from CSF specimens

Counting chambers are used routinely to count the number of white and red blood cells in cerebrospinal fluid (CSF) samples as part of the laboratory diagnosis of meningitis. In cases of bacterial meningitis the numbers of neutrophils are considerably raised, whereas monocytic cells are in the predominance in viral infections. A Gram-stained smear is also prepared and this will show the presence of any bacteria and also give a clearer picture of the type of white cells present (see *Chapter 12* for more on cell counts).

5.3   SPECIALIZED MICROSCOPY

The development of alternative microscopy techniques has enabled more detailed structures to be visualized and additional diagnostic methods to be developed. Fluorescent microscopes have become routine pieces of equipment, whereas confocal microscopes that represent the more recent advances in fluorescent microscopy are principally used in research. Electron microscopes are expensive pieces of equipment, beyond the reach of most routine microbiology laboratories but available in reference laboratories.

Darkground (darkfield) microscopy

The darkground microscope is set up with a specialized condenser that has a peripheral light annulus, effectively a patch over the condenser, causing light to pass outside the periphery of the objective lens. Any small particles in the specimen will deflect light into the optical field and will then appear as bright specks. Darkground, or darkfield illumination is effective because rather like stars in the night sky, the dark background enables unstained cells to be seen, whereas they would be invisible in bright light. This is because the refractive indices of unstained cells are very similar to their surroundings. Darkground illumination can be used to visualize bacteria directly from patient samples, without the need for culture or staining. This is advantageous when looking at the spirochaetes of *Treponema pallidum,* from the initial primary ulcer or chancre of an infected person, because no culture medium has been developed for their *in vitro* growth, and diagnosis is routinely made by demonstrating antibody responses to the infection. In countries where diagnostic tests are more limited, darkground microscopy can be useful in the diagnosis of spirochaetes of *Leptospira* species from plasma or serum specimens, although the test is not always reliable. The technique has also been used in investigations of oral pathogens in cases of periodontal disease. *Figure 5.6* shows the principle of darkground microscopy.

Fluorescence microscopy

Fluorescence microscopy can make an extremely useful contribution to the microbiological analysis of patient samples, especially when few organisms are

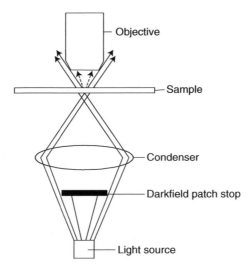

Figure 5.6
Darkground (darkfield) microscopy. The central stop in the condenser prevents light entering the objective. If small particles or microorganisms in suspension are placed above the condenser they will scatter light back into the objective and become visible.

present. Sensitivity is enhanced by the brightness of their localization. Although many types of organisms are auto-fluorescent, the range of fluorescence wavelengths is not selective; however, there are two important approaches for demonstrating a range of organisms:

■   immunocytochemical techniques; these use antibodies that are commercially available and will bind specifically to antigenic targets
■   non-immunocytochemical techniques; acridine orange and calcofluor are two important fluorochromes that bind to nucleic acids and structural components, respectively.

The fluorescence microscope
Setting up a fluorescence facility requires both financial and practical planning. The microscopes are not hugely expensive; a reasonable quality epi-fluorescence microscope with a filter array block to cover three wavelengths of emissions will cost approximately £10 000. In addition to the initial outlay the microscope will require regular servicing, and replacement bulbs become a significant expense with heavy usage. The microscope is best sited in a separate area where there is little through traffic and the room lights can be turned off to aid viewing of the fluorescence signal. There is also the health and safety issue of ultraviolet (UV) emissions. The fluorescence microscope uses short wavelengths of light at the blue end of the spectrum. These provide better resolving power than white light and are generated by a high pressure, high voltage, mercury vapour lamp. The lamp has a standard life of 100 hours and can fail quite unpredictably and in a spectacular fashion, if taken past this point; it is important to keep a careful log of all usage.

Modern fluorescence microscopes operate on the principle of **epi-illumination** where light from the UV source enters the optical system horizontally and is reflected by an angled dichroic mirror (a chromatic beam splitter) to illuminate the specimen after passing down through the objective lens. *Figure 5.7* shows the principle of epi-fluorescent illumination. Any fluorescence that is generated then passes up to the eyepiece for observation via the same objective lens. The wavelength of the incident light reaching the specimen is restricted to a narrow bandwidth that is selected by the **excitation filter**. In a similar fashion, the wavelength of the light being observed after its fluorescent emission is restricted to a narrow bandwidth by the **barrier filter** housed in the filter block. The three filters commonly used will pass light from the fluorochromes, as can be seen in *Box 5.3*. Provision is also made to absorb stray UV light to minimize the risk of conjunctivitis and corneal or retinal injury to the operator.

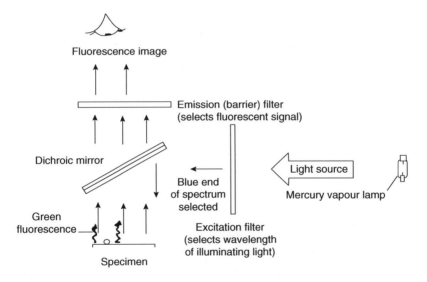

Figure 5.7
Light path in the fluorescence microscope, showing epi-illumination.

Box 5.3 Colour filters used in fluorescence microscopy	
Colour	**Fluorochrome**
Green	FITC
Red	TRITC
	Phycoerythrin
	Texas red
Blue	DAPI
	Calcofluor

The correct selection of filter sets has particular importance as it determines the wavelength of the fluorescent light being emitted. This light could be green, red or orange, depending on the fluorochrome used in the antibody binding system. It has particular relevance to staining and identifying antigen and bound antibody in the following techniques:

■ **direct method** – staining of antigen in the specimen with labelled antibodies, e.g. *Chlamydia trachomatis* elementary bodies in endocervical swabs, urine or eye swabs

■ **indirect method** – staining of bound antibody in patient serum with labelled second antibodies (often anti-human IgG), e.g. *Legionella pneumophila* antibodies in serum detected using *Legionella* bacteria as the substrate; and the binding of autoimmune antibodies in patient serum to tissue substrates such as mouse liver and kidney.

With either of these methods it is possible to double label with different fluorochromes (see *Figure 5.8*).

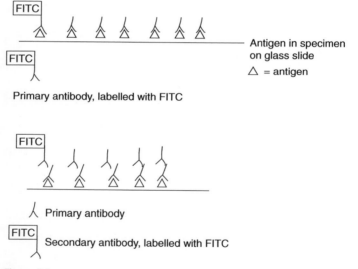

Figure 5.8
Principle of the direct (top) and indirect (bottom) immunofluorescent technique.

Confocal microscopy

Confocal scanning microscopy takes fluorescent microscopy a stage further, using a laser as the light source. The specimen is illuminated in a serial fashion, point by point, as the laser light is rapidly scanned over it, and by saving many digital images, a composite picture is built up. A combination of fluorescent labels can be used within one specimen to give a much clearer picture of constituents and also of cellular changes. Confocal microscopes are much more expensive than epi-fluorescent microscopes, which puts them out of financial range for routine work, although they are valuable in research settings.

Electron microscopy

Transmission electron microscopy (TEM) has enabled structures smaller than the resolution of the light microscope to be visualized. Consequently virus structures and viral identification from clinical samples became possible and also the pathogenic processes of attachment and invasion could be captured. The greater resolution is achieved by using electrons as the energy source rather than light. A beam of electrons is produced from an electron gun consisting of a tungsten filament and focused on to the specimen by a condenser and then the objective lens. The image is magnified again by the projection lens and viewed on either a fluorescent screen or captured photographically. The resultant image is magnified up to 250 000 times.

Electron microscopes are expensive and are housed in dedicated rooms because they need a special electrical supply (high voltages and currents are used), a strong floor to reduce vibration and a plentiful water supply to remove the excess heat. However, they are invaluable for directly confirming the presence of viruses in clinical samples such as faeces, without the need for tissue culture. TEM images have enabled researchers to understand the complex interactions between bacteria and host cells.

Scanning electron microscopy

Scanning electron microscopy (SEM) relies on video technology to reproduce images of the specimen on a television monitor, rather than directly seeing it through the microscope. It is probably most useful for looking at quite large and dense surface structures, as the electrons do not need to go right through the specimen. The images produced are three-dimensional, although the magnification is lower than standard EM. SEM can be used in microbiology research to demonstrate, for example, uptake of bacteria into cells.

5.4   STAINING TECHNIQUES

Staining is an important adjunct to the diagnosis of pathogens in clinical samples. The stains most commonly used in conjunction with the light microscope are cationic or basic dyes. They are positively charged and therefore attracted to the negatively charged cell membranes of most bacteria. The Gram stain provides an ideal starting point for identification of unknown bacteria, whereas the Ziehl–Neelsen or auramine–phenol (fluorescent) stains are used for visualizing the presence of *Mycobacterium tuberculosis*. Other stains are useful for identifying the presence of protozoan parasites: *Trichomonas vaginalis* using the fluorochrome acridine orange, *Cryptosporidia* with either ZN or auramine, and amoebae with Field's stain. A nigrosin (or Indian ink) preparation can be used to demonstrate the presence of a capsule and is particularly useful in the identification of the capsulated yeast, *Cryptococcus neoformans*.

Whenever a staining method is used to demonstrate the presence of acid-fast bacilli, filtered water should be used for all rinsing steps and for making up the stain, to ensure that any environmental mycobacteria cannot contaminate the specimen.

Gram stain

The Gram stain is the most routinely used stain in microbiology laboratories because it distinguishes differences in the structure of cell walls, gives an indication of the morphology of the bacterium and gives the first clues to the identification of an unknown bacterium.

The permeability of the cell wall to the stain differs in different types of bacteria (Gram-positive cells have thicker peptidoglycan walls) and this is exploited in the Gram staining technique. The dye (usually methyl violet or crystal violet) penetrates the cell wall and is then aggregated by adding iodine (it is known as a 'mordant' when it acts in this way). The large dye aggregates are easily removed from the more permeable (because they have a thinner layer of peptidoglycan, with less cross-linking and larger pores) Gram-negative bacteria by a decolorizing agent such as alcohol or acetone, but are retained by the more impermeable Gram-positive bacteria. The difference is only in the rate of removal and so prolonged washing in acetone will decolorize all bacteria.

A smear is prepared by emulsifying a small amount of bacteria into a loopful of distilled water on a clean microscope slide. The slide is left to air dry, at which point the area to be stained should be visible; if there appears to be nothing on the slide the process must be repeated by adding more water and bacteria. This method can also be used to 'build up' samples where there are likely to be few cells, such as a CSF sample. Before staining, the slide is heat-fixed by passing it rapidly through a hot Bunsen flame. Heat-fixing kills the microorganisms, fixes them to the slide and alters them so that they take up the stain more easily. If a wet smear is passed through the flame the bacteria will boil and be destroyed.

Method

- Flood the slide with crystal violet for 30–60 seconds
- Rinse with water
- Add Gram's iodine for 30–60 seconds
- Rinse
- Decolorize with acetone, for a maximum of 10 seconds
- Rinse
- Counterstain with carbol fuchsin, safranin or neutral red for 1 minute
- Blot dry.

View on the light microscope using oil immersion and 100× objective. *Figure 5.9* shows the stepwise staining changes for Gram-positive and Gram-negative bacteria during the Gram stain.

Interpretation

Gram-positive bacteria stain purple, Gram-negative bacteria stain pink/red. Yeast cells are much larger than bacteria and stain Gram-positive. Older bacterial cultures sometimes give a Gram variable result because the cell walls are ageing. Gram-positive bacteria may appear negative if the slides have been over-decolorized.

Ziehl–Neelsen stain

Whereas auramine–phenol staining is more sensitive and therefore preferable for demonstrating the presence of mycobacteria (acid-fast bacilli, AFB) directly from clinical specimens, the original ZN stain (hot carbol fuchsin) is used for confirming the presence of mycobacteria in positive cultures. All cultures and specimens suspected of containing *Mycobacterium* species must be processed in a Class 1 cabinet in a containment level 3 room and appropriate personal protective equipment must

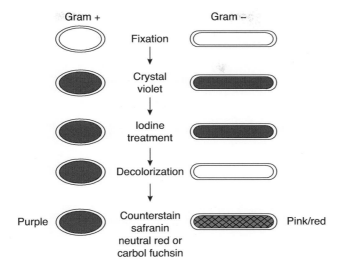

Figure 5.9
Changes during the stages of a Gram stain, showing the difference between Gram-positive and Gram-negative cells. Gram-positive cells contain more peptidoglycan and retain the crystal violet/iodine aggregates.

be worn. A smear of the culture is prepared on a glass slide and dried on a hotplate at 65–75°C inside the cabinet before being placed in a rack for staining. The heat fixing does not kill the bacteria and so care must be used when handling the slides.

Method
- Flood with strong carbol fuchsin
- Heat gently until the slide is steaming and then leave for 3–5 minutes
- Rinse with water
- Decolorize with 3% acid–alcohol solution for 2–3 minutes, rinse with water and then add more acid–alcohol for 3–4 minutes; the slide should then remain a faint pink colour
- Rinse with water
- Counterstain with malachite green for 30 seconds
- Rinse with water and leave to dry.

View the slide using oil immersion at 100×. A positive control slide must be included with each batch.

Interpretation
The acid-fast bacilli stain red and vary from 0.5 to 1 μm in length and some may appear beaded. All other organisms and the background material stain green.

Modified cold Ziehl–Neelsen stain

The cold ZN technique, using Kinyoun's acid-fast stain (3% carbol fuchsin), can be used for confirming the presence of mycobacteria and is often the chosen method for demonstrating the presence of *Cryptosporidium* species in faecal smears. However, many laboratories prefer to use a modified auramine–phenol stain for *Cryptosporidium* species and for the investigation of clinical samples for the presence of mycobacteria. If the auramine–phenol method is used for confirming the presence of mycobacteria, the slide is prepared and heat-fixed, as described in the ZN method above.

Method
- Prepare a medium to thick smear of the faecal sample and air dry
- Fix in methanol for 3 minutes and air dry
- Flood the slide with modified Kinyoun's acid-fast stain and leave for approximately 15 minutes
- Rinse with tap water
- Decolorize with 1% acid methanol for 15–20 seconds
- Rinse with tap water
- Counterstain with 0.4% malachite green for 30 seconds
- Rinse with tap water and air dry.

The slide is then examined using the light microscope and a high power objective. A positive control slide of either mycobacteria or *Cryptosporidium* oocysts must be included in each batch of specimens to demonstrate that the method is working properly.

Interpretation
Cryptosporidium oocysts are 4–6 μm in diameter, spherical, and stain pinkish red. Some of the oocysts may appear unstained. If the purpose of the stain is to demonstrate the presence of *Mycobacteria* species, these will appear as short pink–red rods.

Auramine–phenol stain

Auramine–phenol is a fluorescent stain and requires the use of a fluorescence microscope to examine the slides. If the method is used to detect the presence of *Cryptosporidium* species, a smear is made from the faecal sample and left to air dry and then fixed in methanol for 3 minutes. If the method is used for investigating the presence of mycobacteria, the slide is prepared and heat-fixed as for the ZN method. Stained slides should not be blotted, as some blotting materials themselves may fluoresce.

Method
- Flood the slides with auramine–phenol for 10 minutes
- Gently rinse with tap water (filtered water for acid-fast bacteria)
- Decolorize with 1% acid alcohol for 3–5 minutes
- Rinse gently with water
- Repeat decolorization step until no stain is seen seeping from the smear
- Counterstain with 0.1% potassium permanganate (or thiazine red for acid-fast bacteria) for 15 seconds
- Rinse gently with water and air dry; do not blot.

A positive control slide is included in every batch. After staining, the slides are kept out of the light before examination. The slides are examined using UV epi-fluorescent microscopy at 25× or 40× and scanned thoroughly.

Interpretation

Acid-fast bacilli stain bright yellow–green against a dark background. Oocysts of *Cryptosporidium* species stain as bright yellow–green spheres.

Acridine orange stain

Acridine orange stain is a fluorescent stain used for the demonstration of *Trichomonas vaginalis* in smears made from vaginal swabs and left to air dry. The stains are kept in containers and added to staining baths, kept specifically for that purpose, immediately prior to use. Batches of slides can be placed in staining baskets and dipped into containers of the stains and alcoholic saline for the appropriate times.

Method

- Stain the slides in acridine orange for 5–10 seconds
- Rinse off the stain and then decolorize in alcoholic saline for 5–10 seconds
- Rinse with physiological saline
- Allow slides to dry
- Add a drop of water or saline to the slides and apply a coverslip.

A positive control must be included in every batch. Keep out of natural light before viewing on a fluorescence microscope.

Interpretation

Trophozoites of *Trichomonas vaginalis* stain brick red with a green/yellow banana-shaped nucleus. The average dimensions of the trophozoites are 7–10 μm. Yeasts can also be identified and stain red, epithelial cells fluoresce light green and pus cells (white cells) have bright green nuclei.

Calcofluor stain

Calcofluor is a fluorescent stain which can be used for the identification of microsporidia in faecal specimens, and is also commonly used to stain fungal elements from clinical samples prior to culture. The stain binds to chitin, found in the endospore layer of microsporidia, as well as to polysaccharides, chitin and cellulose in fungal cell walls, and is used at a concentration of 0.5% w/v.

For faecal specimens a thin smear is prepared, air dried and fixed in methanol for 5 minutes prior to the staining method described. For small amounts of any specimen of hair, skin or nail, these are placed on a slide for examination and, as the specimen is not fixed to the slide, a modified staining process is employed where the calcofluor stain is added to the sample and a coverslip applied, rather than adding the coverslip after staining, and no counterstain is used. The slide is then left away from natural light for about 30 minutes before viewing under the fluorescence microscope.

Method

- Stain with one to two drops of calcofluor solution for 2–3 minutes
- Rinse with slow running water
- Counterstain with 0.1% Evans blue solution for 1 minute
- Rinse under slow running water

■ Air dry
■ Add one to two drops of mounting fluid and apply coverslip
■ Examine under fluorescence microscope.

Interpretation

A positive control must be included in each batch of slides stained. Microsporidia fluoresce brilliant blue–white, are ovoid and 1–20 μm in size. Fungal hyphae stain brilliant blue.

Rapid Field's stain and Giemsa's stain

Both the rapid Field's stain and Giemsa's stain may be used in conjunction with the light microscope to demonstrate the presence of *Dientamoeba fragilis* and *Blastocystis hominis* in faeces. For both stains a smear is prepared, air dried and fixed in methanol for 60 seconds.

Method for Field's stain

■ Flood the slide with Field's stain B (diluted 1 in 4 with buffered water at pH 6.8)
■ Add an equal volume of undiluted Field's stain A
■ Mix and leave for 60 seconds
■ Rinse with tap water, drain and air dry.

Method for Giemsa's stain

The stain should be freshly prepared as a 1 in 10 solution in buffered water.

■ Flood the slide with diluted Giemsa's stain and leave for 20–25 minutes
■ Run under tap water to float off the stain and prevent precipitation
■ Air dry.

Interpretation

Parasite nuclei and chromatin stain red with both stains; bacteria and yeasts stain dark blue. A positive control must be included in each batch.

Nigrosin or Indian ink staining to demonstrate capsules

Nigrosin, an acidic dye, and Indian ink are negative staining techniques, i.e. they stain the background rather than the organisms. If an organism is encapsulated, the capsule material displaces the dye and forms a halo around the cell. The method is used to demonstrate the presence of the capsulated yeast *Cryptococcus neoformans* in clinical specimens.

Method

■ Place a drop of nigrosin or Indian ink on to the surface of a slide
■ Add either a drop of liquid culture, or mix in a small amount of the specimen to the ink
■ Apply a coverslip, press down with blotting paper and examine under the light microscope.

Interpretation
Capsulated organisms appear refractile and surrounded by a clear zone against the dark background.

The Schaeffer–Fulton stain for endospores

The spores of Gram-positive bacilli can be visualized by staining with malachite green. A smear of the specimen is prepared and gently heat-fixed. The slide needs to be steamed during the application of malachite green; this can be achieved most simply by placing the slide over a beaker of boiling water. Heating the slide allows the stain to enter the endospores.

Method
- Flood the slide with malachite green; stain for 5 minutes
- Rinse under tap water
- Counterstain with either safranin or basic fuchsin for 30 seconds
- Rinse and dry.

Interpretation
Bacterial spores stain green and bacterial cells stain red.

SUGGESTED FURTHER READING

Goldstein, D. (1998) Inverted microscopes.
    www.microscopy-uk.org.uk/mag/artjul98/invert.html
Smithwick, R.W., Bigbie, M.R., Ferguson, R.B., Karlix, M.A. & Wallis, C.K. (1995) Phenolic acridine orange fluorescent stain for Mycobacteria. *J. Clin. Microbiol.* **33**: 2763–2764.
www.microscopy-analysis.com is a useful website for the latest copy of their journal and innovations in microscopy.

SELF-ASSESSMENT QUESTIONS

1. Which two major innovations improved microscopy techniques in the late nineteenth century?
2. How is the total magnification of a light microscope calculated?
3. What is the maximum resolution of the light microscope and the magnification achieved by the electron microscope?
4. Describe the use of the inverted light microscope in urine microscopy. Which kinds of cells would you expect to see in an infected urine sample?
5. Why is it important to use a graticule for the accurate diagnosis of faecal parasites?
6. Outline four situations where the light microscope is an invaluable tool in the microbiology laboratory.
7. Name two infectious processes where darkground microscopy can help to visualize the infectious bacteria.

8. Name three fluorochromes used in fluorescent microscopy. Distinguish between direct and indirect tests for identifying the presence of antigens and antibodies in clinical specimens.

9. What are the advantages of using electron microscopy and scanning electron microscopy rather than light microscopy?

10. Outline the principal steps in the Gram stain. Why is the timing of the decolorization step so important?

Answers to self-assessment questions provided at:
www.scionpublishing.com/medmicro

CHAPTER
6
General techniques for identifying bacteria from clinical specimens

Learning objectives
After studying this chapter you should confidently be able to:

■ **Explain the need for aseptic technique**
Aseptic technique is necessary when working with microorganisms for two reasons: to prevent contamination of cultures by bacteria and fungi in the environment, and to prevent contamination of the environment and people handling them by the cultures themselves.

■ **Describe the method of spreading bacteria on culture plates to obtain single colonies**
It is important to obtain single colonies, particularly from a mixed culture, in order to be able to perform identification tests on any bacteria of interest. A loopful of liquid culture, or an inoculum from a swab obtained from a patient, is first placed on the culture plate. A sterile loop is then used to spread the initial inoculum at an angle across the plate, which is then rotated and the process of spreading from the second streak repeated until the circumference of the plate has almost been completed, at which point the specimen is spread in a zigzag into the centre. In this way, the initial inoculum is progressively reduced in number and single colonies should be visible after incubation.

■ **Discuss the methods available for enumerating bacteria**
This can be achieved by the following methods: semi-quantitative plate counts; assessing the area of the plate covered with bacterial growth; turbidity of a liquid culture compared with a reference concentration; from liquid cultures by serial dilution of the sample and counting the number of bacteria at each dilution; spread plates to assess the quantity of bacteria growing in a known volume of, for example, environmental water sample; counting chambers where bacteria are counted within a set number of squares and the volume per millilitre calculated; and growth curves using a spectrophotometer to measure turbidity (related to increasing numbers of bacteria) over a period of time.

■ **Discuss the non-molecular methods used for identification of the major groups of Gram-positive and Gram-negative bacteria**
The starting point for identification of unknown bacteria is the Gram stain, which will give vital information on the Gram stain reaction, positive or negative, and the morphology of the bacteria. Further identification tests to indicate the presence of enzymes and specific biochemical reactions can then be performed. More definitive identification can be achieved by the use of commercial identification systems. Staphylococci can be differentiated from streptococci by the catalase test, where a colony of bacteria is added to a drop of hydrogen peroxide. Catalase-positive bacteria such as staphylococci will break down the hydrogen peroxide and bubbles of oxygen will be given off.

■ **Discuss the methods used to determine antimicrobial susceptibility**
The principal methods for detecting the minimum inhibitory concentration (MIC) *in vitro* from clinical isolates are the broth dilution test, the E test and the agar dilution method. The disc diffusion test measures the MIC indirectly by the use of regression lines and relating the size of the zone to MICs. The results are expressed as sensitive, resistant or intermediate. The minimum bactericidal concentration (MBC) is measured by subculture from the MIC broth dilutions or by time-kill curves.

■ **Describe target sites for antimicrobial activity**
Antimicrobial agents inhibit bacterial cell wall synthesis, protein synthesis, dihydrofolate synthesis, nucleic acid and cell membranes.

■ **Discuss the range of antigen–antibody based identification tests**
Antigen–antibody based tests range from simple agglutination tests using red cells or coated latex particles, to the complement fixation test and the monoclonal antibody based tests (such as ELISAs), both manual and automated.

■ **Describe the principles and applications of molecular methods**
Knowledge of the genomic structure of a range of microorganisms and the ability to develop short primers of these sequences, have enabled the development of amplification methods principally based on the polymerase chain reaction (PCR). Real-time PCR using a range of probe technologies has increased the speed and accuracy of detection of a range of pathogens.

■ **Explain the importance of the advent of matrix-assisted laser desorption time-of-flight mass spectrometry, MALDI-TOF-MS, to the identification of clinically important bacteria**
This recent advance in mass spectrometry enables rapid, accurate identification within a short time span. The technique uses laser technology and a matrix solvent to break open cells and ionize them before they migrate according to their mass to charge ratio, creating a unique mass spectral profile for identification. However, the technology can still be expensive for routine use.

6.1   ASEPTIC TECHNIQUE

Infectious disease can be diagnosed by demonstrating the presence of pathogenic microorganisms in a wide range of specimens taken from anywhere in or on the human body. They may be obtained by swabbing an infected area, or from samples of sputum, faeces, urine or blood. If the results of the investigation are to be reliable, the specimen tested in the laboratory must represent as closely as possible the microorganisms present at that site, without contamination from other sources. The use of aseptic technique ensures that the cultures obtained from the patient specimen, the person working with them, and the environment are not contaminated.

Microorganisms are by their very nature invisible to the naked eye, although the macroscopic appearance of the specimen itself may be suggestive of infection, for example, a cloudy CSF, a purulent sputum, a specimen of pus or a liquid stool specimen. If the specimen is spread on to a culture medium containing all the growth requirements for a range of bacteria or fungi, each cell will multiply at a steady rate until they have formed a colony that is visible to the naked eye. The culture plates are incubated at an optimum temperature for cell growth, usually 37°C for 12–18 hours. The atmosphere in which they are incubated is also important and may be aerobic (in air, or air plus carbon dioxide), anaerobic (either in anaerobic jars or a specialized cabinet) or micro-aerophilic. The atmospheres chosen will depend upon the pathogens likely to be present in the specimens being investigated. The culture medium used, whether solid agar or liquid broth, will be sterile and it is important to maintain this sterility during the time it is being inoculated with the patient's sample and during incubation.

Aseptic technique prevents contamination of sterile culture media and bacterial cultures during inoculation and subsequent manipulations. It is also important to ensure that the person carrying out the procedures is protected from contamination from both the initial patient sample and subsequent cultures obtained from them. Cross-contamination from specimens and from liquid culture must also be avoided (see also *Chapter 7*).

Contaminating bacteria and fungal spores are present in the air and on work surfaces. Their presence in the environment can easily be demonstrated by leaving an open Petri dish containing agar on a work surface for a few hours. A variety of airborne bacteria will settle on the surface of the culture medium and after incubation there will be numerous colonies of bacterial and fungal growth.

Aseptic technique is one of the earliest techniques that needs be practised in the microbiology laboratory, whether in the workplace or classroom. If a pure culture of bacteria is inoculated on to culture media, any contamination will be clearly visible after the culture plates have been incubated and the contaminating bacteria have grown along with the initial inoculum.

The first step is to sterilize the metal loop in a hot (blue) Bunsen flame. Always hold the loop almost vertical to the flame; in this way any liquid on the loop will run down into the flame and be sterilized, rather than running back along the handle. Keep the loop in the flame until it is red-hot and then remove it. Allow it to cool slightly before use. If the loop is too hot when it is placed into a liquid culture there is the possibility that aerosols could be formed. If the loop is used to spread a sample on a culture medium when red-hot it is likely that the heat will kill the bacteria. Sterile disposable plastic loops are often routinely used for this purpose, dispensing with the need for sterilization. Keep the bottle of liquid culture upright in a wire rack when it is not being used and make sure the lid is securely in place.

If a liquid culture of bacteria is being used, then it is important to keep the bottle and the contents free from contamination while the loop is used to take out a sample. This is achieved by holding the handle of the sterile loop between the thumb and forefinger of the right hand, and then removing the lid of the bottle or tube with the fourth and fifth fingers. The mouth of the open bottle or tube may be held in the left hand and sterilized in the flame if it is made of glass. After the loopful of culture has been removed, the lid can be replaced and tightened and the bottle replaced in the wire rack. If a sterile plastic loop is used instead of a metal one, it is still important to prevent contamination when the sample is removed from the bottle. When a culture plate is inoculated with a sterile loop, the lid of the Petri dish should be removed for as short a time as possible to prevent airborne bacteria settling on the surface of the medium. Re-sterilize a wire loop or dispose of a plastic one in the appropriate waste container.

6.2   SINGLE COLONIES

The growth of single colonies on a culture plate is essential if further identification is to be carried out. The bacteria causing infection in a particular patient sample may be mixed with normal flora from that site. If the site is normally sterile, for example a swab from a gall bladder, any bacterial growth will be significant, provided that aseptic technique has been used and that the swab did not touch areas containing normal flora during the process of specimen collection. All bacteria present in the sample are inoculated on to the culture medium and have the opportunity to grow and produce visible colonies. The resulting culture plate will therefore give an idea of the numbers of bacteria present in the sample and also of the different types. If all the bacteria or fungi were of the same type there would be a pure growth of similar colonies, whereas if a mixture was present at the original site, different sizes, textures and shapes of colonies are seen.

Identification is achieved by performing further tests on the isolated single colonies of interest and this is much easier to achieve if the colonies are well separated on the spread plate. Spreading a culture plate to achieve single colonies is again a technique that requires practice.

How to obtain single colonies

If the patient specimen is a swab, this is gently applied to the plate surface and rotated so that all surfaces of the swab are represented. If the specimen is fluid, a sterile swab is dipped into the sample and applied to the plate. The culture plate is held in the left hand and inoculated with the swab in the right hand. Further spreading is achieved by using either a sterile disposable plastic loop or a flamed metal one. This is touched on the initial inoculum and spread across the plate, returned to the inoculum and spread again. The plate is then rotated and the second streak spread further as before, followed by rotation and the third streak. Finally the loop is zigzagged into the centre of the plate (see *Figure 6.1*).

It is very tempting, because there is nothing to be seen on the surface of the plate, to return to the previous streak too many times. Experience will show that this is unnecessary.

Initial inoculum

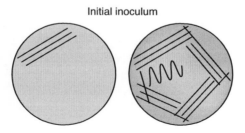

Figure 6.1
The inoculation of a culture plate from a liquid culture. If a swab is used, this is rolled on to the plate at the starting point in order to release as many bacteria as possible. The plate is rotated slightly and new streaks taken from the initial inoculum, ensuring that the loop does not go back in to this more than once or twice. The plate is rotated and spread in this fashion finishing with a zigzag spread into the centre of the culture medium.

6.3   ENUMERATING BACTERIA

There are several ways of counting the number of bacteria in a sample and the method chosen will be dependent on the type of sample and the relevance to the investigation.

Semi-quantitative plate counts

In clinical samples cultured on selective or non-selective culture media, the growth is often recorded in a semi-quantitative form, i.e. 3+, 2+, 1+ and scanty, or heavy, medium and light growth. This is based on how much of the areas streaked on to the plate are covered with bacteria and their density, which of course is related to the quality of the specimen and how much of the original sample was introduced to the culture plate. The purity of growth, the identification of the colonies and the presence of significant pathogens are of greater importance.

Comparison to a set of turbidity standards

For some identification tests (the API strips, described later in this chapter, are a good example of this) a certain density of bacterial suspension is required and this is often referred to as a number on the McFarland scale. The density of the bacteria, observed as the turbidity of the suspension, is related to the number of bacteria present. These standards are supplied commercially and provide a range of concentrations for comparison with working suspensions.

A suspension is prepared by emulsifying bacteria into a diluent, which may be distilled water or a specific buffer, and this suspension is then visually compared with the standard. As with any of these manipulations, care must be taken to prevent the aerosols that will form when loops that are too hot are introduced into the liquid. The droplets of liquid sprayed into the air contain bacteria that could be inhaled by the person carrying out the procedure.

Counting bacteria from liquid cultures

When bacteria are grown in liquid broth there are no colonies to observe for purity and viability. It may be important to know the concentration of cells in the culture, for example if a specific concentration is required for further investigations such as pulsed-field gel electrophoresis (PFGE, a molecular technique used to separate strains of bacteria). The concentration of cells in the suspension may be determined by:

- serial dilution and growing on culture media
- the viable count method, either spread or pour plate
- measuring growth by a turbidometric method such as using a spectrophotometer
- directly counting the bacteria in a counting chamber.

The first two methods also provide a method of checking the purity of the culture.

Serial dilution technique

A series of tenfold dilutions of the sample are prepared using either distilled water, a balanced salt solution or nutrient broth as diluent. The method can be used simply to find out the cell count of the original culture or to demonstrate growth characteristics of bacteria on different culture media formulations. A known volume of each dilution is then added to a whole plate (typically 1 ml), or to a segment of a culture plate (typically 25 µl per segment of a well-dried plate is the maximum volume, to avoid mixing of dilutions). The latter approach is called the Miles and Misra method. After incubation the whole plates, or segments, are observed and counts performed on areas where the colonies are separate and it is possible to count them. The number of colony-forming units (CFU) per ml (the viable count/ml) is calculated as follows:

$$\text{number of colonies counted} \times \frac{1}{\text{vol}} \times \text{dilution} = \text{CFU/ml}$$

Ideally the viable count should be exactly the same in all the calculations, but in practice this is seldom the case because there is a reduction in the level of accuracy, particularly where the number of colonies is small and the multiplication factor is large. It is worth noting that the concentration will be expressed as a negative number, e.g. 1×10^{-3}. The tubes used for the dilutions and the segments of the culture plate are labelled with the concentration. This records that the original bacterial suspension has been diluted a thousand times in that tube and then 25 µl of that concentration has been placed on the segment of the agar plate (the concentration is 1 in 1000), and this is expressed as 1×10^{-3}. The dilution factor, however, represents how many times the bacteria have been diluted, i.e. 1000 or 10^3 times, and to calculate the number in 1 ml it is therefore necessary to multiply by 1000. *Figure 6.2* shows a representative Miles and Misra plate with the calculation of the viable count.

Viable count by spread and pour plate methods

A viable cell will be able to grow on a suitable culture medium and produce visible colonies. After 18–24 hours of incubation each colony represents a clone of approximately 10^6 cells. This method is useful for enumerating bacteria in water samples from environmental sources or from food samples. A known volume is added to the surface of a culture plate and spread evenly across the surface, often

Dilutions

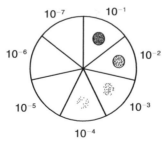

10^{-7} 10^{-1}

10^{-6} 10^{-2}

10^{-5} 10^{-3}

10^{-4}

Figure 6.2
The Miles and Misra method of dilutions and subculture to enable a colony count to be assessed using 25 µl volumes.

Calculation

Colony count $\times \dfrac{1}{\text{volume}} \times$ dilution

$5 \times \dfrac{1}{0.025} \times 10^4$

$= 200 \times 10^4$

$= 2.0 \times 10^6$

using a glass spreader or a commercial spiral plater. If the sample is in a larger volume of water, then this can be filtered through a vacuum pump on to a membrane, which is then placed on the surface of specific culture media. After incubation, the number and different genera of bacteria may be recorded. This technique is useful for detecting *Legionella* species in water supplies.

In the pour plate method a known volume of the sample is pipetted into a sterile Petri dish and then molten agar added. With thorough mixing, the sample will be spread throughout the agar and, after incubation, bacteria growing within it may be counted. Larger volumes of liquid can be tested by this method, but the bacteria present must be able to withstand the temperature of the molten agar, i.e. 45°C.

See *Chapter 14* for other examples of environmental microbiology techniques.

Counting chambers

Counting chambers (see *Figure 6.3*) are used in other areas of biomedical science, and the principles are the same whether counting red cells in dilution, bacteria, or neutrophils and lymphocytes in a sample of CSF. The counting chamber has grid lines marked on the surface of the glass, to provide squares of a known area. A coverslip is applied to the top of the chamber, after slightly moistening the sides, to provide a known volume for counting. The coverslip is applied carefully and firmly by hand until Newton's rings are seen at the sides away from the grid area. Newton's rings are rainbow colours in the liquid, rather similar to those observed in petrol films on water, and are formed when the distance between the chamber and the coverslip is sufficiently narrow to split the light and indicate the correct depth of liquid to be counted. The cell suspension is then mixed thoroughly and applied to the chamber, usually by means of a capillary tube, taking care not to overfill the area. After the contents have settled the count can be performed using the 10× or 40× objective on the light microscope.

There are 16 small squares in each of the five large squares counted, giving a total of 80 squares. The number of cells per mm³ is calculated from the area of the 80 squares counted × the depth of counting chamber. Each set of 16 squares has an area of 1 mm². Multiplied by 5 (the number of sets of 16 squares), this gives an area counted of 5 mm². The depth of the counting chamber is 0.2 mm, which when multiplied by the area gives a volume of 1 mm³. Thus counting the number of cells in 5 large squares gives the count in 1 mm³.

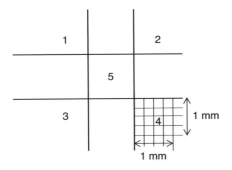

Figure 6.3
A modified Fuchs–Rosenthal counting chamber, showing the detail and position of the squares chosen for counting to provide a representative result.

There are some drawbacks to this method: dead cells cannot be distinguished from viable ones and it is not possible to check the purity of the culture. It is useful, however, if a particular concentration of an overnight culture is needed in the preparation for plugs used in pulsed field gel electrophoresis (PFGE), for example, or for inoculating liquid culture media for growth curve experiments.

Growth curves

Growth curves are conducted as practical demonstrations of differing culture conditions, for example aerobic versus anaerobic, or if it is necessary for research purposes to harvest cells in the exponential, stationary or death phases. Spectrophotometry provides a convenient means of measuring cell density for use in growth curves. Cells growing in suspension scatter light and the greater the number of cells, the more light is scattered, giving the suspension a cloudy, turbid appearance. A spectrophotometer measures unscattered light and this is measured as optical density (OD). Incident light is generated by a prism in a narrow band of wavelengths, usually 625 nm. For single-cell organisms such as bacteria the OD is proportional to cell number and this means that the measured OD can be used as a substitute for direct counting. Plotting OD against time will enable a growth curve to be constructed for the bacteria being studied. Plotting the log value of the OD against time will show a linear relationship in the exponential phase. A typical growth curve, obtained over a time period of 2 hours and a plot of the $\log_{10}$ OD against time are shown in *Figure 6.4*.

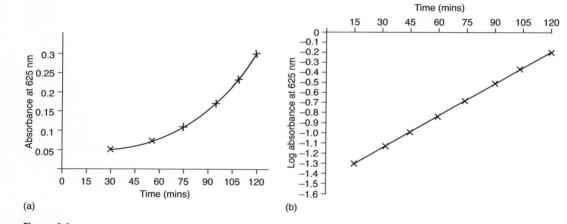

Figure 6.4

The exponential growth phase of *Escherichia coli* in nutrient broth under aerobic conditions over a 2-hour period. (a) The early stages of a typical growth curve. The bacteria were inoculated into the broth at time 0 mins and first sampled after 30 mins. (b) The $\log_{10}$ absorbance is plotted against time and demonstrates the exponential nature of the graph.

6.4   IDENTIFICATION METHODS

The Gram stain provides an excellent starting point for the identification of unknown bacteria. The Gram reaction and the morphology of the cells, e.g. Gram-positive cocci, provide the first step in a schema for identification to the genera and species level using specific tests. There are excellent resources available, such as *Bergey's Manual of Determinative Bacteriology* or *Cowan and Steel's Identification of Medically Important Bacteria*, containing comprehensive tables to aid in the identification and classification of bacteria. The schema provided here, also called dichotomous keys, and the tests described are for the most commonly isolated bacteria only. However, by following the stepwise procedure and then using an appropriate biochemical test system, such as API (analytical profile index) strips, identification to species level is possible.

Identification tests for Gram-positive cocci

The catalase test

This test distinguishes between the major genera of *Staphylococci* and *Streptococci*. Catalase is an enzyme that breaks down toxic hydrogen peroxide, produced during aerobic respiration, into oxygen and water. *Staphylococci* possess catalase, whereas *Streptococci* do not. Lack of this enzyme does not prevent *Streptococci*, classified as aerotolerant anaerobes, surviving in aerobic environments, because they possess other enzymes, superoxide dismutase and peroxidase, capable of catabolizing toxic oxygen and hydrogen peroxide.

The catalase test is simple to perform, requiring only the addition of a bacterial colony to a drop of hydrogen peroxide. If catalase is present, bubbles of oxygen will appear very quickly as the reaction to break down hydrogen peroxide takes place. Blood cells contain large amounts of catalase, and so it is important to test colonies grown on other culture media to avoid false positive tests. Again, care is needed to avoid aerosols when the bacteria are added to the hydrogen peroxide.

Identification of staphylococci

In the presumptive identification of staphylococci, catalase-positive colonies will next be tested for the presence of the enzyme coagulase, which differentiates between *Staphylococcus aureus* and the coagulase-negative staphylococci such as *S. saprophyticus*. Coagulase, or clumping factor, is a virulence factor that can be demonstrated *in vitro* by the ability of the bacteria to clot plasma (free coagulase) and more commonly by latex-coated particles that detect the presence of bound coagulase in conjunction with other virulence factors present in *S. aureus*, e.g. protein A and capsular polysaccharides. These latex agglutination tests are easy to use and give rapid results. If enterococci are mistaken for staphylococci, false positive results may be obtained. Simultaneous detection of the fibrinogen affinity factor, protein A, and capsular polysaccharides provide a more sensitive test capable of detecting the methicillin-resistant strains. The latex test kits provide everything necessary for carrying out the test, including test cards and mixing sticks. A drop of test latex reagent is added to one of the circles on the card and a drop of negative control latex to another. A colony of bacteria is emulsified into both the latex test and control areas and the card is manually rotated for half a minute. If the test is positive, visible clumping, or aggregation, is visible in the test latex area only. If the results are equivocal, it may be necessary to perform a tube coagulase test. The tube coagulase test detects free and bound coagulase. Colonies of the staphylococci are incubated with rabbit plasma at 37°C for up to 6 hours. If coagulase is present, the plasma clots.

Testing for the enzyme DNase will provide further confirmation of the presence of *Staphylococcus aureus*. The activity of DNase, a virulence factor that allows the bacteria to break down cellular DNA and facilitate spread of the organism, can be demonstrated by growing bacteria on culture plates containing DNA. Several patient samples may be stab cultured on to one agar plate. After incubation the plate is flooded with 1 M hydrochloric acid. If DNA is present in the medium it will be precipitated by the acid and the medium will be opaque. If the bacteria have expressed the enzyme DNase the substrate DNA will be broken down and a clear zone will surround the bacterial growth.

S. saprophyticus, a coagulase-negative, DNase-negative staphylococcus, may be further identified by demonstrating resistance to the antibiotic novobiocin. *Figure 6.5* shows a simplified schema for identification of staphylococci.

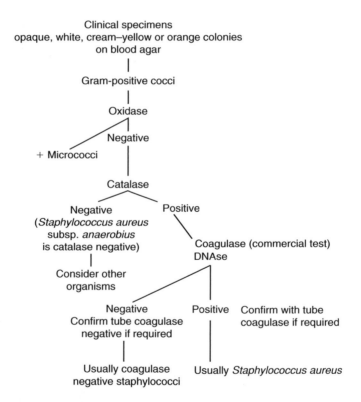

Figure 6.5
A simple schema for the identification of staphylococci from colonial isolates.

Identification of streptococci

Streptococci are initially distinguished from staphylococci by the negative catalase reaction. Two distinct patterns of haemolysis, alpha and beta, will then provide further clues to their identity. Haemolysis of blood agar is the visible effect of protein membrane-acting toxins secreted by the growing cells. Alpha haemolytic streptococcus colonies will have a green colour around the colonies, as will

Streptococcus pneumoniae, denoting some haemolysis of the red cells. *S. pneumoniae* often look like the pieces in the game of draughts, and may appear as dry and non-capsulated, or mucoid and heavily-capsulated colonies. *S. pneumoniae* can be identified by the addition of a disc containing optochin (ethylhydrocupreine hydrochloride). *S. pneumoniae* will show a clear zone of sensitivity whereas other viridans streptococci will be resistant and grow right up to the disc.

Lancefield grouping of beta-haemolytic streptococci

Beta-haemolytic streptococci are grouped (into groups A, B, C, D, F or G) by the Lancefield grouping system, developed by Rebecca Lancefield in 1928. The enterococci were formerly known as group D streptococci, even though they may not exhibit beta haemolysis. The test comes in a kit form with all the materials provided. Differentiation of the groups is based on differences in the cell wall polysaccharide, which is first extracted from the sample by incubation with an enzyme. One drop of the suspension of extracted polysaccharide is then added to latex particles coated with specific antibodies to the major groups, A, B, C, D, F and G. Agglutination of the particles should then occur only with the specific group and thus identify the streptococcal group. Cross-reactions are rare, but may occasionally be seen with groups C and G. The *Streptococcus anginosus* (formerly *S. milleri* group) contains *Streptococcus anginosus*, *S. constellatus* and *S. intermedius*. They may group as A, C, F or G, or no group at all. Many strains have a characteristic caramel odour, universally enjoyed by biomedical scientists as they open the culture plate.

Group B streptococci (*Streptococcus agalactiae*) and the enterococci may also be identified by the use of differential culture media. Group B streptococci will demonstrate characteristic orange colonies when grown on Islam's or Granada medium and incubated anaerobically. The enterococci produce black coloration in bile aesculin media after a relatively short incubation time as they cleave the aesculin to yield glucose and esculetin. Esculetin reacts with ferric ions to produce a black pigment in the medium.

Bacitracin discs are sometimes applied to throat swab plates at the time of culture. Some of the principal pathogens, group A streptococci, are sensitive to this antibiotic and this is demonstrated by a clear zone around the disc where bacterial growth is inhibited. Streptococcal identification can also be confirmed by the use of a commercial test strip such as API Strep. *Figure 6.6* shows a simplified schema for the identification of streptococci.

Identification of Gram-positive rods

The Gram stain reaction, growth conditions, clinical details and the site of infection give valuable clues in the identification of Gram-positive rods. Bacteria growing aerobically without the presence of spores from a blood culture or from an amniotic fluid sample could indicate the presence of *Listeria monocytogenes*. This can be confirmed by a positive catalase test, a positive aesculin reaction and biochemical tests such as with an API strip.

Strictly anaerobic Gram-positive bacilli containing spores, with clinical details suggestive of the disease, could be *Clostridia* species, whereas aerobic spore-bearing Gram-positive bacilli are more likely to be of the genus *Bacillus,* which includes environmental bacteria and the highly pathogenic *B. anthracis.*

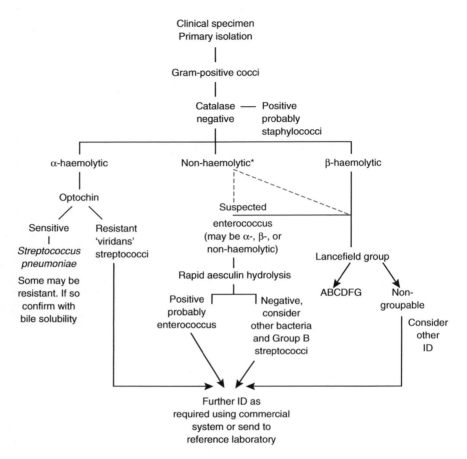

Figure 6.6
A simple schema for the identification of streptococci from colonial isolates. Groups A, C and G will not grow on media containing bile, whereas Group B, the enterococci and the *Streptococcus anginosus (Miller)* groups will. *S. anginosus* group can be F, A, C or G on the Lancefield system. *Non-haemolytic may be Group B enterococcus, *Streptococcus milleri* (ACFG)

Identification tests for Gram-negative bacteria

The tests performed to identify Gram-negative bacteria in a clinical laboratory will, to some extent, be dependent on the specimen type and the culture medium used. For example, a Gram stain is a very useful starting point for the identification of bacteria from a CSF, sputum or wound sample, or a possible campylobacter or *Vibrio* species from a faecal sample. However, it is not of much value for a suspect colony growing on selective media for faecal pathogens such as *Salmonella* species and *Shigella* species where most of the cultured bacteria are likely to be Gram-negative bacilli.

Oxidase test
Oxidase-positive bacteria have cytochrome c (part of the electron transport chain) in their cytoplasmic membrane, and this is able to convert the colourless agent tetramethyl phenylenediamine dihydrochloride to a blue/purple coloured product. Determining

whether bacteria are oxidase-positive or -negative differentiates several large groups of bacteria and is a useful first stage test for the identification of Gram-negative rods, cocci, coccobacilli and curved Gram-negative bacteria. Enterobacteriaceae are oxidase-negative, whereas *Pseudomonas* species, *Neisseria* species, *Haemophilus* species, *Campylobacter* species and *Vibrio* species are positive. *Acinetobacter* species are oxidase-negative and *Moraxella* species are oxidase-positive.

The oxidase test is very simple to perform. Blotting paper is soaked with oxidase reagent, which is an aqueous solution of tetramethyl phenylenediamine dihydrochloride; the suspect colony is picked up and smeared on to the blotting paper. In a positive reaction, the colour develops in less than a minute. Commercial strips or sticks containing oxidase reagent are also available.

Identification of Gram-negative cocci and coccobacilli

Neisseria *species.* Gram-negative diplococci growing on chocolate agar or special media to isolate *N. gonorrhoeae* are strongly suggestive of *N. meningitidis* in a specimen of CSF, but could equally be *N. gonorrhoeae* from a genital or throat swab. Following the Gram stain, the colonies are tested with oxidase reagent; if they are *Neisseria* species they will be oxidase positive. Further diagnostic tests, such as a Gonochek or API NH will give a definitive answer. *N. meningitidis* and *N. gonorrhoeae* are distinguishable by their sugar reactions:

- meningococci ferment maltose and glucose, but
- gonococci ferment glucose only.

Reactions to these sugars can be demonstrated in the API NH strip. The Gonochek method differentiates bacteria of the genus *Neisseria* on the basis of three chromogenic substrates contained in a single tube with paired stoppers (a translucent stopper normally inserted into the tube first and a red stopper on top of that). Four drops of PBS (phosphate buffered saline) are added to the tube and 5–10 colonies of the confirmed oxidase-positive isolates are added. The tube is incubated at 37°C for 30 minutes. If the bacterial suspension is blue or yellow, the bacteria are identified as *N. lactamica* and *N. meningitidis*, respectively. If there is no colour change, both the red and the translucent stoppers are removed and the tube is recapped with just the red stopper. The tube is inverted to bring the diazo-dye coupler reagent contained in the red stopper into contact with the liquid – if this immediately produces a pink/red product it indicates the presence of *N. gonorrhoeae* (see *Table 6.1*).

Haemophilus *species.* *H. influenzae* are Gram-negative, oxidase-positive coccobacilli that grow well on chocolate agar and less well on blood agar because they require both haemin (factor X) and NAD (factor V in the serum) to be available. Heating the blood in the preparation of chocolate agar releases both X and V factors. Confirmation of the presence of *Haemophilus* species, and differentiation between *H. influenzae* and *H. parainfluenzae*, are achieved by the X and V test. The bacteria are spread on to a basic culture medium, such as nutrient agar, that lacks both haemin and NAD. Paper discs containing factors X, V and XV are placed on the bacterial lawn prior to incubation. If *H. influenzae* are present, there will only be bacterial growth around the XV disc, whereas *H. parainfluenzae* will grow around the XV and V discs.

Moraxella *species.* *Moraxella* (previously *Neisseria* then *Branhamella*) *catarrhalis* is a normal resident of the upper respiratory tract and may also be isolated as the causative

Table 6.1 Differentiation of *Neisseria* species by the Gonochek method

Chromogenic substrate	Enzyme activity	Colour of product	Result
5-bromo-4-chloro-indoyl-β-D-galactopyranoside	Hydrolysis of the β-D-galactoside bond by β-galactosidase	Blue	*N. lactamica*
γ-glutamyl-*p*-nitroanilide	Hydrolysis by γ-glutamyl aminopeptidase	Yellow *p*-nitroaniline	*N. meningitidis*
β-naphthyl amino acid derivative	Hydrolysis by hydroxyprolyl aminopeptidase	Colourless free naphthylamine derivative, complexing with a diazo dye coupler in the red stopper gives a pink colour	*N. gonorrhoeae*

organism in respiratory tract infections. The bacteria are Gram-negative cocci and grow on blood and chocolate agar. They are catalase- and oxidase-positive and can be distinguished from *Neisseria* species using the API NH fatty acid hydrolysis test. *Moraxella* species are butyrate esterase positive and penicillin-sensitive, but isolates should be tested for β-lactamase activity.

Acinetobacter species. *Acinetobacter baumannii* is the most likely species to be isolated in the clinical laboratory and will be seen on a Gram stain as Gram-negative cocci or coccobacilli. They can be distinguished from other Gram-negative cocci or coccobacilli bacteria mentioned above, particularly *Moraxella* species, by the fact that although they are catalase-positive, they are oxidase-negative and resistant to penicillin.

The Enterobacteriaceae. Bacteria from this large family of Gram-negative bacilli are found in a variety of clinical specimens, either as part of the normal flora or as significant pathogens. The family contains the enteric pathogens salmonella and shigella, in addition to the enteropathogenic, enterotoxigenic, enteroaggregative and enterohaemorrhagic strains of *Escherichia coli*, responsible for diarrhoea and haemolytic uraemic syndrome. *E. coli* is also a frequent cause of urinary tract infection.

The Enterobacteriaceae are oxidase-negative, which provides a starting point for differentiation from the oxidase-positive genera of, for example, *Pseudomonas* species.

Lactose fermentation
The genera comprising the Enterobacteriaceae are also distinguished by their ability to ferment lactose. *Escherichia coli, Klebsiella* species and *Enterobacter* species ferment lactose and produce acid, whereas *Proteus* species and the enteric pathogens *Salmonella* species and *Shigella* species are non-lactose fermenters.

Lactose fermentation is easily demonstrated by culturing the bacteria on a medium containing lactose and an appropriate pH indicator such as phenol red or Andrade's. When the lactose is fermented, an acid product is formed and the pH change is demonstrated by a change in the colour of the colonies; red if phenol red and yellow if Andrade's is used. Lactose fermentation requires the presence of two enzymes, lactose permease and β-galactosidase. Some bacteria appear to be non-lactose fermenters because they lack the permease enzyme and the reaction is delayed. The ONPG test uses an artificial substrate, *o*-nitrophenyl-β-D-galactopyranoside, to detect the presence of β-galactosidase. ONPG is a colourless compound that is converted to yellow *o*-nitrophenol in the presence of β-galactosidase activity. The reaction can be demonstrated by incubating a bacterial isolate in a small amount of the ONPG substrate and observing any colour change; however, the test is usually incorporated into an identification system such as API strips or the Vitek system. *Shigella sonnei* can be distinguished from other members of the genus by a positive ONPG reaction.

The indole reaction

Bacteria possessing the enzyme tryptophanase are able to break down the amino acid tryptophan to form indole, pyruvic acid and ammonia.

Escherichia coli is indole-positive and *Enterobacter* and *Klebsiella* species indole-negative. The non-lactose fermenting *Proteus vulgaris* is also indole-positive, whereas the more frequently isolated *Proteus mirabilis* is negative. A few drops of bacterial suspension are added to peptone water containing the substrate tryptophan and, after overnight incubation, the presence of indole is visualized by the addition of Kovac's reagent to the surface of the liquid, without mixing or shaking. If indole is present, a red ring is formed around the surface of the liquid as a result of the reaction of the *p*-dimethylaminobenzaldehyde in Kovac's reagent with the indole. 'Spot' indole tests can also be performed by adding a small amount of the culture to a spot of Kovac's reagent on a piece of filter paper and observing a pink colour if the reaction is positive.

Urease activity

When non-lactose fermenters are isolated from faecal samples, the urease test is important to distinguish between the pathogenic genera of *Salmonella* and *Shigella* (urease-negative) and the non-pathogenic *Proteus* species (urease-positive). Suspect colonies are stab cultured into a culture medium containing urea and incubated for up to 4 hours. When urease is present the urea is split and the resulting pH change brought about by the creation of ammonia is demonstrated by the addition of phenol red indicator, which turns red.

The Voges–Proskauer reaction

The Voges–Proskauer (VP) test distinguishes bacteria within the enteric group on the basis of their pattern of glucose metabolism. Most enteric bacteria produce acidic products from pyruvic acid, whereas some produce neutral end products such as acetoin. The VP test identifies the acetoin producers, notably *Klebsiella pneumonia*, *Serratia marcescens* and *Enterobacter aerogenes* and so differentiates them from non-acetoin producers such as *Escherichia coli*. The reagent contains α-naphthol and potassium hydroxide which reacts with any acetoin present to produce a red colour.

glucose → pyruvic acid → acetoin → + α-naphthol + KOH → red colour

The VP test is usually incorporated into a strip identification system instead of being carried out separately.

Citrate utilization

The inorganic molecule citrate can be utilized by bacteria possessing the enzyme citrase. The enzymic activity is demonstrated by the use of culture medium containing citrate and a pH indicator, bromothymol blue. The enzymic activity produces an alkaline end product, detected by a change in the colour of the medium from green to blue. *Salmonella* species and *Enterobacter* species are citrate-positive, whereas *Escherichia coli* and *Shigella* species are negative.

Further biochemical tests

Depending on the type of specimen, simple identification tests including lactose fermentation, indole, and the exclusion of *Salmonella* and *Shigella* may be sufficient. The biochemical tests for identification of the Enterobacteriaceae are conveniently grouped into commercial test strips, allowing identification to species level (for example, the bioMérieux API strips incorporate 20 different microwells, each containing different substrates). A simpler test for the identification of Enterobacteriaceae is often used, utilizing the API 10S strip (containing just 10 wells). These strip tests demonstrate bacterial fermentation patterns of a range of sugars and enzyme reactions, in addition to those already described previously in this section. A unique Analytical Profile Index is derived for the isolate, which can then be compared with the profiles in the relevant API book or entered into the database on the website for identification. A purity plate should always be inoculated at the same time as the API strip because there is no way of assessing purity once the strip has been incubated.

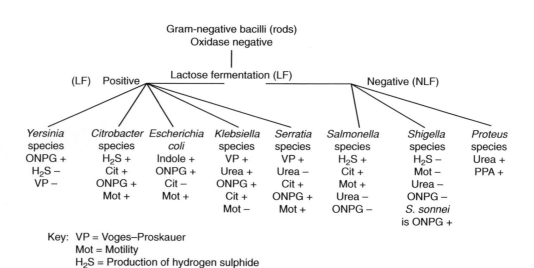

Figure 6.7
Identification schema for Enterobacteriaceae, starting from the confirmation of Gram-negative bacilli growing on a culture plate.

Automated systems such as the VITEK are becoming increasingly popular as the technology combines an identification system with antibiotic susceptibility testing, including the interpretation of extended spectrum β-lactamase enzymes. Molecular methods based on 16S rRNA sequencing are also an option.

A summary scheme for the identification of the Enterobacteriaceae is shown in *Figure 6.7*.

6.5 CHOICE OF CULTURE MEDIA

Culture media remain an essential mainstay of microbiology, with an increasingly sophisticated range available for the growth of a wide variety of pathogens. The principal types of culture media are:

■ transport
■ differential
■ selective
■ formulations for growing anaerobic bacteria
■ media with growth-enhancing additives
■ media containing chromogenic substrates.

In addition there are enrichment and selective broths and agar slopes for storing cultures. The choice of media for the culture of specific pathogens is outlined in Standard Operating Procedures in the laboratory to ensure standardization and reproducibility. The identification of a range of pathogens from different clinical specimens necessitates the use of a combination of enriched, selective and differential media. Full details of the media used are discussed in subsequent chapters in relation to each specimen type.

Transport medium is important to ensure that specimens taken from the patient are representative of the microbial growth at the time they are taken. They must not be overgrown by those with the fastest doubling time but must be able to sustain the viability of more fastidious microorganisms. Swabs taken, for example, for *Chlamydia* testing must be placed in a transport medium compatible with the testing system. Viral swabs must be in a medium that will sustain their viability if they are to be cultured. For the majority of bacteriological specimens, swabs are generally transported in a medium such as Amies modified Stuart's, which contains charcoal to improve the viability of pathogens.

Culture media have been developed to provide all the essential growth requirements *in vitro*, based on knowledge of the growth and metabolic requirements of particular bacteria. Solid culture media have a basis of amino-nitrogen nutrients in the form of peptones, other protein hydrolysates, infusions or extracts and agar as the gelling agent. Energy sources are present in the form of glucose or other carbohydrates, and the media will contain buffer salts to cope with the waste products of metabolism and to maintain a growth-promoting environment. Mineral salts and metals, phosphates, calcium, magnesium, iron and trace elements are included, along with growth-promoting factors in the form of blood, serum, vitamins and NADH.

Blood agar is a good general culture medium used for growing mixed cultures from clinical specimens. Haemolytic colonies are easy to recognize; coliforms are distinctive along with streptococci, staphylococci and anaerobic bacteria. Blood agar is inoculated in conjunction with differential and selective agar as appropriate when the specimens are initially cultured from the patient's swab. MacConkey and CLED agar are good examples of differential agar for lactose fermentation. The addition of bile salts to MacConkey agar makes it selective because some bacteria are unable to grow with even the low level of bile salts in this formulation. Chocolate agar, which contains blood heated to release growth factors haemin and NAD, is added if the specimen, such as sputum or a swab taken from the ear, nose, throat or eye, is likely to contain *Haemophilus* species. XLD and DCA media are used to suppress the normal faecal flora (selective) and differentiate between commensal flora and faecal pathogens such as *Salmonella* and *Shigella* species. More fastidious pathogens such as *Campylobacter* species require special selective and enriched media and incubation conditions in order to grow. Antibiotics are added to culture media to suppress the growth of microorganisms sensitive to them. Chromogenic agar contains substrates linked to a chromogen. When the substrate is broken down by bacterial enzymes, the chromogen is released and gives the bacterial colonies a distinctive colour.

The most challenging bacteria to culture successfully in the laboratory are *Neisseria gonorrhoeae*; the medium contains antibiotics and haemolysed blood, but the exact formulation of the growth-enhancing substances is normally a trade secret. If *N. gonorrhoeae* is suspected, swabs are sometimes cultured immediately in the clinic where they are taken and the inoculated plates then transferred to the laboratory for incubation as soon as possible. No agar has yet been developed that is capable of growing *Treponema pallidum*, the causative bacterium of syphilis, and diagnosis is made by antibody detection or visualization of the bacteria directly from the initial lesion in the patient.

6.6   METHODS TO DETERMINE ANTIMICROBIAL SUSCEPTIBILITY

When a pathogen has been isolated from a clinical specimen, guidance on suitable antimicrobial therapy is given where appropriate. This will be dependent on the site of infection and the clinical significance of the isolate.

A bacterial isolate will be tested *in vitro* against a range of antibiotics selected as suitable for the type of bacteria and the site of infection. For example, antibiotics recommended for treatment of *Staphylococcus aureus* from a skin wound may not be appropriate for *S. aureus* septicaemia or for osteomyelitis caused by the same organism. The *in vitro* susceptibility testing cannot guarantee the success of the drug *in vivo*, but the tests are designed to give the best possible indication of the outcome of therapy. Antimicrobial therapy is guided by a number of factors relating to the uptake of the compound used and its ability to achieve desired concentrations at the site of action. Most laboratory tests are designed for bacteria that grow well after overnight incubation and have unpredictable susceptibilities. Testing would not be necessary if it could be guaranteed that particular bacteria would always be sensitive to the antibiotic of choice. Unfortunately, there are fewer bacteria with predictable susceptibilities as levels of resistance rise.

Antibiotic susceptibility tests are used to determine two important measurements of the effectiveness of the drugs used: the minimum inhibitory concentration (MIC) required and the minimum bactericidal concentration (MBC) (see *Box 6.1*). Most of the tests routinely performed in microbiology laboratories measure the MIC, either directly or indirectly. A drug is considered to be bactericidal if it kills susceptible

> **Box 6.1 Definitions of MIC and MBC**
>
> The MIC is the lowest concentration of antibiotic that results in inhibition of visible growth under standard conditions.
>
> The MBC is the lowest concentration of antibiotic that kills 99.9% of the original inoculum, under standard conditions in a given time.
>
> For an antibiotic to be effective in a patient, it must be possible to achieve the MIC or MBC at the site of infection.

bacteria, and bacteriostatic if it reversibly inhibits the growth of bacteria which are then eradicated by the host immune system.

Measurement of MIC

The earliest method for the measurement of MIC was the macro broth dilution method. The antibiotic is diluted to give a range of concentrations and each dilution placed in a tube prior to the addition of the bacterial suspension, followed by overnight incubation. If the antibiotic has inhibited the growth of the bacteria or killed them, the broth will be clear, but bacterial growth will be visible in the tubes where the concentration of antibiotic is below the MIC. The MIC, or breakpoint, is therefore defined as the concentration of antibiotic in the first tube without turbidity (see *Figure 6.8*). If the tubes are then subcultured on to solid agar, bacteria that have been inhibited rather than killed will grow on the antibiotic-free medium. The concentration of antibiotic showing no growth after subculture is the MBC.

While this is often used as a teaching method to demonstrate the principles of MIC and MBC, the volumes used, apparatus and effort required in a busy laboratory would be prohibitive. A micro broth dilution method in microtitre trays provides a user-friendly alternative, allowing several antibiotics to be tested simultaneously. This method may also be automated using pre-prepared antibiotic dilutions in microtitre wells and inoculating with liquid culture of the clinical isolate.

The agar dilution, breakpoint method

This method is popular, particularly in larger laboratories, as greater numbers of isolates can be tested simultaneously. Agar plates containing specified concentrations of antibiotic around the known MIC are inoculated with test isolates, often using a multiwell inoculator to speed up the process. The sensitivity is visible by the observation of growth or no growth after incubation in a defined concentration of the antibiotic (see *Figure 6.9*). It is, however, difficult to recognize contamination and the result is either sensitive or resistant. If the precise MIC is required for clinical purposes the isolate can be retested by an alternative method such as E test (see below).

Disc diffusion

The disc diffusion method is one of the most commonly used techniques for testing antimicrobial susceptibility and was first standardized in the 1950s following recommendations made by a committee of the World Health Organization. Previously there had been no standard procedures throughout the world, and a wide variety of media, incubation times, inoculation methods and antibiotic concentrations were used which meant that results could not be easily compared.

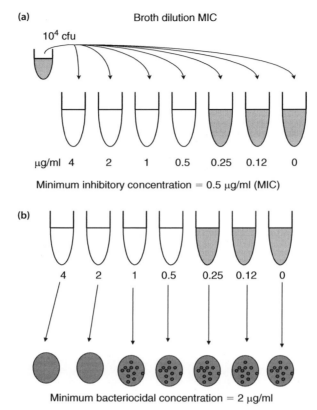

Figure 6.8

(a) The measurement of MIC by broth dilution. Growth is not visible when the concentration of the antibiotic is sufficient to either inhibit growth or kill the bacteria. The dilution of the last tube with no visible growth is the MIC.

(b) The minimum bactericidal concentration (MBC) can be obtained by subculturing loopfuls of the dilutions on to solid agar. Bacteria that have been inhibited rather than killed will grow on the antibiotic-free medium. The concentration of antibiotic showing no growth after subculture is the MBC. An antibiotic is considered bactericidal if the MBC is equal to or less than four times the MIC.

The Stokes method was developed in the UK, whereas the Kirby–Bauer method was adopted in the USA.

The Kirby–Bauer test is performed on Mueller–Hinton agar, whereas the medium of choice for the Stokes method is Iso-Sensitest or a similar formulation, with the addition of lysed blood for more sensitive organisms. In the original Stokes method both test and control bacteria were tested on the same plate, the control being spread around the outside of the plate and the test on the inside. The disc was then placed so that half the zone measured the test and the other the control, allowing differences in zone size to be clearly visible. A modified Stokes method is still widely used, where only the test isolate is spread on to the agar plate (as in the Kirby–Bauer method) and the controls are tested each day on a separate agar plate rather than with each test isolate. The method has been standardized by the British Society for Antimicrobial

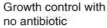

Growth control with no antibiotic

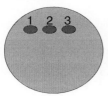

Agar plate with 1 mg/l penicillin

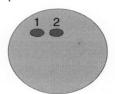

Agar plate with 8 mg/l of penicillin

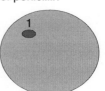

1 = resistant

2 = intermediate

3 = sensitive

Figure 6.9
Demonstration of the agar dilution (breakpoint) method. Agar plates are prepared, each containing concentrations of the antibiotic around the MIC level. Bacteria are then inoculated into the agar and incubated. The concentration of antibiotic where there is no visible growth of the bacteria is the MIC or breakpoint. In practice the plates would be clearly labelled and read over a template indicating which specimens had been inoculated in each position. Specimen 1 is resistant, 2 shows intermediate resistance (resistant at 1 mg, sensitive at 8 mg) and 3 is sensitive.

Chemotherapy (BSAC), the Clinical Laboratories Standards Institute (CLSI), and the German Institute for Standardization, Deutsches Institut für Normung (DIN).

To perform the test, isolates are picked from a culture plate and diluted to give a standard inoculum, as directed by the BSAC method. This dilution is spread evenly on to the surface of a suitable culture medium, for example, Iso-Sensitest agar. Filter paper discs impregnated with antibiotic are then applied. The discs should be applied within as short a time as possible after spreading the plate so that the bacteria do not have time to multiply before the addition of the discs. When the plates are incubated, moisture from the agar passes to the discs and the liberated drug diffuses into the agar and sets up a concentration gradient. If the bacteria are killed or growth is arrested in the presence of the antibiotic, a zone is formed around the disc at a point where the critical concentration of antibiotic meets the critical concentration of cells and inhibits their growth. The zone size is not a direct measurement of the MIC, however; the zone size is compared to data derived from testing large numbers of different bacteria against different antibiotics and plotting the zone sizes against the log of the MIC determined by a direct method. Comparison with the zone size considered sensitive, resistant for a particular bacterium/antibiotic combination enables evaluation of the result. The method is further controlled by using typed culture strains to compare zone sizes.

The advantages of disc diffusion are that it is simple, rapid and economical, and allows simultaneous testing of several antibiotics. The method may be used for cultured bacteria or for testing directly from clinical specimens such as urine, blood culture bottles or CSF. Bacteria have, over time, developed several methods of resistance to antibiotics, one of which is to produce enzymes, β-lactamases, that break down the β-lactam ring of penicillin. Some bacteria, notably Gram-negative rods, have further enhanced their enzymic activity to include newer cephalosporin antibiotics; these enzymes are called extended spectrum β-lactamases (ESBLs). β-lactamase-producing organisms may be identified by enhanced growth at the edge of the zone because, after initial inhibition by the drug, β-lactamase activity is switched on, allowing the bacteria to grow in the presence of the drug at the edge of the zone. Using the disc diffusion method, mixed cultures, and also resistant mutants growing within the zone, may be easily identified. ESBLs may be identified by disc diffusion using a combination of antibiotic discs with and without the addition of clavulanic acid. Clavulanic acid is a β-lactamase inhibitor added to antibiotics to protect the β-lactam ring. Cefotaxime, ceftazidime and cefepime or cefpirome are used, both with and without the addition of clavulanic acid. If the inhibition of the bacteria is greater in the presence of clavulanic acid the bacteria are likely to be ESBLs.

There are also limitations to the method; it is not a direct measurement of the MIC, and care is needed when interpreting the zone size (automated zone size readers are able to give a more precise measurement). A heavy or sparse inoculum may influence the results. BSAC guidelines include the preparation of a suspension of bacteria equal to a 0.5 McFarland standard and then further dilution, depending on the type of bacteria, before inoculation. There is also concern that this method would not identify glycopeptide intermediate resistant *Staphylococcus aureus*.

Several factors will affect the results and reproducibility of the method and these are incorporated into the BSAC guidelines.

- Selection and storage of discs – they should be at the appropriate concentration, stored at 4°C and not left at ambient temperature for any length of time.
- The culture medium should be standardized in content and allow uniform diffusion of the antibiotic. Levels of thymidine are kept deliberately low to prevent bacteria from using an alternative source if exposed to folate antagonist antibiotics.
- After inoculation, culture plates should be incubated as soon as possible, and the time, temperature and atmosphere must be appropriate to the type of bacteria tested and to the antibiotic. Iso-Sensitest agar is often used, with the addition of lysed blood for some more nutritionally dependent bacteria.

The E test

The E (epsilometer) test is useful for directly measuring the MIC of bacteria and is valuable for measuring emerging resistance generally and during specific therapy, in addition to confirming resistance. The E test uses plastic strips impregnated with a gradient of antibiotic concentrations. The strips are placed on to the surface of a culture plate spread with the bacterial isolate. The plate is then incubated at 37°C for 18–24 hours. Diffusion begins immediately the strip comes into contact with the bacteria so it cannot be moved once it has been positioned. As with the disc diffusion method, the inoculum concentration and the spreading of the suspension on the plate are important if an accurate result is to be obtained. After incubation, the MIC of the antibiotic may be measured at the point on the strip where the zone of inhibition crosses.

E tests are used for measuring the MIC of resistant bacteria such as MRSA and *Pseudomonas aeruginosa* and also for assessing high-level aminoglycoside resistance in enterococci. They are also useful as an epidemiological tool to monitor the development of resistance, for example monitoring penicillin resistance in *Streptococcus pneumoniae*. Resistant bacteria growing within the zone can also be identified. The presence of ESBL-producing bacteria can be identified using two E test strips, one containing the antibiotic plus clavulanic acid and the other without clavulanic acid (see *Figure 6.10*). Three antibiotics are used, cefotaxime, cefepime and ceftazidime, all with and without the addition of clavulanic acid. The presence of an ESBL is indicated by one of three observations:

■ The MIC with the addition of clavulanic acid is reduced by 3 log dilutions compared to the antibiotic alone;
■ A deformed zone is seen around the antibiotic without clavulanic acid;
■ A phantom zone is seen in the area of the antibiotic alone.

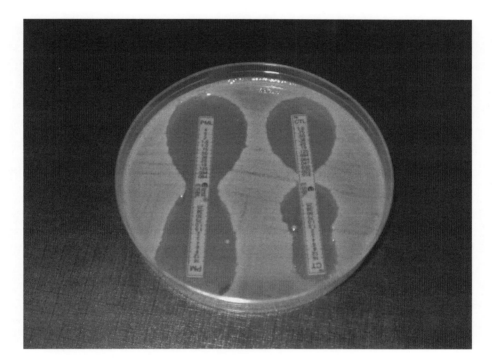

Figure 6.10
Double E test strips used to demonstrate the presence of an extended spectrum β-lactamase enzyme. The cefotaxime CT strip with and without clavulanic acid CT and CTL is showing a deformed zone around the cefotaxime end of the strip, indicative of the presence of an ESBL.

Methods for assessing the MBC

An antibiotic is considered bactericidal if the MBC is equal to or less than four times the MIC. Measurement of the MBC is useful for assessing the efficacy of antibiotic therapy in immuno-compromised patients because their immune system is unable to complete the killing process in conjunction with bacteriostatic drugs. MBC, the lowest concentration of antibiotic required to kill the microorganism, may be measured by extending the broth dilution test. Subcultures are taken from the wells showing no visible bacterial growth and inoculated on to antibiotic-free medium. If the cells are still viable they will be able to multiply and produce visible colonial growth after overnight incubation. The MBC is the highest dilution with no visible growth after incubation.

The MBC results are read at a single point in time, which in most cases is sufficient. For more accurate assessment of MBC, a time-kill curve can be produced which presents the decrease in viability of isolates over a period of time. This process can also be performed on an automatic blood culture machine, where a curve is constructed from reflectance readings taken at 10 minute intervals. An automated system such as the VITEK 2 may also be used to measure MBC.

Target sites for antimicrobial activity

The aim of antimicrobial agents is to either kill, or stop the growth of bacteria at the site of infection while limiting damage to host cells. This selective toxicity is achieved by targeting aspects of the bacterial cell structure, growth and metabolism that are different from our own cells. Antimicrobial activity is therefore targeted at the cell wall, cell membrane, protein synthesis (bacterial ribosomes are different from human ribosomes), and replication processes such as the supercoiling of DNA and nucleic acid synthesis. *Figure 2.13* shows these target sites and some of the antibiotic classes available for use.

6.7 NON-CULTURAL IDENTIFICATION METHODS BASED ON ANTIGEN–ANTIBODY TESTS

Antigen–antibody tests have been in use for many years, based on the principle that specific antibodies recognize the corresponding antigen and when mixed together with gentle agitation, they cross link to form visible clumping. Latex particles are now more commonly used, coated with either antigen or antibody, as described earlier in the coagulase test.

The complement fixation test (CFT)

The CFT was for many years the accepted method for identifying viral antibodies. Enzyme-linked immunosorbent assays (ELISAs) have largely superseded the test, but it is still used in some laboratories. The investigation takes 2 days to complete and relies upon the reagents being carefully controlled. The basis of the test is that if antigen–antibody binding has taken place, complement will bind to the complexes. The patient's serum samples, the first taken in the acute phase of the infection and the second taken 2 weeks later when antibodies will have been formed, are first heated at 56°C for 30 minutes to remove the natural complement. A range of dilutions from 1/10 to 1/320 are prepared in round-bottomed microtitre trays using the serum and CFT buffer. An equal volume of known viral antigen is then added to each well, followed by the same volume of complement. The trays are left overnight at 4°C. Because the reagents in the initial reaction are colourless, the consumption of complement is visualized by the addition of one volume of sensitized sheep cells to each well. Sensitized cells are cells that have been mixed with antibody, but not at a sufficient concentration to form visible clumps. They are, however, sensitive to the addition of complement and will be lysed by it. If the complement that was added in the initial stage has been bound to the antigen–antibody complexes, there will be little or none left to lyse the red cells. The cells fall to the bottom of the well and indicate a negative result. If there is free complement lysed red cells are present, with 50% lysis denoting a positive result. Because the serum was serially diluted it is possible to demonstrate a rising titre of antibodies between acute and convalescent serum samples and retrospectively diagnose the infection. Because the CFT is retrospective and time-consuming, other techniques including latex particle agglutination tests and molecular identification of viral genes are able to provide more timely and accurate diagnoses.

The production of monoclonal antibodies and the discovery of the genomic structure of microorganisms led to the development of sophisticated non-cultural techniques for the identification of antigens, antibodies and specific gene sequences characteristic of bacteria, toxins, viruses, fungi and protozoa.

Monoclonal antibodies and enzyme-linked immunosorbent assays

Naturally occurring antibodies are a heterogenous mix of antibody epitopes from different clones of B cells that together recognize whole antigen structures. Monoclonal antibodies are derived from a single clone and are specific for a particular epitope of the antigen. Monoclonal antibodies were first prepared in 1975 by Milstein and Köhler by combining a normal activated antibody-producing B cell with a myeloma

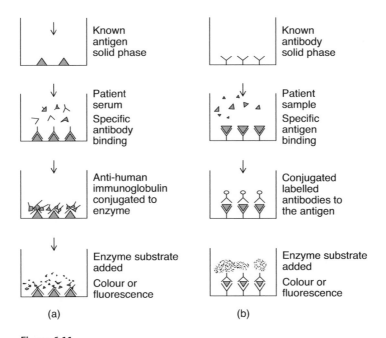

(a)   (b)

Figure 6.11
The ELISA technique can be used in several ways: (a) demonstrates the detection of antibody to a known antigen and (b) shows the detection of an antigen using specific monoclonal antibody as the solid phase. Each step includes an incubation and wash phase to ensure that binding takes place and that unbound antigen or antibody is washed away before the addition of the next reagent. The reactions can be visualized by a colour change or a fluorescent product.

cell (cancerous plasma cell). The resulting cell, a hybridoma, became immortalized and continued to secrete monoclonal antibody. Clones of these hybridomas can be cultured and produce large quantities of specific antibody.

Monoclonal antibodies are used extensively in enzyme-linked immunosorbent assays (ELISAs). ELISAs have a solid phase onto which is coated either an antigen or antibody, to detect antibody or antigen in the patient serum. The solid phase can be a 96-well flat-bottomed plate, or a single-use strip used in an automated machine. The patient serum is added to the wells and left to incubate. After the required incubation time the wells are washed, leaving bound antigen–antibody complexes (see *Figure 6.11*).

An enzyme-conjugated antibody is added to the well, incubated and washed. The addition of a specific chromogenic enzyme substrate yields a coloured product, measured visually or on a spectrophotometer. Automated single-use ELISAs generate a measurable fluorescent or chemi-luminescent signal and are incorporated into automated systems including the VIDAS and Liaison systems. A variation of ELISA is used in the Architect system, where sensitized magnetic beads act as the solid phase to adsorb the target antigen or antibody.

6.8 MOLECULAR-BASED METHODS

The polymerase chain reaction

The polymerase chain reaction (PCR) enables amplification of specific gene sequences to a point where the sequence can be measured, even if it was present in the original sample in very small numbers. An increasing number of laboratory diagnostic tests are using the method as specific primer sequences become available and the technology is affordable, free of contamination and time-saving. Initial extraction of the genetic material can be performed either manually or by an automated extraction method. The latter has the advantages of consistency and reproducibility. The primer sequences used in the amplification technique must be chosen carefully and be unique in order to identify a particular pathogen, for example, *Chlamydia trachomatis* or *Mycobacteria tuberculosis*, or virulence genes such as the verocytotoxin of *Escherichia coli* O157, or a specific resistance gene such as the *MecA* gene in *Staphylococcus aureus*.

Molecular methods involve three essential steps:

- extraction of the nucleic acid
- amplification of the nucleic acid
- detection of the target.

Extraction of nucleic acid

This can be achieved using manual techniques, boiling the sample and adding extraction enzymes. However, it is more frequently achieved by automated methods such as:

- Ampliprep, used for example for HIV and HCV viral loads
- EZ1 Advanced XL, used for example for herpes viruses, screening for respiratory viruses with a panel of primers, adenovirus and enterovirus.

The automated methods use a magnetic separation technology and during the process they add an internal control and buffer.

Amplification of the extracted nucleic acid

Amplification is achieved by a standard PCR, either in one of the light cycler rapid automated machines or at a slower pace using a standard thermal cycler. The latter is useful when multiple primers are used to detect key sequences of up to 20 respiratory viruses. In the PCR reaction the nucleic acid is heated to break open the double-stranded DNA. The primers anneal to corresponding sequences in the DNA strands when the temperature is lowered, and are then extended using Taq polymerase. The process is repeated over many replication cycles until the target is amplified to a detectable quantity. More than one primer can be used in a single amplification technique, in a process called multiplex PCR, capable of identifying more than one target sequence at a time. As mentioned earlier, a multiplex PCR system can be used to identify up to 20 different viruses from clinical specimens.

Reverse transcriptase PCR (RT-PCR) is used to measure RNA sequences and is particularly useful in the detection of viral RNA in blood samples, for example the measurement of HIV and hepatitis C viral load. A reverse transcriptase step is incorporated into the reaction. This generates complementary double-stranded DNA (cDNA) and then an RNA polymerase transcribes the RNA from this and amplification of the RNA follows.

Detection of the target nucleic acid sequences

The amplified products (amplicons) of PCR and RT-PCR can be visualized by separation on an agarose gel. However, the PCR reaction is more frequently performed in an automated system of 'real-time' PCR, where the increasing amount of amplicon is quantified as it is generated.

There are several ways in which the PCR product can be visualized and quantified to give the result in an easily interpreted format. Commercially available amplification systems, examples being the TaqMan48 and the LightCycler 2.0, use a variety of probe systems to visualize and quantify the amplified product.

- Fluorescent dyes: the amplified product is measured as it is produced by a fluorescent detection system. SYBR green is a frequently used fluorescent dye, incorporated into the test system. In solution the dye emits very little fluorescence but as each round of amplification takes place the dye intercalates into the DNA double helix. Fluorescence is enhanced by DNA binding and so the fluorescent signal produced is proportional to the amplified product and recorded on a visual printout. SYBR green is not used extensively in diagnostic assays, as it is not considered specific enough, but it is useful in the developmental work.
- Fluorescence resonance energy transfer (FRET) relies on the transfer of light energy between two adjacent dye molecules. In FRET, one probe has a dye on the 3′ end of the probe and the other on the 5′ end. If both the probes anneal (attach) to a target sequence in the clinical sample, the dyes are brought close to each other. The fluorescent dye on the 3′ end of the probe is absorbed by the acceptor dye on the second, 5′ probe, which becomes excited and emits light at a third wavelength which is detected by the system. Molecular probe systems are used in other disciplines than microbiology, and FRET is used in an assay for clotting factors II and factor V Leiden mutant gene detection. The principle of FRET is shown in *Figure 6.12.*

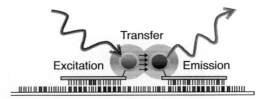

Figure 6.12
The activity of a FRET probe. One probe has a dye on the 3′ end of the probe and the other on the 5′ end. When both probes anneal to a target sequence in the sample, the dyes are brought close to each other. The fluorescent dye on the 3′ end of the probe is absorbed by the acceptor dye on the second, 5′ probe, which becomes excited and emits light at a third wavelength, 640nm, which is detected by the system.

■ The TaqMan probe is a short oligonucleotide that contains a 5′ fluorescent dye and a 3′ quenching dye. When the probe binds to a complementary sequence of DNA at 60°C and *Taq* polymerase cleaves the 5′ end of the probe, the fluorescent dye is separated from the quenching dye and light is emitted.

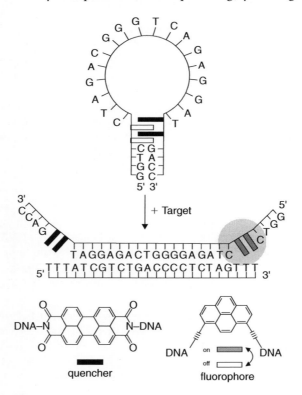

Figure 6.13
Principle of molecular beacons. The hairpin structure keeps the fluorophore and quencher close to each other; no signal is emitted. When the probe binds to the target a rigid structure is formed and the conformational change separates the quencher from the fluorophore and a signal is emitted.

■ Molecular beacons are similar to TaqMan probes but are not cleaved by 5′ nuclease activity. They have a fluorescent dye on the 5′ end and a quencher dye on the 3′ end, and are designed to be complementary to each other, so that at low temperatures the two ends anneal, giving a hairpin-like structure which also means that no light is emitted. The central part of the hairpin probe is designed to be complementary to the PCR product, and so if the probe attaches to its target during the process of heating and annealing, the hairpin opens and the two dyes are separated, allowing the fluorescent dye to emit a signal. This is an example of strand displacement amplification (see *Figure 6.13*).

■ Scorpion probes are used on the LightCycler for the detection of *Herpes simplex* virus, HSV I and II, and *Varicella zoster* viruses. The scorpion probe is so called because its tail coils back on itself (see *Figure 6.14*).

■ Transcription-mediated amplification (TMA) technology can be used to detect either RNA or DNA targets, generating a billion copies in less than 60 minutes. The system incorporates RNA polymerase and reverse transcriptase (RT). The RT generates complementary dsDNA from either RNA or DNA. The RNA polymerase then transcribes RNA from the DNA template and each RNA amplicon generated acts as a template for further rounds of amplification. The method uses a specific gene probe in a hybridization system detected by chemi-luminescence. TMA can be used to detect two pathogens, for example *Chlamydia trachomatis* and *Neisseria gonorrhoeae*, from the same clinical sample. The method is also used for the detection of *Mycobacteria tuberculosis* in clinical specimens.

Many laboratories now have purpose-built molecular suites and throughout subsequent chapters there is reference to the use of molecular-based methods, known as NAATs (nucleic acid amplification techniques) for the diagnosis of a range

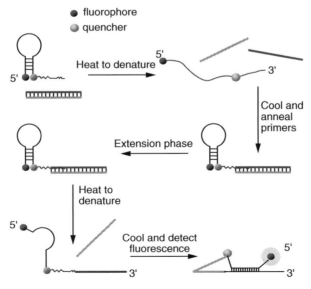

Figure 6.14
The principle of Scorpion probes during the amplification process.

of pathogens. Different technologies and automated systems are used, based on the amplification systems described above. Commercial detection kits are chosen for the detection of different pathogen targets depending on their ability to detect low levels of the target sequence.

Pulsed-field gel electrophoresis (PFGE)

Electrophoresis is a widely-used technique across a range of biomedical disciplines. For example, it can be used for separating immunoglobulin classes in clinical biochemistry in order to diagnose myeloma. In microbiology the technique is used to separate out genomic bacterial DNA. The DNA is first treated with restriction enzymes that cut it into smaller fragments. The treated DNA is applied to one end of an agarose gel through which an electric current is passed. The fragments migrate through the gel according to their size, with smaller fragments being more mobile; they create a pattern of bands that can be compared to standards. PFGE is an improved method using electrical pulses that run at different angles through the gel, and enables more complex DNA analysis. A known concentration of the bacteria to be analysed is prepared in an agarose plug, to which restriction enzymes are added prior to the electrophoresis. The method is useful for analysing different strains of bacteria, for example methicillin-resistant *Staphylococcus aureus* isolates. Different clones of epidemic strains will have a unique DNA fingerprint (DNA separation band patterns). This is useful for the investigation of hospital-acquired infections; if the different isolates all have the same PFGE bands, they are likely to be from a single source, whereas the presence of several different clonal groups is indicative of multiple sources of infection.

Matrix-assisted laser desorption ionization time-of-flight mass spectrometry (MALDI-TOF-MS)

MALDI-TOF-MS has been used in research laboratories for several years, but is a recent addition to some diagnostic laboratories. The equipment is, however, very expensive and beyond the budget of many laboratories. The technique provides fast, accurate, reliable and cost-effective identification of bacterial and yeast isolates from culture and from clinical isolates, for example blood cultures. Widespread introduction of the technique will considerably reduce the time taken for more conventional methods of identification and render many of the methods described earlier unnecessary. The technique has produced consistent results when compared with conventional and molecular methods. The system does not distinguish *Escherichia coli* from *Shigella* species, or *Streptococcus pneumoniae* from other *Streptococcus mitis/oralis* group bacteria, or MRSA from MSSA (methicillin-sensitive *Staphylococcus aureus*). Simple biochemical tests and selective culture, however, resolve these issues.

Mass spectrometry is used to provide accurate measurements of molecular weights of compounds and by fragmenting molecules helps to give valuable information on their molecular structure. MALDI-TOF mass spectrometry analyses intact cells such as bacteria or yeast cells by their ribosomal and membrane-associated proteins (see *Figure 6.15*). The reaction takes place in nanoseconds. The principal steps of the analytical technique are:

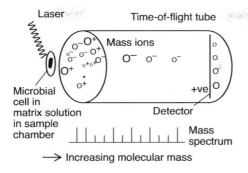

Figure 6.15
The principle of MALDI-TOF mass spectrometry. The microbial cell is surrounded by matrix solution and placed in the sample chamber. When the laser is fired the sample is ionized. The ions move rapidly along the time-of-flight tube towards the oppositely charged detector. This movement is dependent on their mass/charge ratio. A unique mass spectrum is created.

- 1 µl of intact cells are added to a 96-well target plate and placed in the machine.
- A crystalline matrix admixture which includes organic solvent is added to the cells and breaks open the cell wall, crystallizing the proteins within nanoseconds. Alpha-cyano-4-hydroxy-cinnamic acid is used as the matrix for Gram-negative species and 5-chloro-2-mercaptobensothiazole for Gram-positive species.
- The laser is fired at the cells surrounded by the matrix in a vacuum chamber, causing ionization in the sample chamber and rapid movement of the mass ions towards the detector.
- Smaller ions with a low m/z ratio (mass to charge) travel faster than larger ions.
- Differences in m/z ratios result in different times of flights of each ion.
- A mass spectral profile is determined, which gives unique biomarkers for bacteria and yeasts.
- Comparison with stored profiles provides identification.

In common with many advances in diagnostic methods, including molecular methods, the routine use of MALDI-TOF-MS has been dependent on the introduction of bench-top machines, reference data banks and affordable technology at an affordable price. However, because of the rapid results obtained using MALDI-TOF, other biochemical tests would not be necessary.

SUGGESTED FURTHER READING

Andrews, J.M. (2001) BSAC standardized disc susceptibility testing method. *J. Antimicrob. Chemother.* **48**: 43–57.

Andrews, J.M. (2001) Determination of minimum inhibitory concentrations. *J. Antimicrob. Chemother.* **48**: 5–16.

Benagli, C., Rossi, V., Dolina, M., Tonolla, M. & Petrini, O. (2011) Matrix-assisted laser desorption ionization – time of flight mass spectrometry for the identification of clinically relevant bacteria. *PLoS ONE*, viewable at www.plosone.org

Brown, A. (2007) Chromogenic media: bacteriology in colour. *The Biomedical Scientist*, **6**: 458–461.

Espy, M.J., Uhl, J.R., Sloan, L.M. *et al.* (2006) Real-time PCR in clinical microbiology: applications for routine laboratory testing. *Clin. Microbiol. Reviews*, **19**: 165–256.

Eydmann, M. (2011) Introduction of MALDI-TOF: a revolution in diagnostic microbiology. *The Biomedical Scientist*, **55**: 5.

Kader, A.A., Angamuthu, K.K., Kamath, K.A. & Zaman, M.N (2006) Modified double-disc test for detection of extended spectrum β-lactamases in *Escherichia coli* and *Klebsiella pneumoniae. Br. J. Biomed. Sci.* **63**: 51–54.

Macrae F. (2006) Multidrug resistance in Gram-negative bacteria. *The Biomedical Scientist,* **10**: 891–893.

Myers, F. (2008) Biocidal agents: modes of action and correlation with antibiotic resistance. *The Biomedical Scientist*, **3**: 227–231.

Turnidge, J. & Paterson, D.L. (2007) Setting and revising antibacterial susceptibility breakpoints. *Clin. Microbiol. Reviews*, **20**: 391–408.

www.bsac.org.uk – current British Society of Antimicrobial Chemotherapy guidelines are found here, along with valuable information on all aspects of antimicrobial testing.

SELF-ASSESSMENT QUESTIONS

1. How would you ensure that a culture of pathogenic bacteria does not infect the work station and the biomedical scientist who is subculturing the bacteria on to a sterile culture plate?

2. How is the viable count per ml calculated? What would be the viable count/ml of a culture dilution using the Miles and Misra method and 25 μl aliquots, where six colonies are counted at a dilution of 10^5?

3. Why are the catalase and coagulase tests useful for further identifying Gram-positive cocci?

4. What is the basis of the streptococcal grouping test? Why is it important to differentiate between the β-haemolytic streptococci?

5. The oxidase test is important because it distinguishes between some major groups of Gram-negative bacteria. Give some examples of this.

6. Gram-negative diplococci are observed on a Gram stain. How could they be further identified?

7. Which two genera of non-lactose fermenting Gram-negative bacteria can be separated by the urease test? Why is this important when investigating the faecal sample of a patient with diarrhoea?

8. Describe the main components of culture media.

9. Explain the terms MIC and MBC.

10. Outline the principal methods for determining the MIC of a particular antibiotic with a clinical isolate.

Answers to self-assessment questions provided at:
www.scionpublishing.com/medmicro

Organization of the microbiology laboratory

Learning objectives
After studying this chapter you should confidently be able to:

■ **Describe the principal areas of a clinical microbiology laboratory**
Most laboratories will have a separate specimen reception area, where the specimens are sorted, checked and given a unique identification number before being distributed to specific areas of the laboratory for culture and microscopy. Typical work stations will include: an enteric area, or in some cases a suite of rooms; a urine bench; general swabs; ear, nose and throat swabs; and screening swabs. There may perhaps be a separate area for genital specimens, blood cultures, sputa and fluids, TB specimens, serology and possibly a molecular suite. There will also be dedicated waste disposal areas.

■ **Outline specimen requirements, reception, storage and disposal**
All samples accepted by the laboratory must be clearly labelled and packaged in a sealed bag along with a corresponding request form. The minimum information required on this form is the patient's full name, date of birth / hospital number, address, GP or consultant and the report destination. Clinical details will further guide the investigations required. In specimen reception the samples are given a unique identifying number and then transferred to the appropriate area of the laboratory for testing. After testing the specimens are stored at either 4°C or –20°C in numerical order, following appropriate guidelines. Clinical specimens are removed in sealed plastic bags and autoclaved prior to disposal as clinical waste.

■ **Describe the principles of quality assurance and quality control**
Quality assurance covers every aspect of the service provided by a clinical microbiology laboratory and assures all employees and users that quality requirements are continually met. All laboratories partake in internal and external quality assurance schemes and undergo accreditation. Quality control is part of this and ensures that all equipment and tests are regularly checked and controlled.

■ **Explain the requirements and importance of working safely in the laboratory and hazards associated with equipment**
Safe working practices are essential when working with clinical specimens containing pathogenic microorganisms. Safety at work is governed by health and safety legislation and is an integral part of the planning, organization and running of a microbiology laboratory. The health and safety executive in the UK (the HSE) enforces the regulations, and safe working is enshrined in accreditation standards.

■ **Explain the development and use of standard operating procedures**
Standard operating procedures (SOPs) are integral to the quality assurance of the laboratory and ensure that all specimens are treated consistently by different biomedical scientists and that an analytical procedure is performed in the same way on every occasion. SOPs provide a comprehensive guide to the likely pathogens to be isolated, the culture media to be inoculated, the procedure to be performed and further identification tests required, and also give reporting, storage and disposal guidelines.

7.1 DESIGN AND ORGANIZATION

All clinical microbiology laboratories in the country appear to be different. Some are new and represent the latest in design, build and equipment, while others still deliver a high quality service from old buildings with less sophisticated equipment. The number and type of specimens processed will also differ considerably between a large laboratory in a teaching hospital offering a wide range of routine and specialist tests, and a smaller one dealing with routine work from a local hospital with mechanisms to send away specialist requests. Reorganization within the NHS involves the merging of pathology services with a central 'hub' laboratory, where many of the routine tests are performed, and satellite laboratories. What is important is that they are all quality assured and provide reproducible results that meet the service user's need.

Most laboratories have discrete areas for dealing with different types of specimen, from receipt to storage and disposal. Microbiology specimens vary in terms of the nature of the specimen and the body site from which they are taken. The first important area is therefore specimen reception, whether this is in the laboratory itself or a central reception area for pathology, where all specimens are initially sorted, given a unique identifying laboratory number or barcode, and then transferred to the area in which they will be tested. Some specimens are always urgent, for example cerebrospinal fluid specimens, and these are prioritized and taken immediately for testing. All specimens marked urgent are dealt with in a similar way and the results telephoned to the requesting doctor as soon as they are available.

Generally the organization of the areas would reflect the following types of specimen:

- Bacteriology: urines; faeces; blood cultures; Category 3 specimens such as sputa, TB requests, fluids; general bench for wound swabs, ENT and genital swabs, MRSA screening; mycology specimens; sensitivity testing.
- Blood samples for serology; molecular techniques.
- Virology specimens.

There will also be areas set aside for waste disposal, autoclaving and wash-up. The work areas described for different sections are sometimes in an open plan arrangement or may be in separate rooms. Category 3 facilities will always be separate, as will the molecular area. The former is a containment facility and the molecular techniques require an uncontaminated environment.

The introduction of MALDI-TOF mass spectrometry (see *Chapter 6*) also provides opportunities for reorganization of the workflow, where isolates from a range of clinical specimens are identified by the system, negating the need for discrete bench areas in general bacteriology (with the exception of Category 3 and mycology specimens) and extensive biochemical testing.

Molecular techniques must be performed in an environment where amplified DNA or RNA amplicons cannot contaminate other specimens. Ideally the molecular suite should contain three rooms, or at least clearly designated areas: one for sample reception and preparation, the second for pre-analytical preparation where the DNA or RNA is extracted, and finally the amplification area. Once analysed, the products must be disposed of in a way that does not allow them to come into contact with unprocessed specimens, as small amounts of contaminating amplicon could affect the results of other patient samples.

The role of these different areas of the laboratory in the diagnosis of infectious disease is discussed in more detail in the subsequent sample-specific chapters.

7.2 SPECIMEN RECEPTION, STORAGE AND DISPOSAL

Receipt and labelling

Samples arrive at the laboratory from a variety of sources: hospital wards, GP surgeries and residential homes. Sometimes patients deliver their own specimen directly to the laboratory. All clinical samples should be clearly labelled and packaged, preferably in a sealed bag attached to the request form. Before a sample is accepted it must meet certain minimum criteria to ensure that it is correctly matched to the right patient. Every pathology department must have a standard operating procedure (SOP) describing the correct procedure for labelling and sample identification; these are also laid out in the IBMS leaflet *'Patient sample and request form identification criteria'*. The minimum requirements for information are shown in *Table 7.1*.

Table 7.1 The information required on patient samples and accompanying request forms

	Essential information	Desirable information
Patient sample	NHS or CHI number* Full name Date of birth and/or hospital number	Date and time Report destination
Request form	Patient's full name Date of birth NHS number Patient's address Patient's GP or consultant Report destination	Clinical information Type/site of specimen Date and time collected Patient's address Patient's sex Signature of clinician Bleep number if appropriate

*The CHI (Community Health Index) number is used as a unique identifier for the Health Service in Scotland.

Hospital inpatients often have self-adhesive typed labels on the request card providing all of the identification required. The use of NHS numbers on all patient records and request forms was made mandatory under the NHS operating framework for 2008–9. The NHS number provides a unique identifier for patients across the NHS provision and the Community Health Index (CHI) is used by the Health Service in Scotland. If the samples or request cards are inadequately labelled or completed, they must be referred back to the requesting clinician, not amended by laboratory staff. Samples or request forms that do not provide the minimum essential information may be rejected without analysis. However, if a sample is received from a patient who cannot easily be recalled for a repeat, the sample may be processed at the discretion of a senior biomedical scientist, with the condition that the report contains a disclaimer.

Quality and results

For microbiology samples the quality of the specimen sent for investigation will have a great influence on the quality of the result obtained. The laboratory can only work with the specimens they are sent, and there are several factors that influence the quality of the specimen and the result obtained:

■ the specimen must be taken at the optimal time
■ the specimen must be of the correct type for the investigation requested
■ the specimen must be taken with care to avoid contamination from the patient's normal flora and from the person collecting it
■ there must be a sufficient quantity for the investigation required; this may include sequential samples
■ all specimens must be clearly labelled, in the correct container and safe for transport and handling within the laboratory.

Optimal timing

In clinical conditions the causative organisms may only be present intermittently in the specimen chosen for investigation. They may peak at a particular stage of the infection, or be killed if successfully treated before the specimen is taken. Timing is important and the following examples illustrate considerations to be taken.

Any specimen suspected of a bacterial infection should be taken before antibiotics are given. Even small doses of antibiotic substances could be enough to affect the subsequent culture. One important exception to this is a patient with suspected bacterial meningitis. Evidence-based practice has demonstrated that the sooner antibiotics are administered to the patient, the better the outcome. This may mean that no viable bacteria are left in the cerebrospinal fluid (CSF) or blood culture specimen for subsequent culture. However, the macroscopic and microscopic appearances of the CSF will still be suggestive of bacterial infection. The identification of the bacteria can be successfully achieved by using molecular techniques to detect bacterial DNA and should a further specimen of blood be needed for the test, this can be requested.

Specimens for the isolation of viruses using electron microscopy should be obtained when the disease is acute and the pathogens are shed in the greatest numbers. Serum samples taken at the acute and convalescent stages of respiratory disease enable a more accurate diagnosis as antibody titres will show a significant rise, indicating that the disease was recent and not a chronic condition. If only an acute specimen is submitted, a report can be sent requesting a convalescent sample and indicating that the acute sample will be retained and tested in parallel with the later one.

Specimen type

Specimens need to reflect the situation at the exact site of the infection and if the microorganisms are not present in the specimen collected, the result will be meaningless and an important diagnosis may be missed. *Neisseria gonorrhoeae* infects the columnar epithelial cells of the endocervix and this is where the swab must be taken, as a high vaginal swab may not contain the bacteria. Urethral and rectal swabs should also be cultured.

A CSF (cerebrospinal fluid) specimen will correctly indicate the presence of *Neisseria meningitidis* meningitis, but a blood culture is needed to indicate meningococcaemia and septicaemia, and a further blood sample is required for molecular identification of the bacteria.

Pus samples, rich in dead neutrophils and trapped bacteria, are always preferable to swabs if there is a choice, and are essential when mycobacterial infection is suspected. Sputum samples must be representative of the area of respiratory infection and so salivary specimens are unacceptable, as they will only contain mouth or upper respiratory tract flora, whereas the mucopurulent specimen is more likely to be diagnostic of pneumonia. *Bordetella pertussis* attaches to pernasal epithelial cells and a swab from this area is essential for the diagnosis of whooping cough.

All of these potential problems can be identified when the specimen is received and can often be rectified easily by alerting the requesting clinician to the problem and requesting a repeat or additional specimen as necessary.

Minimum contamination of specimens

This is particularly important if the specimen is taken from a normally sterile source such as blood for culture, swabs from a gall bladder operation, peri-operative specimens from an orthopaedic site, joint, pleural or ascitic fluid, or CSF. Any pathogen isolated from these areas should be significant, but there is also the possibility that other flora will grow on culture media, especially if an enrichment step or prolonged incubation has been included in the investigation. These floras may include those on skin from inadequate cleansing of a venepuncture site, normal flora touched by a swab on mucous membranes after swabbing a sterile site, and skin flora shed into the air or on the needle used for aspiration. For the diagnosis of infection from deep sites, more invasive procedures are sometimes necessary, for example bronchial lavage, or lung biopsies for some opportunistic infections such as *Pneumocystis carinii*. Drainage of pus from abscesses and bone biopsies in a case of osteomyelitis may be necessary to diagnose the causative organisms.

For the relatively uncomplicated investigation of urine it is important for the patient to be given clear instructions about how to obtain a good midstream specimen to minimize the contamination of skin and urethral flora and in females, vaginal flora. However, for the detection of *Chlamydia trachomatis* from urine a first-catch specimen is required to ensure that any bacteria within the epithelial cells are detected.

It is important to be aware of these potential contamination problems when dealing with microbiological samples. Once the sample has been received by the laboratory, the aseptic procedures used are designed to minimize the risk of further contamination. Even this is difficult if the specimen requires complex testing procedures and prolonged incubation, for example, tissue or bone samples from potentially infected prosthetic joints. It is always worth remembering that biomedical scientists have no control over the initial taking of the clinical specimen and have to rely on the expertise of others to provide a non-contaminated, representative sample.

Sufficient quantity for the investigation

If the sample is too small, the chances of identifying the causative organism are minimized and there may also be dilution problems if the sample is taken into liquid. This is true of blood cultures where it is important to add the required volume of blood to the liquid culture medium in the bottle to maximize the isolation of bacteria. The sensitivity of detection is also increased if two sets of blood culture samples are taken over several days. If there is a clinical suspicion of endocarditis and previous bottles have given negative results, up to four additional sets over several days are advised in order to detect the bacteria shed into the blood from the infected heart valve.

If the pathogen is only present in low numbers, as in some *Salmonella* and *Shigella* or *Giardia lamblia* infections, this will also affect the subsequent results. This problem is addressed by the inclusion of an enrichment step in the bacterial culture, and concentration techniques are carried out to maximize the isolation of parasites and ova from faecal specimens. Samples taken on consecutive days will also be of benefit. This is true of specimens for mycobacterial culture, as adequate specimens taken over three consecutive days are necessary for sputum and early morning urines.

Clearly labelled and safe specimens in the correct container

All specimens accepted for testing by the laboratory must conform to national and local guidelines for safe collection and transport. The request card should be attached to a sealed plastic bag containing the specimen in a leak-proof container. Leaking specimens must be discarded as they present a potential contamination hazard for any staff handling them. All specimens should be regarded as potentially infectious and treated as such. If the sample is in a known high-risk category, such as from a person with hepatitis B or who is HIV positive, it is labelled with yellow biohazard labels and not opened until placed in an appropriate containment area. This would also apply to sputum specimens and all specimens to be tested for mycobacteria.

Every laboratory will provide their users with a guide to the correct sample containers required for different types of specimen and if the specimen is not in the correct one, it is likely to be rejected. Examples of this would be a urine sample in a non-sterile jar, heparinized blood when a clotted sample is required for serum, and requests for viral culture submitted as a charcoal swab.

Storage and retention of samples

The Royal College of Pathology and the IBMS have issued guidelines for the storage and minimum retention times for pathological samples in their report '*The Retention and Storage of Pathological Records and Archives*'. The World Health Organization (WHO) guidelines, '*Use of Anticoagulants in Diagnostic Laboratory Investigations*', include information on the storage of blood, urine and CSF. Medical, legal and public interests have to be considered when advising on minimum retention times. Plasma and serum may be disposed of 48 hours after the final report has been issued. In practice most laboratories will have a facility for storing frozen serum samples in case they need to be re-examined at a later date to observe a rise in titre of antibodies, or to check HIV status, or in the case of needle-stick infections to provide a baseline sample at the time when the incident occurred. The specimens are stored in numerical order. When the storage system is full, the earliest samples are discarded. Body fluids, aspirates and swabs are stored in racks at 4°C on a rotational basis and may be discarded 48 hours after the final report. Urine is an exception and may be discarded earlier, as the sample may be easily and non-invasively repeated. Microbiological culture plates may be discarded 24–48 hours after the issue of the final report.

All specimens for discard are removed in approved, sealed plastic bags and autoclaved before final disposal as clinical waste.

7.3   QUALITY ASSURANCE AND QUALITY CONTROL

Quality assurance covers every aspect of the service provided by the microbiology laboratory, including recruitment, health and safety, organization, administration, procedures and results.

Quality control ensures that all laboratory tests meet their quality requirements in terms of accuracy, precision, consistency and reproducibility. This is measured by internal quality assurance schemes and participation in external quality assurance schemes. Clinical Pathology Accreditation (CPA), which merged with the United Kingdom Accreditation Service (UKAS) in 2009, encompasses both total quality assurance and quality control, ensuring that services are of a sufficiently high standard to meet user requirements in line with current developments. CPA is important for clinical laboratories and is required for training purposes, particularly when the laboratory is involved in placements as part of professionally accredited and approved higher education courses.

All accredited laboratories participate in National External Quality Assurance Schemes (NEQAS) for a range of samples tested and the results are displayed on laboratory notice boards. The NEQAS samples should be treated in the same way as any routine specimen. In addition to their role in quality assurance, NEQAS specimens are valuable for educational purposes, as the pathogen isolated may rarely be seen in clinical specimens received in some laboratories. This is certainly true of some faecal ova and parasites, bacterial isolates of cholera or diphtheria and unusual fungal pathogens. Laboratories also operate an internal quality assurance scheme. Urine and other samples may be split so that one is tested routinely and the second processed later as an internal quality assurance specimen.

Quality assurance procedures encompass all *in vitro* diagnostic tests in use and any new procedures introduced into the laboratory. New diagnostic procedures are regulated by the Medical and Healthcare products Regulatory Agency (MHRA), and the Royal College of Pathologists has issued guidelines and criteria. All diagnostic tests must comply with European Union regulations, and CE (*Conformité Européenne*) marking confirms that health and safety regulations have been met.

Quality control procedures are an integral aspect of the day-to-day running of the laboratory. They include systems to ensure incubators and refrigerators are constantly running at the right temperature. Every test kit and all culture media are quality controlled by the manufacturer and further controlled by the inclusion of positive and negative controls. Automated systems are regularly quality-controlled according to the manufacturer's instructions; every batch of slides to be stained includes a positive control; susceptibility tests use control organisms every day.

7.4   WORKING SAFELY IN MICROBIOLOGY

The culture of working safely is so well embedded into microbiology laboratories that it becomes second nature to everyone working there. Achieving this safe working environment does, however, involve a considerable amount of planning, effective training, due regard to legal requirements and continuous monitoring and audit. The very nature of the specimens and investigations dictates that:

■ personnel must be protected from the infectious agents likely to be present in the clinical specimens
■ appropriate precautions and containment must be available for working with the more hazardous pathogens
■ effective disposal systems must be in place to prevent further contamination of individuals and the environment.

Safety is a responsibility for all and a legal requirement

An employee's safety at work is protected by both civil and criminal law. Health and safety civil law is based on an employer's 'duty of care' and obliges them to provide a safe place of work with systems and training to ensure the health, safety and welfare of all employees as far as is reasonably practicable. Any legal action is based on an accusation of negligence.

Criminal law encompasses many aspects of health and safety legislation. One of the earliest pieces of legislation, 'The Health and Safety at Work Act (1974)', states that all members of staff have a duty "to take care for the health and safety of themselves and of other persons who may be affected by their acts or omissions at work". This Act established the Health and Safety Commission (now the Health and Safety Executive), which defined the duties of employers and employees and the roles of workplace safety committees and union safety representatives. Health and safety at work is also regulated by European EC directives including the Management of Health and Safety at Work regulations of 1992 and 1999.

Employers are obliged to "ensure, as far as is reasonably practicable, the health, safety and welfare of all employees". They must provide:

■ safe plant and safe systems of work
■ safety in the use, handling and storage of articles and substances (Manual Handling Operations Regulations 1992, amended 2002)
■ information, instruction, supervision and training
■ a safe place to work with safe access to and egress from
■ a safe and healthy working environment (including provision of personal protective equipment)
■ management of occupational illness and accidents, reporting as appropriate under RIDDOR (Reporting of Injuries, Diseases and Dangerous Occurrences Regulations).

They must also prepare a written organizational health and safety policy and a local health and safety policy. In every laboratory it is mandatory to display a poster outlining the main responsibilities of the employer and employees.

The Health and Safety Executive (HSE) provides enforcement action by inspection and has a legal right of entry to workplaces. It can issue improvement or prohibition notices and prosecute under health and safety law. It also publishes approved codes of practice, advice and guidance; the Advisory Committee on Dangerous Pathogens (ACDP) is a good example of their activity. The HSE maintains a useful website and produces numerous publications to help staff comply with the current UK regulations.

The Control of Substances Hazardous to Health (COSHH) regulations introduced in 2004 have had a considerable impact on practice in microbiology. It is therefore important that everyone working in the laboratory engages with the documentation and the processes and their role in their implementation. All chemicals and other hazardous substances must be risk assessed and appropriate safety measures for their use put into place. Initially this was a daunting task, given how many different chemicals and reagents are used within the average working day. Now it is incorporated into practice and the process is less laborious, as all new test kits and reagents have COSHH assessments included.

Quality policy also includes commitments to the health, safety and welfare of all staff and visitors to the laboratory. CPA accreditation includes specific standards relating to health and safety. Standard C5 states that "a health and safety statement, and procedures to implement it, are required to ensure a safe environment in the laboratory for staff, patients and visitors". Subsections of this standard outline the requirement for containment facilities conforming to ACDP guidelines appropriate to the type of investigation, and the requirement that work areas must be clean, uncluttered and well-maintained with evidence of "good housekeeping procedures". Most of the pathogens and specimens encountered in the microbiology laboratory are Category 2, with the notable exceptions of tuberculosis, *Escherichia coli* O157 and mycobacteria. *Box 7.1* outlines the four categories of biological agents. The ACDP of the HSE provides a full approved list of biological agents on its website. All laboratories should have a Health and Safety Officer and the laboratory management has a responsibility for defining and implementing appropriate procedures and all staff must be aware of them.

Box 7.1 Classification of pathogens into hazard groups

The Advisory Committee on Dangerous Pathogens (ACDP) supplies a list of the four hazard groups of microorganisms. This is based on how pathogenic the microorganisms are to humans, the risk to laboratory workers, how easily they are transmitted in the community and whether there is any prophylaxis (protection by immunization or antimicrobials) available:

- Group 1 organisms are most unlikely to cause human disease.
- Group 2 organisms are the most often encountered group in clinical microbiology. Laboratory exposure to them rarely causes infection and prophylactic treatment is usually available. Group 2 are the most frequently encountered in clinical specimens submitted to the clinical microbiology laboratory. They are cultured and tested on the bench with due consideration to health and safety regulations, for example personal protective equipment, provision for their safe disposal of equipment and cultures. They include *Staphylococci*, *Streptococci* and *Salmonella* species (but not *Salmonella typhi*), *Campylobacter*, *Escherichia coli* (excluding cultures of *E. coli* O157), herpesviruses, adenoviruses and picornaviruses.
- Group 3 includes organisms that cause severe human disease and are serious hazards to laboratory workers, and may present a risk to the community. There is usually prophylactic treatment available. Samples suspected of containing these pathogens are dealt with in appropriate containment level 3 facilities. Examples include any specimen suspected of containing tuberculosis, HIV, hepatitis B, *Escherichia coli* O157, *Salmonella typhi* or *Histoplasma capsulatum*.
- Category 4 organisms cause severe human disease and are a serious hazard to laboratory workers. This category includes Lassa fever, filoviruses, smallpox and Crimean Congo haemorrhagic fever. Any clinical specimen suspected of containing one of these viruses is sent to an appropriate Category 4 containment laboratory and the HSE is informed.

Working safely within the law

The culture of working safely begins as soon as employees start to work in the laboratory, with health and safety training that includes laboratory policy and instruction in every area in which they work. They must be shown where all the policies are kept and made aware of safety notices and equipment for dealing with broken samples or spillages. There will be procedures for decontamination of equipment and work areas, disposal and handling of contaminated waste, safe working practices incorporated into SOPs, and the provision of personal protective equipment. Periodic inspections will be made to identify any unsafe working practices and all visitors will be supervised effectively. Hazardous substances will be handled and stored in a safe manner.

A further important aspect of working in microbiology is a visit to the Occupational Health department, where a record of the individual's vaccination status is kept and further courses of injections given as necessary. All microbiology personnel must be vaccinated against rubella, tuberculosis, and hepatitis B in addition to the normal childhood vaccination schedule. They may also be offered influenza and typhoid vaccinations. There is no prophylactic protection for HIV and therefore all specimens must be treated as potentially infectious and handled appropriately. Employees must also take reasonable care for their own and other people's safety and cooperate with their employer and others to improve health and safety. They also have a responsibility to report unsafe equipment and working practices, accidents and near misses.

Personal protective equipment (PPE)

Laboratory coats must be worn at all times when working in the laboratory and removed when leaving the work area, for whatever reason. Howie coats should be worn closed up to the neck and with safety cuffs on the sleeves. Howie coats are full length, designed to offer the same protection when sitting, have quick-release studs or Velcro, are absorbent to protect clothing underneath and should not shrink with autoclaving. Laboratory coats should be stored separately, away from uncontaminated clothing, usually on a set of hooks within the laboratory near

---

Box 7.2 A typical microbiology laboratory scenario

It is a busy Monday morning in specimen reception. A nurse on Nightingale ward phones to say that she is sending two specimens from a patient, Mr Reginald Ramsbottom. One is a faecal sample to test for the presence of *Clostridium difficile* toxin as the patient has diarrhoea after taking antibiotics, and the other is a set of blood cultures as he has a raised temperature. She comments that he is very difficult to venepuncture.

The specimens arrive. The faecal sample has leaked into the plastic bag and the container is unlabelled. The blood cultures have been labelled 'Archie Rowe', although the request card has a typed hospital label with all the appropriate information for Reginald Ramsbottom. When the ward is telephoned to report that the faecal specimen is unlabelled and unfit to test for health and safety reasons, and that the blood cultures are inconsistently labelled, the ward sister sounds very irritated and says she is very busy and short staffed; of course the specimens were taken from Reginald – was her word being doubted? Archie is in the next bed and she certainly did not take blood from him and anyway, he hasn't got diarrhoea.

What would be the correct course of action in a situation like this?

hand washing facilities. The hand-basin should ideally be sited near the exit; taps should be operated without using the hands, with liquid soap and paper towels available. Disposable gloves are also worn when dealing with clinical samples, but should be removed to work at the computer or answer the telephone, as they are potential contaminants for other people using the equipment. Personal protective equipment will also include goggles to prevent splashes to the eye when dealing with liquid cultures. At the end of the working day all laboratory work surfaces must be decontaminated using an appropriate disinfecting agent. This will vary between laboratories but will usually be a chlorine-based compound such as Tristel. The active compound of Tristel, chlorine dioxide, is selectively toxic to microorganisms, reacting with the basic molecular structure of the cell proteins. Any disinfecting agent used in microbiology must be sporicidal (able to kill spores), mycobactericidal, bactericidal and virucidal.

Separate gowns and protective equipment are used when working in the containment level 3 room. Sometimes this facility comprises a suite of rooms with a controlled entry system. There are clear guidelines governing the design and use of Category 3 facilities and these form an important part of the CPA.

7.5   STANDARD OPERATING PROCEDURES

SOPs are developed by combining knowledge of the likely pathogens to be isolated from a particular specimen and site, the optimum identification methods, and a recognition of evidence-based practice.

SOPs are integral to the quality assurance process of laboratories and ensure that all specimens are analysed by the same methods on all occasions and by all biomedical scientists. SOPs cover all aspects of the sample journey from receipt to disposal. They form part of the evidence for CPA accreditations and a record of signatures is kept to demonstrate that everyone involved in carrying out the procedures has read and agreed to follow them. They provide an extremely useful source of information for on-call work, especially if the biomedical scientist has not been working in the section recently. For bacterial culture, each SOP is based on knowledge of the most likely pathogens to be isolated from the site or specimen type and outlines the range of culture media to be inoculated. This will also be related to the patient's clinical history; for example, extra culture plates would be required for a sputum specimen from a cystic fibrosis patient, or for a faecal sample where the patient has a history of travel to an endemic area. The SOP will also contain details of incubation time, atmosphere and temperature, and give guidelines on the reading of the culture plates the following day. It will specify which bacteria will require susceptibility testing and with which antibiotics, and then give guidelines on the reporting of the results. There will also be an SOP for susceptibility testing of all specimens. SOPs for automated methods, for example in virology or molecular techniques, will describe the specimen requirements and the detailed method and interpretation of results. The HPA Standards Unit in the Evaluation and Standards Laboratory develops detailed and comprehensive national standard methods which are used throughout their laboratories in the UK.

New techniques and methods are introduced as appropriate, often as a result of evidence-based practice, and these necessitate the updating of SOPs or the introduction of a new one. Research may demonstrate that a novel culture medium, perhaps a chromogenic one, will give better identification and separation of mixed cultures of urine samples or enhanced recognition of faecal pathogens. The new medium is then tested in parallel with the existing method, prior to replacing it. The introduction of automated continuous monitoring for culturing mycobacteria from clinical specimens, rather than the gold standard of culture on Lowenstein–Jensen slopes, was based on sound evidence that the bacteria grew better in liquid culture medium and that the time to detection was reduced.

SOPs are important for quality management, but should not be used as a limited 'recipe' for success. They may not represent the only method available, but the one selected for their particular laboratory. Registered biomedical scientists should also be aware, through their continued education and training, of the advantages, limitations and interpretation of the procedures, the theory behind them and also the alternative methods available.

SUGGESTED FURTHER READING

Ajeneye, F. (2007) Pre-analytical quality assurance: a biomedical science perspective. *The Biomedical Scientist*, **51:** 86–87.

Ames, D. (2009) Do CPA standards reflect ISO quality management principles? *The Biomedical Scientist*, **53:** 472–474.

Eydmann, M. (2011) Introduction of MALDI-TOF: a revolution in diagnostic microbiology. *The Biomedical Scientist*, **55:** 5.

Health and Safety Executive (2002) *COSHH: a brief guide to the regulations.* Available from www.hse.gov.uk/pubns/leaflets.htm.

Health and Safety Executive (2003) *Health and Safety regulation, a short guide.* Available from www.hse.gov.uk/pubns/leaflets.htm.

Institute of Biomedical Science (1996) *Code of Professional Conduct and Code of Practice for Biomedical Science Laboratories.* Institute of Biomedical Science.

Report of the working party of the Royal College of Pathologists (1995) *Retention and Storage of Pathological Records and Archives.* Royal College of Pathologists.

Royal College of Pathologists (2006) *Evaluating and introducing new diagnostic tests: The need for a national strategy.* Royal College of Pathologists.

Talbot, G. (2007) Accreditation or certification – implications for the laboratory. *The Biomedical Scientist*, **51:** 267–270.

Womack, C. (2008) Human Tissue Authority regulation: the impact on tissue research. *The Biomedical Scientist*, **52:** 387–390.

Clinical Pathology Accreditation details available from www.cpa-uk.co.uk

NHS operating framework 2008–9 available from www.dh.gov.uk

The Human Tissue Act (2004) available from www.parliament.the-stationery-office.co.uk

Tristel's biocidal action available from www.tristel.com/laboratories.html

HMSO publications: HSE ACDP, the approved list of biological agents. Available from www.hse.gov.uk

SELF-ASSESSMENT QUESTIONS

1. What are the minimum requirements for patient identification on a specimen sample and request form?
2. Describe some of the factors that will influence the quality of the result obtained from a clinical sample.
3. What is the role of NEQAS in quality assurance and quality control?
4. Why is it important to have clear guidelines for the storage and disposal of microbiological specimens?
5. Employers have a duty under the Health and Safety at Work Act to provide a safe working environment. Outline the main requirements.
6. What do the initials COSHH stand for? What impact does this have on daily work in the laboratory?
7. What essential items of personal protective equipment (PPE) are required for safe working with a microbiological sample?
8. Why are standard operating procedures so important to the overall quality assurance of a laboratory?
9. What is meant by the term 'evidence-based practice'?
10. Why is it important to ensure that the correct type of clinical specimen is received for culture and diagnosis of infection?

Answers to self-assessment questions provided at:
www.scionpublishing.com/medmicro

The laboratory investigation of urinary tract infections

Learning objectives
After studying this chapter you should confidently be able to:

■ **Outline the types of urine specimen received in clinical microbiology laboratories**
Urine samples can be midstream (which avoids contamination with normal flora and epithelial cells), catheter urine taken from the collection bag, specimens taken from babies into bags, suprapubic aspirates where urine is aspirated directly from the bladder, and conduit urines. Early morning urine samples are required for testing for mycobacteria.

■ **Describe the structure of the urinary tract in males and females**
The urinary tract comprises the kidneys, ureters, urinary bladder and urethra. Valves at the distal ends of the ureters prevent reflux. The detrusor muscle at the bladder / urethra junction forms the urethral sphincter to prevent leakage, and the external urethral sphincter allows urine to be passed.

■ **Explain the normal flora of the area and the natural defence systems in place to protect the individual from infection**
Defence of the area is provided by the flushing mechanism whenever urine is voided, by high levels of urea and variable pH, by the presence of the resident flora on the mucosal surfaces, and by secretions on to the mucosal epithelium.

■ **Discuss the causes of urinary tract infections (UTIs)**
Infections of the upper urinary tract and of the kidneys are most commonly the result of structural abnormalities, urinary reflux, spread of bacteria to the kidneys in the bloodstream, renal calculi (stones) and ascending infection from the bladder. Lower urinary tract infection is more common and arises from bladder obstruction, bladder tumours, autoinfection, pregnancy, catheterization, anatomical abnormalities, and neurological defects. Diabetic patients are also more prone to urinary tract infections.

■ **Describe the causative organisms and their laboratory diagnosis**
The bacteria most commonly associated with urinary tract infections are *Escherichia coli*, other coliforms, *Pseudomonas* species, staphylococci (coagulase-positive strains including MRSA and coagulase-negative strains), enterococci and Group B streptococci, and *Candida* species. Laboratory diagnosis includes the use of microscopy for visualizing cells and casts in the urine, culture on to media that will grow and differentiate the principal pathogens, and tests for antibiotic susceptibility where indicated.

8.1   SPECIMEN COLLECTION AND TRANSPORT

Urine specimens usually constitute the highest volume of requests in routine diagnostic laboratories and originate from all departments of the hospital – wards, outpatients, specialist units and antenatal clinics. Large numbers are also sent by GPs and from residential nursing homes. Urine samples are non-invasive specimens and in the majority of cases are collected by the patients themselves.

Types of specimen

Midstream urine

Midstream urine (MSU) is the ideal specimen for testing as it most closely represents the composition of the urine in the bladder. The patient is advised not to collect the first volume of urine passed as this will contain more epithelial cells with their normal flora attached, and may give a false impression of the bladder flora. The midstream specimen is then collected in the sterile container provided.

Catheter urine

Catheter samples of urine (CSU) are taken from patients with indwelling urinary catheters, where a tube passed through the urethra drains urine directly from the bladder into a collection bag attached either to the patient's leg or hooked onto the side of the bed. Urine samples are taken from the tap at the end of the collection bag into an appropriate sterile container. It is important that the request form clearly indicates that the sample is from a catheter because this type of specimen is more likely to contain mixed organisms and lead to misinterpretation of the results. Bacteria may be colonizing the catheter itself and forming biofilms on the surface rather than causing a genuine urinary tract infection (UTI).

Bag urines, suprapubic aspirates and conduit urines

Young babies sometimes have urine collected in a bag fitted inside the nappy instead of an attempt being made to collect a midstream specimen; however, this can be prone to contamination. A suprapubic aspirate (SPA), where urine is collected directly from the bladder by means of a needle and syringe, is seen as the gold standard for the diagnosis of UTI, as this procedure significantly reduces the risk of contamination.

Where patients have undergone procedures to drain their urine by means of a conduit from the ureter, the request form will indicate that the specimen is a conduit urine. Again it is important to be aware of this, as any bacteria found in conduit urine are likely to be significant.

Early morning urine for tuberculosis investigation

If a clinical diagnosis of tuberculosis is suspected, three consecutive early morning urines are requested. These specimens are processed along with other specimens to be investigated for the presence of mycobacteria in a Category 3 containment area.

Urine specimens for chlamydia testing

Urine testing for *Chlamydia trachomatis* is usually performed in a different section of the laboratory and the sample required would be a clean catch first specimen of the morning. This is to ensure that if chlamydia elementary bodies are present, they will be in sufficient concentrations to be detected.

Specimen containers

Bacteria are able to multiply rapidly; the doubling time of *Escherichia coli*, for example, is about 20–30 minutes and this is encouraged in warm conditions. If a sample takes a long time to reach the laboratory it is not difficult to calculate the increase in the number of bacteria and to realize this is likely to result in a falsely elevated result. For this reason specimen containers containing a preservative, usually boric acid, are used. The boric acid is present as soluble granules and these are usually contained in red-topped universal bottles. Urine specimens in boric acid remain stable for between 48 and 96 hours. For some urine tests in other areas of pathology, boric acid samples are not appropriate; for example pregnancy tests, when a plain universal bottle has to be used. Delays in testing will have an adverse effect on the validity of the results reported. Refrigeration will help to stabilize the bacterial count but cannot prevent the breakdown of white cells.

Specimen reception

All samples are checked for their points of identification and to ensure that the specimen sample matches the accompanying request card (see *Chapter 7*). Patient

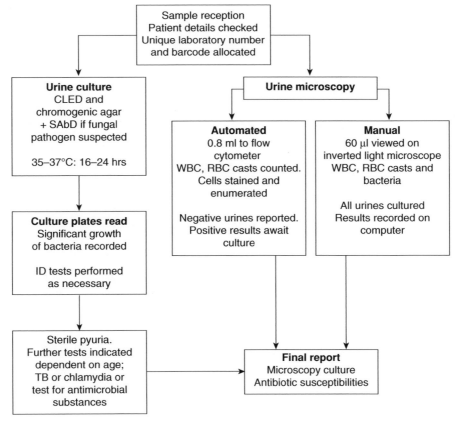

Figure 8.1
Principal steps involved in investigation of UTI.

details are then entered on to the computer system and the specimens placed into racks and taken to the urine section. A flow diagram for the processing of urine specimens is shown in *Figure 8.1*.

8.2   SOURCES AND SYMPTOMS OF INFECTION

UTIs occur relatively frequently in the population. Before exploring the reasons for this it is useful to be aware of the structure of the male and female urinary tracts, the normal defence mechanisms and the definition of a UTI (see *Figure 8.2*).

Structure of the urinary tract

The urinary tract consists of the kidneys, ureters, urinary bladder and the urethra. Urine created from filtration and absorption in the kidneys passes via the ureters to the bladder. Reflux (backflow) into the ureters is prevented by the closing of the distal ends of the ureters via the cysto-ureteric valves when there is an increase in bladder pressure during filling. The urethra, a thin-walled muscular tube, drains the urine from the bladder to the outside of the body. The detrusor muscle, part of the bladder wall, is thicker at the junction between the bladder and urethra and forms

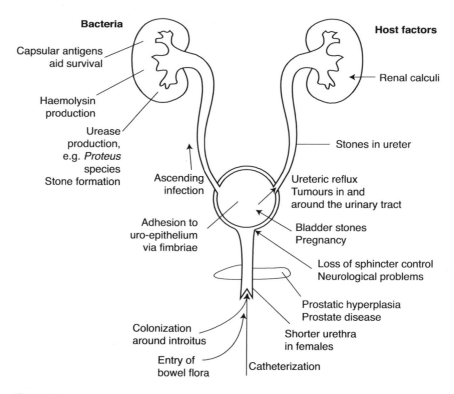

Figure 8.2
Factors influencing the development of urinary tract infection.

the internal urethral sphincter. This is an involuntarily controlled sphincter that prevents urine leaking out, and together with the external urethral sphincter, which is under voluntary control, allows urine to be passed.

In males the prostate gland surrounds the bladder neck and the urethra serves the double purpose of carrying semen as well as urine out of the body. The male urethra is considerably longer than in females (20 cm in total compared to 3–4 cm), passing through the penis before opening at the external urethral orifice.

These anatomical differences are important in understanding the differences in occurrence and frequency of UTIs in males and females.

Defence mechanisms

There are several discrete defence mechanisms that together protect the area from infection most of the time: mechanical methods, the presence of normal flora, protection given by the mucosal epithelium and the presence of Tamm–Horsfall protein.

Bacteria have to be able to reach the bladder in order to cause infection and to do this they have to ascend the urethra. Every time urine is voided the flushing mechanism will wash them from the epithelial surface. Small numbers of bacteria present in the bladder would also be phagocytosed by neutrophils. Any bacteria that make a successful attachment to the epithelial cells also risk being shed along with the uppermost layer of these cells. Attachment itself will also be made more difficult by the presence of normal flora occupying the receptor sites on the epithelial cells.

Tamm–Horsfall protein (THP) is present in large quantities in normal urine. The glycoprotein, also known as uromodulin, is produced in the ascending limb of the loop of Henle and is the protein constituent of renal casts and stones. THP is involved in the defence of the urinary tract in two ways; first, the protein inhibits the crystallization of calcium in the tract, and secondly it helps prevent the attachment of key uropathogens to the mucosa. Uropathogenic *Escherichia coli* possess variant type 1 fimbriae. THP binds to these fimbriae and traps them via its mannose molecules. The protein is also thought to be a defence factor against *Proteus mirabilis*. Defective protein, or low levels thereof, may lead to the formation of renal stones and THP is also deposited in areas of necrosis and inflammation.

Colonization by invading bacteria is further deterred by the secretion of secretory IgA and bacterial peptides from the mucosal epithelium. The presence of high levels of urea and varying levels of pH and osmolarity also help to discourage bacterial colonization (see *Chapter 4*). Prostatic fluid in males has also been shown to prevent the growth of some of the common pathogens and provides a further protective mechanism.

Definition of a UTI

The generally accepted definition of a UTI is the presence of microorganisms in the urinary tract with significant bacteriuria (bacteria in the urine) of $>10^8/l$, or $10^5/ml$ in pure culture. This figure was determined from studies performed by Kass, who counted the number of bacteria in large numbers of normal and infected urines. As with many definitions this is a general guide, as experience working in the urine section of the laboratory will provide exceptions to the rule. Non-infected urines will contain a mixture of bacteria that are representative of the normal flora acquired as the urine passes through the urethra. Genuine UTIs are usually characterized by the presence of a single causative organism rather than mixed growth.

Predisposing factors and symptoms of UTI

Microorganisms are able to cause infection in all areas of the urinary tract although they most commonly occur in the lower part, the bladder. The causes and predisposing factors are different for the upper urinary tract (infection of the kidneys) compared with the lower part of the tract. However, the difference between the two becomes blurred because an infection originating in the lower urinary tract may ascend via the ureters and cause symptoms in the upper tract. Acute pyelonephritis is the result of an infection and inflammatory process involving the kidneys.

Bacterial cystitis, or acute uncomplicated cystitis, is a bladder infection characterized by significant bacteriuria, pyuria (white cells in the urine) and sometimes haematuria (presence of blood in the urine). There is also pain associated with the lower abdomen and back, the onset is abrupt and it occurs most often in women.

Predisposing factors

Upper UTIs are most commonly caused by structural abnormalities, urinary reflux, haematogenous spread of bacteria, the presence of renal calculi and ascending infection from the bladder.

Any congenital abnormality that tends to obstruct the flow of urine will predispose the person to recurrent UTIs. If frequent UTIs occur in young children the possibility of anatomical abnormalities should be investigated to avoid future damage to the kidneys. Abnormality in the structure of the kidney itself will affect the normal renal outflow from the pelvis of the kidney. Ureteric reflux is the result of urine flowing back up the ureters, and may be caused by a ureteric abnormality, such as reduced length or presence of an extra ureter, or malfunction of the junction between the bladder and the ureter. Similarly, abnormalities in the structure of the urethra will prevent adequate emptying of the bladder.

If the patient is suffering from septicaemia, infection of the kidney may occur from bacteria arriving in the bloodstream. Renal calculi will also provide a surface on which bacteria can adhere and multiply. Renal abscesses located in the renal cortex may occur as a result of *Staphylococcus aureus* bacteraemia and may also arise as complications of pyelonephritis caused by Gram-negative bacilli. Perinephric abscesses may also be a complication of a UTI, occurring in patients with one or more anatomical abnormalities. They are, however, uncommon; the abscess forms in the perinephric space and may extend to adjacent structures.

Infections of the lower urinary tract may arise because of bladder obstruction, bladder tumours, autoinfection, pregnancy, catheterization, anatomical abnormalities and neurological defects. *Schistosoma haematobium* is a significant cause of damage to the bladder and urethra in populations without access to clean water in tropical and subtropical countries.

In males, an enlarged prostate will cause pressure and squeezing of the urethra and will impede the passage of urine. This can lead to over-distension of the bladder and acute or chronic urinary retention, which can be relieved by the insertion of a urinary catheter. Inflammation of the prostate may have an infectious cause if bacteria ascend from the urethra or if there is some reflux of infected urine into the prostatic ducts. Infection may arise from haematogenous spread or from the rectal area, giving rise to genitourinary symptoms. Prostatic hyperplasia is a significant cause of urinary reflux and renal complications.

Pregnant women are monitored regularly for the presence of UTIs; susceptibility is increased in pregnancy partly because of some down-regulation of the immune system and also the physical presence of the fetus pressing on the bladder. Asymptomatic bacteriuria occurs in up to 5% of pregnant women and may lead to pyelonephritis and pre-term birth if undetected.

A lower UTI is usually the result of autoinfection. The short urethra in females means that bacteria find it easier to ascend and reach the bladder, and there are already skin, vaginal and rectal bacteria and yeasts present in the area. However, there are other factors that influence the higher incidence of UTIs in women: sexual activity increases the opportunity for bacteria to access the area, and diaphragms and spermicidal creams are a further predisposing factor. Uropathogens appear to bind preferentially to vaginal epithelial cells and those around the female urethra; this binding is higher when oestrogen levels are at their peak. The majority of lower UTIs originate from the patient's own body (so-called endogenous UTIs or autoinfection). Heavy colonization of the urethral area by normal flora will increase the opportunity for infection.

Bladder stones and bladder tumours alter the surface of the bladder and increase bacterial adherence.

The introduction of a catheter not only bypasses the natural defences of the area but also provides a surface to which bacteria can adhere and form biofilms (complex groupings of microorganisms formed on a solid surface), facilitating their access to the bladder. When liquid containing bacteria comes into contact with an inert surface, the adherent bacteria produce a glycocalyx around them and develop a micro-environment rich in nutrients. Bacteria leaving this biofilm can then gain access to the bladder. The nature of the biofilm makes it difficult for antibiotics to penetrate and kill the bacteria.

Diabetic patients are at risk of developing infection, because of the high levels of glucose in the urine, and diabetic neuropathy, causing bladder dysfunction. The glucose provides nutrients for any bacteria present and particularly for yeasts. Neurological problems resulting in loss of sphincter control will predispose to infection. If the nerves controlling the bladder and sphincters are not functioning correctly, stale urine remains in the bladder and any bacteria present are able to multiply.

Age and sex of the individual

There are clear differences in the distribution of UTIs between the sexes. Males are more predisposed in the first 3 months of their lives, which may be due to structural abnormalities, and again in old age as a result of physiological and anatomical changes. They may develop chronic, sometimes asymptomatic, bacteriuria as a result of prostate problems, impaired immune systems and the presence of catheters. Age-related changes, with the exception of prostate problems, affect females in a similar manner. UTIs are rare in males below about 50 years of age but more prevalent in females. Between 10 and 20% of women will experience a UTI at some time (see *Figure 8.3*).

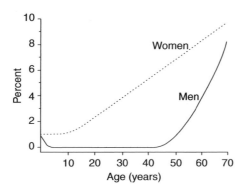

Figure 8.3
Prevalence of bacteriuria according to age and gender.

Urethritis is common in both male and female patients, often associated with a UTI and with bacterial prostatitis. Male urethritis may also be caused by sexually transmitted diseases (see *Chapter 10*), such as those resulting from infection with *Chlamydia trachomatis, Neisseria gonorrhoeae* and *Ureaplasma urealyticum,* and is often accompanied by a urethral discharge. Hospitalized patients are also more susceptible to UTI because of their general debilitated condition and the effect of drugs, instrumentation and possible catheterization.

Symptoms

The presence of dividing and dying bacteria produces an intense inflammatory response. The innate immune response is activated by the presence and shedding of bacteria on the mucosal surfaces. In an immuno-competent patient, immune cells, particularly neutrophils and lymphocytes, are attracted to the area and inflammatory cytokines are released. Evidence of this inflammatory process is seen in infected urine, which will contain white cells, red cells, and protein. If the infection involves the upper urinary tract, casts may be present, where the normal functioning of the kidney is disturbed and protein is forced through the tubules. Renal infections such as pyelonephritis are characterized by fever, chills and pain in the area of the kidneys. Cystitis and lower UTIs generally produce symptoms of urinary frequency, pain on passing urine (dysuria) and sometimes the presence of blood in the urine. The normal capacity of the bladder is about 500 ml but the acute inflammation accompanying an infection reduces this, leading to greater frequency of micturition (passing of urine). In elderly patients the inflammatory response may not give rise to these symptoms and they will present with confusion, or in the case of long-term catheterized patients, the bacteria may already have entered the bloodstream and resulted in a fever. Similarly, newborn babies may have the less obvious symptoms of poor feeding or failure to thrive.

Urine specimens are often sent to the laboratory for investigation when the patient is suffering from the need to empty the bladder at night (nocturia), bed wetting (nocturnal enuresis), incontinence, prostatism and renal colic, all of which may have an infectious cause.

8.3 PRINCIPAL PATHOGENS

In comparison with other sites of the body, relatively few types of bacteria are associated with causing infection in the urinary tract. Females in particular are easily colonized by bacteria from the urethra, including skin bacteria and microorganisms from the vaginal area and rectum.

Bacteria causing ascending infection in the urinary tract must be motile, have good adherence mechanisms and be able to survive in the presence of the innate immune defence systems. For this reason they are usually capsulated organisms.

There are several bacteria commonly associated with urinary tract infections:

- *Escherichia coli* are the most commonly isolated urinary pathogens. *E. coli* associated with UTIs (uropathogenic strains) possess K polysaccharide capsular antigens. Uropathogenic strains are also able to exhibit enhanced adhesion and ascend to cause pyelonephritis as they possess P fimbriae (pyelonephritis-associated pili), allowing enhanced adhesion to a specific galactose residue in the glycolipids of epithelial cells. Thus only certain serotypes of *E. coli* are associated with UTI.
- **Other coliforms such as *Klebsiellae, Enterobacter* species and *Proteus* species** cause infections in the bladder and are also associated with renal calculi.
- *Pseudomonas* **species infection** is often associated with infection in patients who have long-term catheters *in situ*.
- **Staphylococci,** both coagulase-positive (*Staphylococcus aureus*), MRSA and coagulase-negative staphylococci are associated with infection in all areas of the urinary tract. *S. saprophyticus* is very efficient at attaching to uro-epithelial cells and is responsible for about one-fifth of acute UTIs in healthy, sexually active young women.

Box 8.1 Case study

A 30-year-old woman presents to her GP with symptoms of frequent micturition and dysuria which she says have been getting worse over the last 7 days. She has been drinking copious amounts of cranberry juice, as advised by her mother, to try to 'flush it out' and 'not bother the doctor with it'. She now has pain in her back and abdomen and feels sick and feverish. The doctor checks her temperature, which is 38.8°C, and tests a sample of her urine for protein and blood cells, both of which are positive. He sends her urine specimen to the microbiology laboratory and prescribes trimethoprim.

The laboratory results show >100 white blood cells per high power field, and ++ red blood cells. There is a significant growth of a Gram-positive coccus, coagulase-negative and resistant to novobiocin. Antibiotic sensitivity testing confirms that the isolate is sensitive to trimethoprim.

After taking the 5-day course of antibiotics she began to feel better and made a full recovery.

Questions:

1. Why would the patient's mother have advised her to drink large amounts of fruit juice?
2. Why did the GP test her urine in the surgery for protein and blood?
3. How would you interpret the microscopy result?
4. Suggest the identity of the bacteria isolated.
5. How could you explain the fact that over the period of a week her symptoms have progressed from frequent micturition and dysuria to back pain, nausea and fever?

- **Enterococci and Group B streptococci** are both found occasionally as the cause of UTI. Enterococci are often associated with instrumentation and catheterization.
- *Candida* **species** are found particularly in diabetic urines, and in catheterized and immuno-suppressed patients.

The role of fastidious organisms such as lactobacilli, *Gardnerella vaginalis*, the more fastidious streptococci and anaerobes has been the subject of controversy for a long time and remains unresolved.

8.4   LABORATORY DIAGNOSIS

Laboratory diagnosis relies on microscopy, culture and sensitivity, and request forms received with the urine specimens will usually ask for these tests, abbreviated as 'm c & s'. The number of urine specimens sent for analysis can be so high that in some laboratories there is a screening process to exclude those falling outside certain criteria.

Biochemical testing

Biochemical urinalysis used to be routinely performed on all urine specimens along with microscopy and culture. Some laboratories may still carry out biochemical strip tests, but the practice is much less common. Often the tests will have already been performed in the ward or doctor's surgery and the additional expense is not considered beneficial to the laboratory diagnosis.

Various combinations of test strips are available to detect the presence of protein, glucose, white cells, red blood cells and haemolysis, as well as the metabolic breakdown products of bacteria such as nitrites, although the latter are not necessarily a reliable indicator of infection. The strips contain small squares of filter paper impregnated with chemicals that will change colour after immersion in urine if the analytes are present. The colour changes are then interpreted as positive or negative by comparison with information provided on the side of the strip container.

Microscopy

The macroscopic appearance of the urine can give some hints to the presence of infection; a urine sample with a high white cell count will be very cloudy and if there is a large amount of blood present, this too will be obvious. Appearances can, however, be deceptive and macroscopically clear urines will sometimes have a high level of white cells when examined microscopically; conversely, very cloudy urines may contain amorphous debris and few white cells.

Urine microscopy is performed with an inverted microscope (see *Chapter 5*) using flat-bottomed wells. Urine (60 μl) is pipetted into each of the 96 wells and allowed to settle for at least 5 minutes. Several fields of each well are then scanned to ensure the contents are evenly distributed and a count of the cells performed. The results are recorded on to the computer system, either manually or via a voice recognition system. Disposable counting chambers are sometimes used for laboratories handling low volume numbers of urine specimens.

White cells (pus cells). The number of white blood cells is recorded as <10 or >10 per high power field, usually by entering the result into the appropriate computer screen and using the parameters and codes relevant to the laboratory system. White cells are present in very low numbers in urine from healthy patients but are usually present in large numbers in infected urine.

Red blood cells. Red cells will appear either as intact discs or as crenated (having a notched edge) red cells. The presence of red cells in urine (haematuria) may be indicative of trauma associated with infection, renal damage, endocarditis, immune complex disease, renal calculi and non-infective pathological conditions, but may also be due to contamination from menstruation in women.

Epithelial cells. The presence of squamous epithelial cells is an indication of the level of contamination of the sample, as they are shed with the first flush of urine and coated with skin flora.

Figure 8.4 shows the presence of red cells, white cells, epithelial cells and bacteria in a urine sample.

Casts. These are formed from protein forced through the renal tubules and, depending on the nature of the casts, their presence can be highly suggestive of renal damage. Identification of the type of cast is therefore important and if a urine sample is found to contain a large number of casts the result is telephoned to the requesting doctor.

■ Hyaline casts appear as hollow cylinders and may be indicative of renal disease, but may also be present after strenuous exercise or in patients with a fever (see *Figure 8.5*).

■ Granular casts (see *Figure 8.6*) and cellular casts are found in cases of pyelonephritis and glomerulonephritis. Cellular casts may contain white or red blood cells. Red cell casts are associated with post-streptococcal nephritis.

Crystals. With the introduction of boric acid as a preservative, the pH of the urine is lower, and so crystals associated with alkaline urine are rarely seen. Boric acid

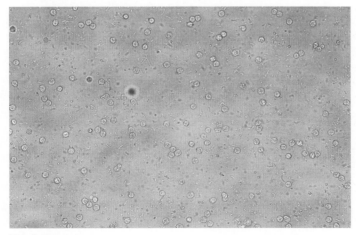

Figure 8.4
Infected urine.

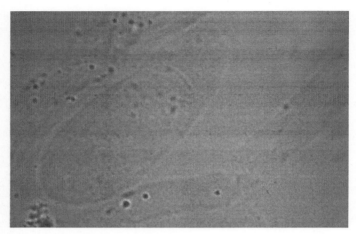

Figure 8.5
Hyaline casts.

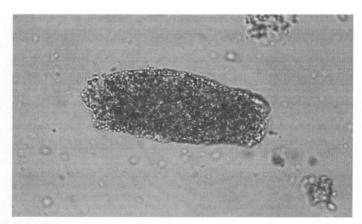

Figure 8.6
Granular casts.

crystals may be present and sometimes those of uric acid. Uric acid crystals may be an indication of dehydration, rhubarb consumption or the presence of renal calculi.

Flow cytometry has replaced conventional microscopy in some laboratories, and the principle of this procedure is explained in *Box 8.2*.

Urine culture

The range of culture media and techniques has increased considerably in recent years. The guiding principles in urine culture are to provide a means of easily identifying the bacteria of significance, to suppress the growth of other bacteria such as diphtheroids, lactobacilli and micrococci, and to prevent the swarming of *Proteus* species.

Other considerations will include the cost-effectiveness and efficiency of the system chosen, particularly as large numbers of urine specimens are processed daily.

Box 8.2 The use of flow cytometry for analysing urine samples

The principle of flow cytometry is measurement of light scattered by particles as they pass through a laser beam. The system can be used in a variety of laboratory settings and disciplines, differentiating blood components in haematology, detecting cells labelled with specific antibodies, or in urine analysis by the size and nature of the different particles. Using the Sysmex UF-1000i analyser as an example, the urine sample is automatically mixed and 0.8 ml is aspirated and stained in two channels of the machine with two specific fluorescent polymethine dyes, one for bacteria, the second for the components of the sediment of the urine, blood cells, epithelial cells and casts. The samples are then delivered to the flow cell using a system of hydrodynamic focusing to ensure that each particle passes through the laser beam individually. The scattered light from each particle is detected by a photo diode at two different positions, to measure forward and side scatter. This is converted into electric signals along with intensity of fluorescence. The forward scatter measures the size of the particle and the side scatter provides information on the surface and internal complexity. The intensity of the fluorescence gives information on the nucleic acid content. The system combines all the signals, and classifies and counts all bacteria, yeast-like cells, red and white blood cells, different types of casts, epithelial cells, spermatozoa and crystals.

Because they are stained separately the system can detect bacteria to a level of 10^2–10^3 per ml. This level of accuracy, accompanied by the white cell count, allows laboratories to make decisions about whether to culture all urines regardless of their flow cytometry result, or whether to set cut-off limits, allowing negative urines to be reported earlier.

CLED medium

CLED (cystine, lysine, electrolyte deficient) medium has been routinely used in diagnostic laboratories and while it is still the medium of choice for many, the development of chromogenic agar has provided an alternative. One disadvantage of CLED is that it is possible to miss the fact that a specimen may contain mixed organisms rather than a pure culture, as several genera of bacteria have similar colour colonies on this medium. However, it is useful for the diagnosis of urinary pathogens as it suppresses the growth of diphtheroids, lactobacilli and micrococci, and the electrolyte deficiency prevents the swarming of *Proteus* species. Andrade's indicator (acid fuchsin) is often added to the medium to differentiate between lactose fermenting and non-lactose fermenting bacteria.

The urine may be directly inoculated on to the medium with a 1 µl sterile loop, using a quarter of the plate for each specimen. Alternatively the medium can be inoculated by an automated multipoint method such as the Mastascan system.

Chromogenic agar

Chromogenic agar has been introduced into urinary culture relatively recently. The agar contains various substrates specific to different bacteria. As the substrate is broken down by enzymes present in the growing bacteria, chromophores are released and a characteristically coloured colony produced, allowing presumptive identification of the bacteria. An example of this is the Oxoid chromogenic UTI medium that contains two chromogens. The first of these is X-gluc, a chromogen cleaved by the enzyme β-glucosidase and present in enterococci, with the formation of blue colonies; the second is Red-Gal cleaved by β-D-galactosidase in *Escherichia coli*, resulting in pink colonies. Other coliform bacteria cleave both chromogens and are visualized as purple colonies. The activity of tryptophan deaminase, produced by *Proteus*, *Morganella* and *Providentia* species, uses tryptophan in the media as a substrate and brown colonies are produced (see *Table 8.1*).

Table 8.1 Colour changes produced by Oxoid chromogenic UTI medium

Organism	β-D-galactosidase	β-glucosidase	Tryptophan deaminase	Colony colour
Enterococci		+		Blue
Escherichia coli	+			Pink
Coliforms	+	+		Purple
Proteus, Morganella and *Providentia* species			+	Brown
Pseudomonas				Fluorescence
Staphylococcus				Normal pigmentation

Chromogenic agar is more expensive to use than conventional agar and the cost may to some extent be offset by testing a greater number of samples on each culture plate or by using commercially prepared strips of agar in individual wells. There are also differences in the product specificity from different manufacturers. One method of making each culture plate more cost-effective is to dip a small piece of filter paper into the urine and then place this on to the culture medium, allowing more samples to be tested. Alternatively, commercially supplied strips of wells containing agar can be inoculated as part of a multipoint inoculation procedure.

The Mastascan system is an example of a combined identification and antibiotic susceptibility system, carried out in microtitre trays. The multipoint inoculator transfers 1 µl of urine from the microtitre plate used for the microscopy. Each urine is tested on: chromogenic agar, GPOS to identify Gram-positive organisms, and one containing a phenylpyruvic acid (PPA) plate for identifying *Proteus* species by the deamination of phenylalanine. The urine is also tested against a panel of antibiotics. The plates are photographed by the Mastascan and the result recorded. The antibiotic susceptibilities are recorded as growth (resistant) or no growth (sensitive).

The decision to culture all urines, whether or not the microscopy or flow cytometry results suggest infection, is constantly under study and review.

Incubation, reading and interpretation of results

The culture plates are incubated at 37°C overnight and then read either manually or by a plate reader and checked manually. Growth, categorized as heavy, significant (>100 colonies), moderate (10–100 colonies), scanty (1–10 colonies), mixed, or no significant growth, can be recorded manually, or entered into the relevant field on the computer. The identification of the bacterial growth is also recorded along with the antibiotic susceptibility profile. The interpretation of the number of colonies is dependent on the volume of urine inoculated on to the culture medium. Using the Kass interpretation of >10^8/l, with 10^5/ml of pure growth being a significant

UTI, *Table 8.2* gives guidance on the significance of colony counts using different inoculum sizes (this does not apply to the filter paper technique). For example, if a 2 µl loop is used to inoculate a culture plate, 200 CFU of a pure culture of bacteria suggests a significant infection.

Table 8.2 Interpretation of colony counts from urine culture

Number of colony-forming units (CFU) counted using volume of:					
	0.3 µl	1 µl	2 µl	5 µl	10 µl
10^6 CFU / l	-	-	-	5	10
10^7 CFU / l	3	10	20	50	100
10^8 CFU / l	30	100	200	500	1000

Sometimes further tests may be necessary to confirm the identity of the bacteria, and these may include coagulase and DNase for staphylococci. The coagulase-negative species *Staphylococcus saprophyticus* and *S. epidermidis* may be distinguished by testing with novobiocin; *S. saprophyticus* is resistant to the antibiotic. The presence of MRSA will be detected by the sensitivity pattern of a *Staphylococcus aureus*.

If CLED agar is used, coliforms can be differentiated by lactose fermentation. Non-lactose fermenting Gram-negative rods suspected of being *Pseudomonas* species can be further tested for oxidase (they are oxidase-positive). *Proteus* species are oxidase-negative and urease-positive. *Pseudomonas* species are intrinsically resistant to some of the antibiotics routinely used for UTI and so require susceptibility testing against a further selection of antibiotics suitable for their treatment in urinary infection.

Streptococci can be Lancefield grouped; identification of groups B and D enterococci can be achieved by inoculating Islam's or Granada medium and using aesculin plates. The majority of group B will have orange pigment after overnight anaerobic incubation on Granada or Islam's media, both of which demonstrate the carotenoid pigment produced by these bacteria, and enterococci will have black pigment around the growth on an aesculin culture plate.

At this point, significant growth of bacteria can be identified and reported along with the microscopy results. Interpretation of the significance of the results is not always straightforward and will include consideration of the age of the patient, the age of the specimen, purity of the bacterial growth, the microscopy results, the type of urine specimen and any significant clinical details. For example, a urine sample from a child may grow a single type of bacteria, but at a growth level normally considered insignificant, and along with the microscopy result and clinical details this may be reported as a significant infection with accompanying antibiotic susceptibilities. A catheter urine may well have a high level of mixed growth, indicative of colonization rather than infection.

Sterile pyuria
Large numbers of white cells (pyuria) excreted in the urine and observed on microscopy may sometimes be accompanied by no growth on the culture plate.

Possible explanations for this include the presence of antimicrobial substances in the urine because the patient has already started taking antibiotics. Some laboratories will test for antimicrobial substances by inoculating urine on to a culture medium containing a lawn of *Escherichia coli* and *Staphylococcus aureus* and observing the plate for a zone of inhibition after incubation, indicating that chemicals in the urine are killing the bacteria.

Sterile pyuria can also be investigated by centrifuging a sample of the urine in a small micro centrifuge tube and staining the pellet to look for the presence of bacteria.

If no organisms are isolated and no antimicrobial substances are present, sterile pyuria may, depending on the age of the patient, be the result of either a *Chlamydia trachomatis* infection or may indicate the presence of mycobacteria. The suggestion of further appropriate testing may be added as a comment to the final report.

Antigen testing

Individual test kits are used for the detection of specific antigens of *Streptococcus pneumoniae* and *Legionella pneumophila* in urine samples. Urine is added to the strip according to the manufacturer's instructions. The test strip contains immobilized specific antibody and substrate. If the antigen is present it binds to the antibody and a coloured product is visualized by the use of bound substrate and enzyme activity.

Schistosoma haematobium

Schistosoma haematobium ova which attach to the bladder wall may also be detected in urine samples. Haematuria is one of the most common presentations and chronic infection can lead to bladder cancer. The sample is preferably taken after exercise and between the hours of 10 am and 2 pm to ensure the maximum number of eggs are dislodged from the wall of the bladder and excreted. Specimens are collected into a boric acid container and processed as soon as possible after collection. The urine is centrifuged gently at 500 rpm for 2 minutes to minimize breaking-up of the schistosomes; the supernatent is discarded and all the deposit viewed in a flat-bottomed well normally used for urine microscopy. Alternatively the deposit can be viewed by adding drops to a microscope slide, adding a coverslip and viewing under a normal light microscope.

Automation

The sheer volume and number of urine specimens makes a fully automated procedure appear very attractive. Some automation is available for urine analysis; the Mastascan system, described above, cultures the urine by a multipoint method, and incorporates several different media types. A fully automated screening method would be extremely welcome in laboratories with a high throughput of urine specimens. Automated screening tests are based on various techniques, using the principles of particle counting, electrical impedance, photometry, or bioluminescence. There are several commercial systems that analyse particles in urine and classify them according to size, using flow cytometry (see *Box 8.2*). These machines can be used to indicate a low predictive possibility of a UTI, as they are able to detect the presence or absence of white blood cells, red blood cells, bacteria casts, etc. If infection is not likely due to the absence of white cells, bacteria, etc. then no further culture is required. Machines can be interfaced with the laboratory computer and results rapidly produced for the requesting clinicians. However, automated systems are expensive and variable in their performance and may not provide the sensitivity and level of interpretation of each specimen available (compared with current microscopy methods) to detect all clinically significant infections.

Antibiotic susceptibility testing

Identification of the causative organism in a UTI must be accompanied by appropriate guidance for antibiotic treatment. The choice of antibiotics to be tested is influenced by the efficacy of particular agents for use in UTI, and by the antibiotic policy of the hospital and the community clinicians. SOPs will then be developed and followed routinely. In a semi-automated system involving a set of media and antibiotics, such as described earlier, the breakpoint system of testing is used. Other methods include multipoint inoculation of breakpoint plates and the disc diffusion method (see *Chapter 6*). If antibiotic testing is not part of the SOP for all urine samples, the presence of large numbers of white cells in the microscopy may be used as an indication that testing should be carried out directly from the urine. This allows positive urine samples to be reported after only 24 hours. Alternatively, colonies may be taken for testing from a pure culture of significant bacteria in the absence of indicative microscopy.

Examples of antibiotics in use for the treatment of UTI include trimethoprim, amoxicillin, nitrofurantoin, nalidixic acid, ciprofloxacin, mecillinam, cephalexin and cefpodoxime. Nitrofurantoin and nalidixic acid only achieve adequate concentrations in urine and are therefore used solely in this context. *Pseudomonas* species will be resistant to many of the first-line antibiotics and will need to be tested against gentamicin and ceftazidime.

If the coliform bacteria isolated are resistant to amoxicillin and cefpodoxime, further testing is required to exclude infection with extended spectrum β-lactamase-producing bacteria. Further testing is indicated with ceftazadime, cefotaxime and cefepime, or cefpirome with and without clavulanic acid. The isolate is classified as an extended spectrum β-lactamase producer if the zone size of the antibiotic with clavulanic acid is >5 mm larger than that of the antibiotic alone. E tests with the above combinations may also be used to confirm the presence of extended β-lactamase production.

When the results of the microscopy, culture and sensitivity are complete, a report can be issued detailing the findings. This would typically record the bacteria isolated and give a list of the antibiotics tested and their sensitivities.

SUGGESTED FURTHER READING

Ivancic, V., Mastali, M., Percy, N. *et al.* (2008) Rapid antimicrobial susceptibility determination of uropathogens in clinical urine specimens by use of ATP bioluminescence. *J. Clin. Microbiol.* **46:** 1213–1219.

Jacobsen, S.M., Stickler, D.J., Mobley, H.L.T. & Shirtliff, M.E. (2009) Complicated catheter-associated urinary tract infections due to *Escherichia coli* and *Proteus mirabilis. Clin. Microbiol. Rev.* **21:** 26–59.

Manoni, F., Fornasiero, L., Ercolin, M. *et al.* (2009) Cutoff values for bacteria and leukocytes for urine flow cytometer Sysmex UF-1000i in urinary tract infections. *Diagnostic Microbiology and Infectious Disease,* **65:** 103–107.

SELF-ASSESSMENT QUESTIONS

1. Describe the different types of urine specimen that may be sent for investigation to a clinical microbiology laboratory.
2. Why are catheterized patients more prone to UTI?
3. The majority of people do not suffer from recurrent UTIs. Outline the defence systems of the body that protect the individual from such infections.
4. What would you expect to see microscopically in a) a normal urine sample, and b) infected urine?
5. Outline the principal pathogens associated with UTI.
6. Describe the factors that will guide the choice of culture media used in the investigation of urines for infection. Give two examples.
7. Chromogenic agar is used increasingly for urine culture. Describe the basis of the differentiation of the significant pathogens.
8. A pure growth of a lactose fermenting coliform of at least $10^8/l$ is observed on a CLED culture plate. What are the most likely pathogens? If the culture was a non-lactose fermenting coliform, which simple test would distinguish between *Pseudomonas* species and *Proteus* species?
9. Explain the term 'sterile pyuria'. Suggest some reasons for this and further tests that may be advised for certain patients.
10. Outline the factors influencing the choice of suitable antibiotics for urinary infections.

Answers to self-assessment questions provided at:
www.scionpublishing.com/medmicro

The laboratory investigation of gastrointestinal infection from faecal samples

Learning objectives
After studying this chapter you should confidently be able to:

■ **Discuss the sources and symptoms of gastrointestinal (GI) infections**
There are two main sources of infection: the ingestion of pathogens within contaminated food or water, or the transfer of pathogens from an infected individual to a non-infected individual by the faecal–oral route. The symptoms generally include diarrhoea, vomiting, abdominal pain, fever, passing of blood in the faeces or a change in bowel habit. Not all symptoms are experienced by all people and in all types of infections. Diarrhoea and vomiting can lead to dehydration and, if the bacterial pathogen is able to survive in the blood, susceptible patients may develop septicaemia.

■ **Describe the principal bacterial, viral, protozoan and parasitic infectious agents**
The bacterial pathogens most commonly isolated from faecal samples include *Campylobacter* species, *Salmonella* species, *Shigella* species and *Escherichia coli*. Less commonly isolated bacterial pathogens in the UK include *Vibrio* species and *Yersinia enterocolitica*. Viral pathogens include rotavirus, adenoviruses and noroviruses. *Giardia lamblia*, *Cryptosporidium parvum* and occasionally *Entamoeba histolytica* are protozoan causes of gastrointestinal infection. The ova of eukaryotic parasites may also be seen in patients with appropriate exposure in endemic areas.

■ **Discuss the pathogenesis of the microorganisms involved in infection**
Any infectious agent causing disease in the GI tract must be able to survive the extreme pH changes of gastric acid and bile. Receptor sites for attachment must be available in the GI tract. After attachment to the mucosal epithelium, gastrointestinal pathogens disrupt the normal function of the cells, by inducing uptake into normally non-phagocytic cells, releasing toxins, or destroying the villus tips. Damage to the cells induces several aspects of the host immune response and the symptoms of GI infection.

■ **Explain the current methods available to diagnose and treat gastrointestinal infection**
Bacterial pathogens are isolated on differential and selective culture media, designed to suppress as much of the normal flora as possible and to clearly differentiate colonies of interest for further identification. Microscopy and staining are used to visualize white and red blood cells in the sample and to diagnose protozoal infections, e.g. *Giardia lamblia* cysts, *Entamoeba histolytica* cysts, oocysts of *Cryptosporidium parvum*, and the ova of eukaryotic parasites.

9.1 SPECIMEN COLLECTION, TRANSPORT AND RECEPTION

In the majority of cases, faecal samples are collected by patients themselves into sterile pots provided by the requesting doctor, and sent to the laboratory as soon as possible. One exception requiring rapid transfer to the laboratory is if the presence of amoebae is suspected, as the amoebae will encyst. On arrival in the laboratory faecal samples are checked for their essential identification points – full name, date of birth, NHS number – and to ensure that the specimen sample matches the accompanying request card. The request card and specimen are then given a unique laboratory number and the patient's details are entered on to the computer system and the specimens placed

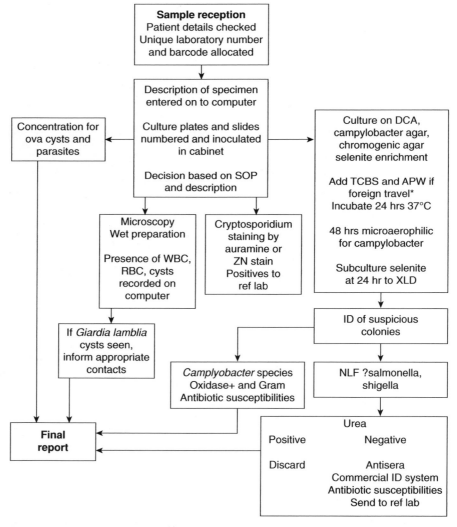

*Add selective media as necessary if possible food poisoning by *Clostridium perfringens* or *Bacillus cereus*.

Figure 9.1
Flow diagram for investigation of gastrointestinal infection from faecal samples.

into racks. The numbering and entering of the data takes place either in specimen reception or in the enteric section.

After checking that the details on the screen match the request card, a description of the faecal sample is then entered on to the relevant screen, using pre-defined codes to describe the consistency, e.g. soft-formed, watery, and whether mucus or blood are visible macroscopically. Specimens are usually processed in a Class 1 cabinet, although some laboratories will use the open bench. Personal protective equipment is worn wherever the specimens are handled. *Figure 9.1* shows a flow chart for the investigation of faecal specimens.

9.2   SOURCES AND SYMPTOMS

The majority of pathogens causing GI infection originate from ingesting contaminated food or water and may also be acquired by direct contact from an infected person. The method of transmission is usually referred to as the faecal–oral route. Some bacterial pathogens are able to grow in food or water whereas viruses require human cells in which to multiply. Protozoa and parasitic ova are ingested in an environmentally protected form, often as cysts, and require the gastrointestinal environment to change into the active, reproductive form. Bacterial toxins are also powerful infectious agents, notably those produced by *Clostridium botulinum*, *C. difficile* and *C. perfringens*, as well as *Staphylococcus aureus* and *Vibrio cholerae*. *Clostridium difficile* is associated with antibiotic use and is a significant hospital- or health care-associated infection. *Helicobacter pylori*, transmitted by the oral route, is associated with gastric ulcers and chronic infection may lead to the development of gastric carcinoma and MALT (mucosa-associated lymphoid tissue) lymphoma.

Successful pathogens of the GI tract require effective survival and attachment mechanisms and this limits the range of microorganisms. The infectious dose also varies considerably, as demonstrated by *Salmonella* species (10^6 organisms, although may be considerably fewer) and *Escherichia coli* O157 (2–3 organisms), or the low numbers of norovirus required (between 10 and 100 viral particles). In the UK the most prominent bacterial intestinal pathogen is *Campylobacter* species, followed by *Salmonella* species and *Shigella* species. Viruses such as norovirus cause more infections and outbreaks, but they are often not specifically diagnosed and are consequently under-reported because the symptoms are of a shorter duration. A patient's travel history is important, particularly if it involves tropical areas of the world where *Vibrio cholerae* is endemic, and areas where parasitic infections are more likely to occur. It is important to remember that gastrointestinal infections are a considerable cause of morbidity and mortality worldwide, with millions of children under the age of five dying annually of diarrhoea. This is often related to water supplies contaminated with human effluent, and with contaminated water supplies in overcrowded refugee camps resulting from natural disasters and conflict.

Epidemiology

The epidemiology of gastrointestinal infections varies. Some are spread from a single source and affect several people simultaneously, for example following a restaurant meal or a wedding reception. Others are sporadic, affecting one person or a family. Hepatitis A viruses, particular strains of *Escherichia coli* and some parasitic infections may be endemic to a country or geographical area with high sero-prevalence of specific antibodies, elevated levels of childhood illness and chronic parasitic infestation. When large numbers of people are affected in an outbreak situation, the disease may reach epidemic proportions, demonstrated in cholera epidemics throughout history. In the UK, incidences of gastrointestinal disease are reported to the Health Protection Agency (HPA), where epidemiological data are recorded. Incidences of a specific pathogen above the expected levels will trigger investigation. The HPA website (www.hpa.org.uk) provides an extremely useful source of data for individual types of infection. Additionally, some infections are reported locally to the Environmental Health Officer who will interview the patient to try to pinpoint the source.

Symptoms

The symptoms of gastrointestinal infection generally include diarrhoea, with or without vomiting, abdominal pain, fever, passing of blood in the faeces, or a change in bowel habits. Diarrhoea is defined as change in the frequency of bowel movements, with the passage of loose, unformed stools. Severe diarrhoea may lead to dehydration and if the pathogen is a bacterium able to survive in the bloodstream, septicaemia may be a complication in susceptible patients.

Defences

Any pathogen infecting this area must have adapted to the harsh conditions and possess virulence factors for attachment and survival. The alimentary canal from the mouth to the anus is protected by the mucoepithelial cells lining its entire surface and from specialized anatomical and physiological features of the area. The oral cavity contains high numbers of normal flora and is protected by the secretion of saliva at a neutral pH, which is able to neutralize bacterial acids. The saliva is rich in antibacterial substances including lysosyme which attacks the β1–4 linkages in the bacterial peptidoglycan. The low pH of the stomach is inhibitory to most pathogens unless they are protected by a hard outer coat, such as the cysts of *Cryptosporidia* species or *Giardia lamblia* or the spores of *Clostridia* species. Bacteria able to survive the journey beyond the stomach have acid tolerance mechanisms or, as demonstrated by the success of *Helicobacter pylori*, the ability to secrete a urease enzyme to neutralize their immediate surroundings. They also use flagellae to allow them to access their receptor sites on the gastric wall beyond the mucosal layer. Secreted enterotoxins of *Staphylococcus aureus, Streptococcus pyogenes* and *Bacillus cereus* are acid tolerant. Gastrointestinal viruses show a similar disregard for the acid conditions. Beyond the gastric area pathogens must survive the presence of bile salts and a further change in pH. This again distinguishes between those able to cause infection in the GI tract, and is used *in vitro* to select for intestinal bacterial pathogens by the addition of bile salts (sodium deoxycholate) to culture media.

The gastrointestinal area is well protected from insults by the covering of mucus over the villous surface and the specially adapted lymphoid cells of the area, known as the gastric-associated lymphoid tissue (GALT) in the Peyer's patches. Foreign antigens are sampled and appropriate antibody in the form of IgA is secreted in the mucus to protect the lumen of the tract as the food passes through. The area is one of the most densely populated with normal bacterial flora, providing colonial resistance and occupation of receptor sites. Of the normal bacterial flora, 99.9% are anaerobes, principally *Bacteroides* species and *Peptostreptococcus* species, and some *Clostridia* species, with the remaining 0.1% composed of coliforms and enterococci. The metabolic by-products, particularly of the anaerobic bacteria, make the environment unfavourable for exogenous bacteria. The normal flora comprises about 10^{11} organisms per gram of faeces and they may be the cause of endogenous infection if, through leakage or rupture of the intestine, they gain access to the peritoneal cavity.

Gastrointestinal infection is usually the result of ingestion of the infectious agent via food, in the form of bacterial contamination, viruses, spores, cysts, ova or pre-formed toxins, often in previously healthy immuno-competent individuals. There are, however, certain situations in which some people are more predisposed to infection through changes in their anatomy and physiology or by their age or immune status. Reduced stomach acidity is associated with chronic infection with *Helicobacter pylori* and a reduction in the numbers of *Vibrio cholerae* needed to cause disease. Diverticulitis, where herniated pouches of intestine are formed, may predispose to a diverticular abscess. Cholecystitis can lead to biliary sepsis and liver disease may compromise the activity of Kupffer cells to clear bacteria entering the area. Severely immuno-compromised patients are at greater risk from infection with *Cryptosporidia* as their immune systems are unable to clear the protozoan infection, resulting in chronic debilitating diarrhoea. One of the important changes leading to infection is the effect of taking antibiotics that kill the normal flora of the colon on their passage through the GI tract. This leaves more antibiotic-resistant bacteria and yeasts and also allows important receptor sites to be occupied by *Clostridium difficile* or occasionally *C. perfringens,* leading to antibiotic-associated diarrhoea, a leading cause of hospital-acquired infection and associated morbidity and mortality.

9.3 THE PRINCIPAL PATHOGENS AND THEIR PATHOGENESIS

The principal bacterial pathogens isolated from faecal samples in the UK are *Campylobacter* species, *Salmonella* species, *Shigella* species and *Escherichia coli* O157. Travellers to endemic areas must also be tested for *Cholera* species and specific strains of *E. coli*. Patients presenting with appropriate symptoms would also be tested for the presence of *Helicobacter pylori*. *Yersinia enterocolitica* is associated with mesenteric adenitis, the symptoms of which may mimic appendicitis, and may be isolated from faecal samples if suspected, using specific culture media. Bacterial infections diagnosed by toxin detection will be covered in *Section 9.7*.

Campylobacter species

These bacteria are flagellated curved Gram-negative bacteria that resemble seagull shapes in the Gram stain. Birds and poultry of all types carry the bacteria in their GI tracts and become zoonotic sources of human infection. Other animals including cats and dogs also carry the bacteria. The infection may follow the ingestion of minced meat such as hamburgers and chicken which has been insufficiently cooked, as well as infected dairy products, particularly unpasteurized milk. *Campylobacter* infections account for the largest numbers of GI infections reported to the HPA annually; almost 58 000 in 2009 and 63 000 in 2010 (HPA data). Surprisingly, the bacteria have only been recognized as an important pathogen and routinely investigated in cases of diarrhoea since the late 1970s and early 1980s; prior to that time culture media and conditions had not been optimized. A choice of selective culture media is now readily available and testing for the bacteria is part of routine faecal investigation. Human infections are usually caused by *Campylobacter jejuni* or *C. coli*. In the laboratory these may be distinguished by the hippurate test, although this is not routinely performed, and the isolates are reported as *Campylobacter* species.

The bacteria are ingested with the infected food and have an infectious dose of 10^6 organisms, although much lower numbers can also cause infection. They are able to survive the stomach acid and bile salts before reaching their receptor sites in the jejunum. The flagellae and LPS are both thought to facilitate adhesion to the mucosal epithelium. Adhesion to the mucosa, as in many bacteria, triggers the production of further virulence factors and it has been shown that as many as 14 new proteins are synthesized within 60 minutes of attachment. Toxins are released and damage to the mucosa follows, with resulting diarrhoea. The initial symptoms are not, however, of diarrhoea (which may take 4 to 5 days to occur), but of general malaise, headache, limb pains and flu-like symptoms. When the diarrhoea does occur it is frequently blood-stained. Symptoms may last for up to 2 weeks, during which time the patient is likely to visit their GP and give a stool sample for analysis. The bacteria are able to survive in the bloodstream and *Campylobacter* infection may lead to bacteraemia and septicaemia in susceptible patients. In 1999, 117 cases were recorded in the HPA data with a figure of 75 for 2004. Complications may occasionally develop after infections with certain serotypes, leading, for example, to acute demyelination of the peripheral nervous system in Guillain–Barré syndrome.

Testing for *Campylobacter* species using specialist culture media forms part of the routine investigation of faecal samples. Antibiotic susceptibility tests are carried out on all isolates and the patient will often be prescribed antibiotics (usually erythromycin or ciprofloxacin) before the result is available.

Salmonellae

There are over 2300 serological varieties (serovars) of salmonellae as a result of the ability of these Gram-negative bacilli to undergo antigenic variation. Two species of salmonella infecting animals and humans are recognized, *Salmonella enterica* and *S. bongori*. There are six subspecies of *S. enterica* containing multiple serovars. The majority of human pathogens are in the subspecies *S. enterica enterica*. Serotyping is performed as part of the identification process and can provide valuable epidemiological evidence, especially if a rare serotype is isolated, in pinpointing the source of the infection. In practice, there are a few predominant serotypes that are more commonly isolated in the UK, with more unusual serotypes sometimes being acquired from foreign travel. Of the total numbers of salmonella infections reported to the HPA in 2009 (just under 10 000) and 2010 (in the order of 9000), around 20% of isolates were *S. typhimurium*, and 33% *S. enteritidis*. Incidences of infection are at their highest in the summer and autumn and this is related to food preparation and storage in the warmer months. Serotyping is performed using antibodies specific to the O somatic antigen, H flagellar antigen and the K capsular antigen. The letter O, being the antigen on the oligosaccharide moiety of the LPS, originates from the German *ohne Hauch*, meaning 'without film', and H comes from *Hauch*, meaning a waft or aura and referring to the flagellar antigens, while K is derived from *Kapsel*, the German word for capsule. *Figure 9.2* shows the positions of these antigens on *Salmonella* species and on other Gram-negative bacteria.

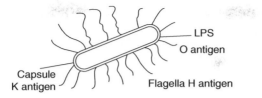

Figure 9.2
Position of antigens used for typing *Salmonella* species and other Gram-negative bacteria.
Salmonella species are typed by their O and H antigens, and classified accordingly, for example
Salmonella enterica serovar Typhimurium is O:4 H:l.

Salmonella infections are zoonotic, and are acquired from contact with infected food, usually by ingestion; it may then be passed by the faecal–oral route from person to person. Salmonellae are found as normal flora of many animals and have become associated with infection caught from chicken, cattle, eggs and dairy products. Since these form the ingredients and constituents of many other foods, the variety of sources of infection is vast. Infection may also be acquired from handling pet turtles that harbour the bacteria and incidences have even been reported from handling various pet treats made from contaminated ingredients. *Salmonella typhi* (not to be confused with *S. typhimurium*) is a human pathogen passed by infected carriers, famously Typhoid Mary, with the route of transmission being food and water infected by the carrier.

The infectious dose of salmonellae is high (between 10^6 and 10^8 organisms, but as few as 15–20 cells may cause infection in susceptible individuals) and the bacteria are more acid-sensitive than shigellae, and are able to cause infection more easily in individuals who have lower levels of stomach acid. However, they are able to sense the acid levels of the stomach by a two component regulatory system and via the expression of their *atr* (acid tolerance regulator) genes which produce proteins to protect them from the low pH. The virulence genes are located on a pathogenicity island on the genome and are expressed and switched off in a coordinated manner. They then attach to and invade the microvilli of the mucosal epithelial cells lining the small and large intestines. Invasion has been demonstrated *in vitro* via the apical surface of the epithelium and also via the M cells associated with Peyer's patches. Contact is made by the expression of bacterial fimbriae; a type III secretion system is expressed to inject the expressed proteins inside the cell and characteristic membrane ruffling of the enterocyte is induced, with cytoskeletal rearrangements and subsequent uptake of the bacterium into the cell. The characteristic symptoms of abdominal pain and diarrhoea are the result of the production of inflammatory cytokines and the influx of white cells. Cell damage also triggers the arachadonic acid cycle with the production of leukotrienes and prostaglandins, leading to abdominal pain. The electrolyte balance of the infected cells is disturbed, leading to the symptoms of diarrhoea. Salmonellae may also pass through the subepithelial layers into the bloodstream and are capable of causing bacteraemia and septicaemia. The incidence of salmonella infection in immuno-compromised patients is significantly higher than in healthy individuals. The pathogenesis of *S. typhi* is more complex, leading to the systemic disease of typhoid fever, involving the liver and gall bladder. It is therefore important in laboratory investigations to serotype all salmonella isolates. If *S. typhi* and *S. paratyphi* are isolated they must be handled as Category 3 organisms.

All faecal samples are routinely tested for *Salmonella* species using selective and differential media. Antibiotic susceptibility testing is performed on all isolates for treatment (ciprofloxacin or chloramphenicol are often used) and for epidemiological purposes to monitor resistance levels.

Shigellae

Shigellae are also Gram-negative bacilli and four species are associated with human disease, causing dysentery-like gastrointestinal infections (also called bacillary dysentery). The resulting diarrhoea is characterized by the presence of blood and mucus from the cell damage, and sloughing off of dead cells in severe cases may lead to ulcer formation. The four species, *S. flexneri*, *S. boydii*, *S. dysenteriae* and *S. sonnei* are distinguished by serology using specific antibodies to O antigens. Genetically, shigellae are closely related to *Escherichia coli*. *S. sonnei* is the most common in developed countries but all species are isolated in the UK, whether acquired here or from travel to endemic countries. Of just over 1700 isolates reported to the HPA in 2010, *S. sonnei* accounted for 1123, *S. flexneri* for 496, *S. boydii* for 85 and *S. dysenteriae* for 42; although the figures vary slightly each year, the distribution of species is similar. The infection can be fatal and is a major cause of death in children in developing countries where multiresistant *S. dysenteriae* type I is more common. In contrast to salmonellae, they are principally human pathogens, transmitted from person to person and by the faecal–oral route in contaminated food and water. The infectious dose is small (in the range of 10–100 organisms) allowing easy transmission between hosts.

Box 9.1 Type III secretion systems – molecular syringes

In common with eukaryotic cells, bacteria have secretion systems to transport molecules from the inside to the outside of the cell. The ATP binding cassette (ABC) transporters are common to eukaryotes, bacteria and archaea. Gram-negative bacteria have two membranes to cross, which adds to the complexity. Six types of specialized secretion systems have been identified in Gram-negative bacteria. Simple type I systems have three protein subunits; the ABC protein, a membrane fusion protein and an outer membrane protein. Ions, drugs and proteins are transported and secreted in this way. Types II, V and VI are different systems used for protein transport.

Type III secretion systems, however, are virulence factors of *Salmonella*, *Shigella*, *Bordetella* and *Pseudomonas* species, enteropathogenic *Escherichia coli* and *Chlamydia* species, and were first discovered in *Yersinia pestis*. Once the bacteria have attached themselves to the surface of a eukaryotic host cell, the Type III secretion system allows them to inject bacterial proteins across the two bacterial membranes and the host cell membrane to either destroy or change the cytoskeletal arrangement of the host cell. A molecular syringe of 25 proteins is formed along with a range of proteins to be 'injected' into the cell – there are similarities in structure to the flagellar basal body. The effector proteins injected act on either the cytoskeleton of the cell to enhance uptake or attachment of the bacteria, or interfere with intracellular cell signalling. Similar systems operate in plant pathogens.

Type IV secretion systems, which also appear on EM preparations as syringe-like structures, are capable of transporting both DNA and proteins from bacteria to host cells. *Helicobacter pylori* uses a type IV secretion system to deliver the toxin CagA into gastric epithelial cells; pertussis toxin of *Bordetella pertussis* (whooping cough) is partially delivered in this manner and *Legionella pneumophila* translocates numerous effector proteins into the host cell in this way.

The bacteria have well-developed acid tolerance mechanisms, expressed and then switched off after passage through the stomach. Invasion of the intestinal cells is effected by crossing the epithelium via the M cells, as they are unable to enter enterocytes on their apical surface. Ingestion by macrophages and subsequent escape after inducing their apoptosis usually follows. The bacteria then invade the basal surface of the cells, inducing cytoskeletal rearrangement and the formation of pseudopods that surround the bacterium and take it into the cell in a membrane-bound vacuole, a process that takes a matter of minutes. All of this is effected and controlled by more than 30 genes, including the *ipa* (invasion plasmid antigen) genes, and a type III secretion system to ensure the export of the proteins into the cells. Inside the cell the bacteria escape from the vesicle and move into the cytoplasm where they can multiply. They are then able to move from cell to cell, propelled by actin tails resulting from further cytoskeletal rearrangement. The cells die and are sloughed off into the lumen of the intestine, resulting in erosion of the epithelial layer. Neutrophils accumulate in the area as a result of the damage and are excreted in large numbers; blood is also excreted, giving rise to the characteristic microscopic appearance of shigella infection seen in the wet preparation of the faecal sample. *S. dysenteriae* type I produces a Shiga toxin, which has a cytotoxic effect on intestinal epithelial and endothelial cells and affects the 60S ribosomal subunit and therefore protein synthesis, further contributing to diarrhoeal symptoms and causing the most severe illness of the four species. Isolates of *S. dysenteriae* type I must be handled in a Category 3 containment area. *S. sonnei* is most commonly associated with watery diarrhoea without the symptoms of dysentery.

All faecal samples are routinely tested for *Shigella* species using selective and differential media. Antibiotic susceptibility testing is performed on all isolates, and used in severe cases.

Escherichia coli

Escherichia coli are Gram-negative bacilli – they are ubiquitous members of the normal flora and may also be the cause of infection in most areas of the human body. They are part of the normal intestinal flora, yet specific serotypes are capable of causing serious gastrointestinal illness. They are characterized by their interactions with the epithelial cells and the production of toxins. The majority are responsible for severe childhood diarrhoea in developing countries and may cause traveller's diarrhoea in non-immune hosts. Enterohaemorrhagic *E. coli, E. coli* O157:H7 has emerged as a significant pathogen in the UK and has been responsible for several major outbreaks and many sporadic cases. On average up to 1000 cases of *E. coli* O157 are recorded annually, and there is growing evidence of their becoming reservoirs for extended spectrum β-lactamase enzymes.

The bacteria are zoonotic Gram-negative bacilli, part of the normal flora of animal intestines, and are transmitted through infected meat, milk and dairy products. They are extremely infectious with single numbers of bacteria able to cause infection, and so there is a high risk of person-to-person secondary infection after the initial food-borne transmission. For this reason they are treated as Category 3 organisms once isolated from clinical specimens in the laboratory. Transmission is often from infected meat, for example undercooked burgers. Because the meat is minced, infected outer surfaces of the animal muscle are present throughout the product, and unlike meat with solid muscle such as steak, the product requires thorough cooking to kill the bacteria. Cross-contamination between cooked and raw meat is another source of infection. Raw or inadequately processed milk may be infected by faecal matter during milking and transmit infection, as will cheese and other dairy products made from it. *E. coli* O157 has the ability to cause serious disease, particularly in children and elderly people, because of the production of Shiga toxin that can enter the blood stream, damage the glomeruli of the kidneys and lead to haemolytic uraemic syndrome. The associated diarrhoea is frequently bloody.

The bacteria are acid-resistant, enabling safe passage through the stomach, and on arrival in the lower regions of the intestine they interact with the epithelial cells, forming characteristic attaching and effacement lesions, with pedestal formation. The virulence genes responsible for this are carried on the LEE (locus of enterocyte effacement) pathogenicity island and control the bundle-forming pili expressed prior to attachment. They also activate a type III secretion system to deliver proteins, including a bacterial receptor, into the cell. The bacteria do not invade the cells after attachment but evoke a strong inflammatory response from the host. The Shiga toxin released leads to haemorrhagic diarrhoea and, in conjunction with the cytokines, damages the small blood vessels in the area. Complications arise in 5–10% of patients infected, and can lead to acute and chronic renal failure. Given the low infectious dose and the possible consequences of the infection it is important for laboratories to diagnose cases of *E. coli* O157 quickly and accurately. Most of the strains do not ferment sorbitol, providing an identification method when sorbitol is incorporated into the test media. However, sorbitol-fermenting strains have now been isolated.

In May–June 2011 a new variant of *E. coli* (*E. coli* O104:H4) was responsible for over 3800 cases and over 40 deaths in Germany and among those who had visited the country. The source was believed to be sprouted seeds. The emergence of this variant, which contains the Shiga toxin and is also non-sorbitol fermenting, demonstrates that new strains continue to appear as a result of horizontal gene transfer.

Screening for *E. coli* O157 is part of the routine investigation of faecal samples, and is carried out using specialist culture media. Antibiotic testing is performed on all isolates. Testing for other specific toxigenic strains would only be performed if requested.

Vibrio cholerae

Vibrio cholerae and *V. parahaemolyticus* are Gram-negative, comma-shaped, oxidase-positive bacteria causing acute infection and severe diarrhoea that is toxin mediated. Cholera has a long history of causing pandemics throughout the world and was endemic in the UK prior to the introduction of public health systems to ensure clean water supplies. It is now confined to SE Asia, parts of Africa and South America and is spread in contaminated water. It is therefore important that travel details are included on patient request forms so that the correct culture media can be inoculated if cholera is a possible diagnosis.

The infectious dose is high, about 10^6–10^8 organisms per ml; the bacteria are acid-resistant and pass through the stomach and attach to the GM1 ganglioside on intestinal epithelial cells. The bacteria do not invade the cells but produce cholera toxin, a classic A–B toxin where the binding portion B attaches to the target cell and the active portion A enters the cells where it causes ADP ribosylation of a G protein involved in cell signalling. The result of this is to 'freeze' the activity of this protein into stimulating adenylate cyclase. This leads to high levels of cAMP within the cell and a large loss of fluid into the intestinal lumen, producing the classic watery diarrhoea of cholera, often referred to as a rice water stool. The resulting loss of fluid and electrolytes can lead to death in untreated patients.

Specific culture for the presence of *V. cholerae* is only performed if the travel details or the nature of the specimen (rice water stool) suggest the possibility. Antibiotic susceptibility testing is also performed.

Yersinia enterocolitica

The bacteria are zoonotic and are acquired through consumption of infected food, such as pork, milk or water. The symptoms may be varied and include diarrhoea, mesenteric lymphadenitis, pseudo-appendicitis and septicaemia.

Yersinia enterocolitica culture is only performed on request, if there is clinical suspicion that the bacteria may be the cause of infection. Isolation is achieved by enrichment and culture on specific selective media and susceptibility tests are performed.

If treatment is considered necessary for bacterial gastroenteritis, ciprofloxacin is the usual antibiotic of choice.

Yersinia pseudotuberculosis, *Aeromonas* species, *Clostridium septicum* and *Plesiomonas shigelloides* may also be the cause of bacterial gastrointestinal disease.

9.4 VIRAL CAUSES OF GASTROENTERITIS

Viral gastroenteritis is more common than that from other causes, but tends to be under-reported because of the shorter duration of symptoms. Viruses are ingested with contaminated food and water or by contact with infected animals and then passed easily from person to person via the faecal–oral route. The principal viral pathogens diagnosed in a routine microbiology laboratory are rotavirus and norovirus. Hepatitis A is also transmitted by the faecal–oral route; the laboratory diagnosis is discussed in *Chapter 3*. Laboratories with facilities for electron microscopy are able to identify a greater variety of viral pathogens, including caliciviruses and astroviruses.

Rotavirus

Infection with rotavirus causes acute febrile gastroenteritis in children, although it can occur in adults, and tends to be seasonal, usually occurring during the winter and spring months. Following ingestion there is an incubation period of 2–3 days and the virus is shed for up to a week after the onset of symptoms. The symptoms may lead to hospitalization and approximately 15 000 children aged up to 4 years (HPA data for England and Wales) are admitted each year. The picture in underdeveloped countries is much more severe, with 400 000 to 600 000 deaths annually from dehydration and delays in access to treatment.

The virus gets its name from the Latin for wheel, *rota*, as the structure visible under EM resembles this. Rotaviruses are double-stranded RNA viruses with 11 segments and complex antigenic properties, grouped A–F. Group A infections are the most commonly isolated. The virus invades and replicates in the microvilli of intestinal epithelial cells, leading to cell death, villus tip desquamation and loss of water, salt and glucose. The child becomes febrile and has symptoms of vomiting and diarrhoea. Neutralizing antibodies are formed after infection, but this does not prevent infection with a different serotype. Rotavirus infection is diagnosed in the laboratory from a faecal sample using an ELISA technique.

Adenoviruses

Adenoviruses are double-stranded non-enveloped DNA viruses associated with respiratory infection and they are also an important cause of acute diarrhoea in young children. They are detected by EM or ELISA techniques.

Norovirus

Norovirus is a member of the Caliciviridae family. Norwalk virus, also known as small round structured virus and Norwalk-like virus, was the first norovirus identified; it was the cause of an outbreak of winter vomiting disease in Norwalk, Ohio in 1968. Noroviruses are responsible for large numbers of sporadic cases and outbreaks in otherwise healthy individuals. The virus is a naked (non-enveloped) RNA virus that survives well in the external environment. Outbreaks have notably occurred on cruise liners, from a common source and thence by person-to-person transmission, and within other semi-closed communities such as schools, nursing homes and hospitals. The symptoms are short-lived but the virus is highly infectious, has a very low infectious dose and may be transmitted by food and water, via contaminated surfaces as well as aerosols from projectile vomiting. Transmission can be prevented by good hygiene, abstinence from food preparation until at least 48 hours after the symptoms have subsided, and restriction of visitors and movements of infected people. The incubation period is 24–48 hours, during which time the virus infects intestinal epithelial cells. The viruses attach to the cells by binding to the histo-blood group antigens, with different viral genogroups expressing a preference for different blood group antigens. Blood group type and the status of the individual as a secretor or non-secretor (secretors have antigen and immunoglobulins in their saliva and gastrointestinal secretions) are closely linked with susceptibility; non-secretors are less likely to become infected. During an infection the intestinal villi appear blunted and there is a transient malabsorption of D-xylose and fat; however, the precise mechanisms of pathogenesis are not fully understood. There are five distinct genogroups of noroviruses, GI–GV. GI, GII and GIV infect only humans, and epidemiological studies have demonstrated that the rise in the incidence of norovirus worldwide is linked to the emergence of two novel GII strains, GII.4 variants: 2006a and 2006b.

9.5 PROTOZOA

The protozoan pathogens most frequently isolated from faecal samples in the UK are *Giardia lamblia* and *Cryptosporidium parvum* and amoebic dysentery caused by *Entamoeba histolytica*. They are transmitted by ingestion of contaminated water, or food that has been in contact with contaminated water, where the protozoa are present in an environmentally protected cyst form. Once inside the human host they are able to change into metabolically active protozoa, replicate and then are shed once again in the cyst form.

Giardia lamblia

Giardia lamblia was the first microorganism to be visualized under the light microscope, by Anton van Leeuwenhoek in 1681. There are two life cycle stages; the 4-nucleate cyst and the binucleate flagellate form.

Giardia lamblia cysts are shed into lakes, streams and ground water by wild animals (beavers building dams are sources of infection, hence the term 'beaver fever' sometimes used to describe the infection). In this way the cysts may find their way into drinking water supplies through cracks in sewage and water systems, where they are fairly resistant to treatment with chlorine. The cysts are metabolically inert and are able to survive for long periods in the environment. The incidence in the UK is around 3000 cases a year, some of which are acquired during foreign travel to areas with a higher incidence. *Giardia lamblia* may also be sexually transmitted as a result of anal intercourse.

After ingestion, the cysts change into the trophozoite form after contact with the gastric acid, and the motile flagellates move to the duodenum and jejunum, using a sucking disc on the ventral surface to attach to the brush border of the intestinal mucosa. The attachment damages the cells, triggers a host immune response and affects the cell's absorptive capacity, which leads to dehydration and fatty stools as a result of the malabsorption. The patient suffers from unpleasant, foul-smelling and sometimes fatty diarrhoea, abdominal pain, discomfort and excess gas. Samples arriving in the laboratory may also contain gas, as many a biomedical scientist who has not heeded the hissing sound on opening the specimen container can attest.

Laboratory diagnosis is made by visualizing the cysts or trophozoites in a wet preparation or faecal concentration method. The trophozoites can be stained with Field's stain (described in *Chapter 5*). A recently developed molecular amplification method using primers to the cyst wall protein 1 present in both cysts and trophozoites can detect antigen even if the microscopy is negative. The infection is self-limiting after 7–10 days but is usually treated, often with metronidazole, and family members are also tested for infection.

Cryptosporidium parvum

Cryptosporidiosis is a zoonotic infection resulting from ingestion of cysts shed into the environment by animals, particularly calves. In recent years there has been a greater awareness of the risks associated with farm visits where children pet and feed animals, as young children are particularly susceptible. Publicity of the risks and the provision of hand washing facilities have helped to reduce the infection rate. While direct contact with infected animals is one source of infection, the cysts also drain into the water supply. This has the potential to infect large numbers of consumers. Significant outbreaks have occurred, notably in Milwaukee in 1993 where 403 000 (of a total of 1.6 million) residents were infected following an ineffective filtration process, which led to inadequate removal of oocysts, in two treatment plants. Over 4000 people were hospitalized and around 100 died. Small outbreaks and sporadic cases are reported in the UK with on average 4000–5000 cases annually. Outbreaks have also been associated with inadequate removal by sand filters in swimming pools, of cysts shed from infected people. Walkers and campers are also at risk from drinking apparently clean water from rivers and streams.

Sporozoites are released from the cysts after contact with intestinal cells. These sporozoites then develop into structures containing merozoites, which can undergo sexual reproduction to form more oocysts; these infectious forms are then shed in the faeces. The infection is self-limiting after one or two cycles of reproduction in immuno-competent hosts, and resolves within a month. The infectious dose is less than ten organisms. For immuno-suppressed patients the consequences are far more severe, leading to debilitating chronic diarrhoea. Paromomycin, azithromycin or nitazoxanide can be used to treat immuno-compromised patients but are not fully effective. Screening for cysts in water supplies is a challenge akin to looking for needles in a haystack, as it is difficult to identify all the particles of a similar size. Screening has only become mandatory in recent years; flow cytometry is currently used and if there is any concern that cysts may have entered the domestic water supply residents are advised to boil their water, as the cysts are chorine resistant.

The cysts may be visualized in stained preparations of faecal samples by using a fluorescent, auramine or Ziehl–Neelsen stain.

Other oocysts acquired from endemic areas of the world include *Cyclospora cayatanensis* and *Isospora belli*.

Entamoeba histolytica

Entamoeba histolytica is a major cause of morbidity and mortality in developing countries where it causes amoebic dysentery and hepatic abscesses. Following attachment by the cysts, the amoebae destroy the cells, leading to ulceration of the intestinal epithelium. Hepatic abscesses may form if the amoebae enter the bloodstream and travel to the liver. Of the six species of *Entamoeba*, only *E. histolytica* is associated with disease. Human hosts may also carry very similar-looking amoebic cysts, called *E. dispar*, asymptomatically, which complicates the interpretation of their significance in the faecal sample. The cysts of *E. histolytica* can be seen in wet preparations of faecal samples and need to be distinguished from the cysts of *Escherichia coli*.

9.6   PARASITES

The ova of eukaryotic parasites are shed in the faeces of infected patients and may be seen in wet preparations, or concentrations made from the sample. Concentrations are performed on request if the clinical history and travel details of the patient are indicative of possible infection. In some laboratories the isolation of ova from nematodes (roundworms), trematodes (flukes) and cestodes (tapeworms) is an extremely rare occurrence and most experience in their identification is gained from the National External Quality Assessment Samples (NEQAS). Occasionally an entire worm is received for identification; these are generally preserved in formalin and provide an ideal future teaching aid. The ova of *Enterobius vermicularis,* pinworms or threadworms in children, are visualized by examination of a Sellotape slide under the microscope.

A range of treatments including piperazine, mebendazole, thiabendazole and praziquantel are available for treating parasitic infections.

9.7   TOXIN-MEDIATED GASTROINTESTINAL INFECTIONS

Toxin-mediated infections are not dependent on the culture of the causative organism, as they are diagnosed by the presence of the toxin in a faecal sample. Occasionally, however, it may be necessary to confirm the presence of the bacteria. Where a patient has antibiotic-associated diarrhoea caused by enterotoxigenic strains of *Clostridium difficile*, the presence of the toxin can be detected using an ELISA method, and the presence of the bacteria confirmed by culture on selective media and specific typing by molecular methods. Some intoxications give rise to vomiting and diarrhoea symptoms of relatively short duration and specimens are not routinely sent for laboratory investigation, unless the infection leads to an outbreak, for example with *Staphylococcus aureus*, *Bacillus cereus* and *Clostridium perfringens*. The number of outbreaks reported annually is low (between 1 and 10 a year in the UK) but these figures do not represent sporadic self-limiting cases. However, compared with the figures for the major bacterial and viral pathogens the incidence is low. *Clostridium botulinum* has a powerful neurotoxin and, depending on the infectious dose, may lead to mild or life-threatening illness caused by the flaccid paralysis. Although the infection may be food-borne, it does not cause the typical symptoms of gastroenteritis. Incidences are fortunately rare. Intoxication by scromboid toxins in fish and the investigation of contaminated food is covered in *Chapter 14*.

Staphylococcus aureus

The toxins of *Staphylococcus aureus* gain access to food from human sources during food preparation and through poor storage. An example of this would be ice cream that is left out and allowed to thaw, then becomes contaminated and is refrozen, or a chef with an open wound handling cooked meat. *S. aureus* produce bacterial enterotoxins that are capable of surviving the freezing process, and are ingested with the food. The toxins are heat-stable and protease-resistant and cause symptoms of vomiting, nausea, abdominal cramps and diarrhoea. The genes encoding the enterotoxins have been cloned and sequenced and can be divided into two groups, SEA and SEB, both of which act as superantigens to produce an exaggerated immune reaction. The precise mechanisms by which the symptoms of food poisoning occur are, however, incompletely understood. *S. aureus* intoxication is characterized by a short incubation period of a matter of 1–6 hours and does not last for longer than 12–24 hours.

Bacillus cereus

Bacillus cereus is a Gram-positive aerobic spore-bearing bacterium classically associated with infection of cooked rice that has been allowed to cool, kept at an ambient temperature and then inadequately reheated. The bacteria get into the food from the environment and multiply. The spores are not killed during the reheating process and can then germinate. The emetic toxin takes effect 2–3 hours after consumption and lasts for up to 24 hours. A second toxin produced by these bacteria causes diarrhoea and is more frequently associated with meat sauces and soup. The incubation period is longer and the symptoms last for 24–48 hours.

Clostridium perfringens

Food poisoning is caused by these Gram-positive bacteria contaminating food products, often meat stews, that are held at room temperature and then inadequately reheated. The bacteria are killed when the food is cooked, but they produce heat-resistant spores that vegetate into viable cells as the food cools. If the food is not thoroughly reheated, the bacteria continue to multiply. The symptoms appear between 8 and 14 hours after the food has been eaten and cause watery diarrhoea lasting 24 hours. The symptoms are more severe for the elderly and can cause death in rare cases. Outbreaks tend to have a high attack rate, and are often associated with institutions and large gatherings of people, where greater quantities of food are prepared in advance and kept warm. If the conditions are optimal, *C. perfringens* has a generation time of as little as 10–12 minutes, allowing a great opportunity for growth in a nutrient-rich stew. *C. perfringens* Type A is associated with infections and has a high infectious dose (10^8 organisms); toxin is produced from the viable cells as they sporulate. Commercial kits are available for toxin testing in outbreak situations.

Clostridium difficile: antibiotic-associated diarrhoea

The development of antibiotic-associated diarrhoea is linked to the use of most broad-spectrum antibiotics. The antibiotic treatment disturbs the normal flora of the bowel and allows spores of *C. difficile* acquired from the environment to germinate, reproduce and produce toxins A and B. Patients may suffer varying degrees of diarrhoea or develop life-threatening pseudomembranous colitis. The pseudomembrane consists of fibrin, mucin and dead neutrophils as a result of the intense inflammatory process and damage to the mucosal cells following toxin activity. *C. difficile* has become a leading cause of hospital-acquired infection, with 55 498 cases in 2007 when mandatory reporting was introduced (HPA data for England, Wales and Northern Ireland) and a significant number of deaths associated with certain serotypes; 027 has been responsible for several outbreaks. Since 2007 there has been a significant reduction in these figures; there was a 29% reduction in 2008–9. Even lower numbers (25 600) were recorded in 2009–10, which represented a reduction of 54% on the 2007 figures. This is encouraging and reflects a growing awareness and implementation of control of infection measures. A vaccine targeting both toxins is being developed. Traditionally, cell culture was used to detect the presence of the toxin and currently toxin detection is achieved using an ELISA method, either using an automated system such as VIDAS or a solid phase system. These are described in more detail in *Chapter 6*. However, a toxin AB test may not be sensitive enough to identify all patients who are infected and so a screening test for *C. difficile*-specific glutamate dehydrogenase (GDH) enzyme in the faeces, followed by a toxin AB test on positive samples, improves the diagnosis of infection. The GDH test only identifies the presence of the bacteria in the intestine, not whether they are producing toxin; however, a positive GDH test followed by a toxin test ensures that any patients who are GDH positive and toxin negative can be monitored carefully.

9.8 LABORATORY METHODS

The SOPs for examining faecal specimens include culture, serological and microscopy methods chosen to identify the range of pathogens most likely to be present, with the addition of further investigations where relevant clinical and travel details suggest their likelihood. *Figure 9.1* shows a flow diagram for the routine laboratory investigation of a sample of faeces, from reception to reporting.

All faecal samples routinely undergo microscopy and culture for the major pathogens discussed in *Section 9.3*: *Campylobacter*, *Salmonella* and *Shigella* species and *Escherichia coli* O157. If the clinical history and travel details suggest it, further culture is included for *Vibrio cholerae* or *Yersinia enterocolitica* and a concentration specimen prepared for ova cysts and parasites.

Microscopy and staining

A small amount of the faecal sample is added to a drop of saline or iodine on a microscope slide. The selection of diluent is a matter of choice and some laboratories may choose to use both. A coverslip is applied and the slide viewed at low (10×) and then medium (40×) magnification. The specimen will be full of artefacts and practice is required to become competent at identifying significant features, particularly cysts. The presence of white blood cells, red blood cells, cysts of any kind and protozoa such as *Giardia lamblia* is recorded. A trophozoite can be seen in *Figure 9.3*. The microscope will most probably have a means of measuring the size of any cysts or protozoa, by replacing one of the eyepieces with a graticule (as described in *Chapter 5*). Measurement is essential for the identification and differentiation of cysts and ova. *Figure 9.4* shows a cyst of *Entamoeba histolytica*.

A smear on a slide is made at the same time for staining for the presence of *Cryptosporidia*. The slides are stained either with Ziehl–Neelsen (ZN) acid-fast stain or by a fluorescent stain, auramine–phenol. ZN stains are viewed using a light microscope and 100× oil immersion lens with the oocysts stained red, whereas auramine–phenol slides are viewed on a fluorescent microscope at 100×, showing fluorescent yellow circular oocysts. *Figure 9.5* shows a cyst of *Cryptosporidium parvum* stained with ZN.

Culture media

There are 10^{11} organisms per gram of faeces, and although many of these are anaerobic and therefore not cultured on the range of media used, those that do replicate and

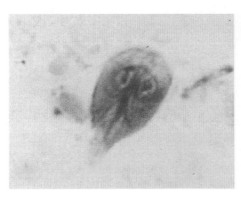

Figure 9.3
Giardia lamblia trophozoite.

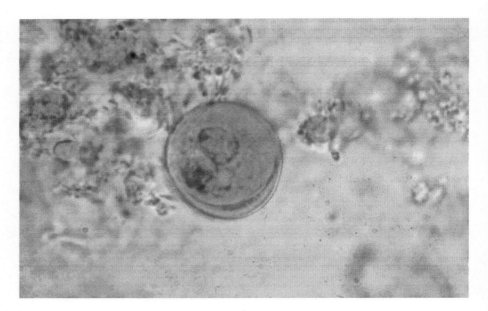

Figure 9.4
Cyst of *Entamoeba histolytica*, 10–15 μm in diameter.

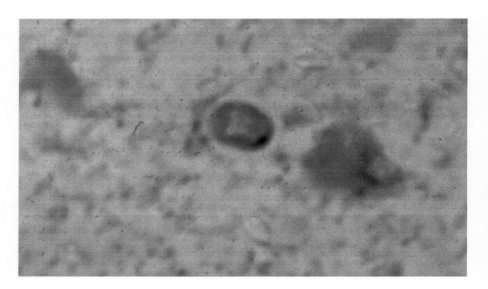

Figure 9.5
Cyst of *Cryptosporidium parvum*. The cysts measure 4–6 μm and are visualized using the 100 ×
magnification objective.

produce colonies are largely Gram-negative bacilli, many of them commensal flora.
Selective and differential media are therefore required to isolate and subsequently
identify faecal pathogens. There are a wide variety of media available, as inspection
of any of the manufacturers' catalogues and manuals will demonstrate, with new

products being continually developed. For routine faecal culture, the following are most commonly used: DCA, XLD, and a selective enrichment broth for *Salmonella* and *Shigella* species, MacConkey agar for purity plates, sorbitol MacConkey for isolation of *Escherichia coli* O157, and a selective medium for isolating *Campylobacter*. Chromogenic agar may also be used.

Isolation of *Salmonella* and *Shigella* species

DCA agar
Selectivity and differentiation of these two genera on deoxycholate citrate agar (DCA) is achieved by the addition of bile salts and sodium deoxycholate, for selectivity, and the inclusion of lactose, for differentiation. Lactose fermentation lowers the pH and this is indicated by the addition of phenol red. Gram-positive and some Gram-negative bacteria, including *Escherichia coli*, are inhibited by the bile salts. *Salmonella* and *Shigella* species are non-lactose fermenters and appear as colourless or straw-coloured colonies, sometimes with black tops, whereas lactose fermenting colonies appear pink.

XLD agar (xylose lysine decarboxylase)
XLD agar is often the medium of choice if only one selective agar is to be inoculated. The agar contains inhibitory bile salts, xylene, lysine and an indicator for hydrogen sulphide. Most enteric bacteria, with the exeption of *Providencia*, *Edwardsiella* and *Shigella* species, ferment xylose and form yellow colonies while the non-xylose fermenters form pink/red colonies. Salmonellae exhaust the xylose and then decarboxylate the lysine in the medium, changing the pH back to alkaline and mimicking the *Shigella* reaction. The presence of *Salmonella* and *Edwardsiella* species is indicated by the incorporation of hydrogen sulphide, and either red colonies with black centres, or entirely black colonies are formed. The medium also contains lactose and sucrose that is fermented by some of the coliforms, resulting in an acidic pH. The complex interactions and pH changes serve to maintain the difference in colonial appearance between the various bacteria for at least 24 hours after incubation.

An enrichment broth containing the sugar mannitol and sodium selenite is inoculated at the same time and subcultured on to a further XLD culture plate after 24 hours. The broth encourages the growth of salmonella that may be present in the original sample in small numbers, and further inhibits the growth of commensal bacteria. Selenite should be handled with care as it is toxic. All of these culture media and the enrichment broths are incubated for 16–24 hours in air at a temperature of 35–37°C.

Chromogenic agar
Several chromogenic agars designed to distinguish colonies of *Salmonella* species are available and used in routine screening of faecal specimens along with standard agar or enrichment. ABC (alpha-beta chromogenic) incorporates two substrates (3,4-cyclohexenoesculetin-β-D-galactoside and 5-bromo-4-chloro-3 indolyl-α-D-galactopyranoside). *Salmonella* species are distinguished from other members of the Enterobacteriaceae by their α-galactosidase activity in the absence of β-galactosidase activity, to form green colonies. Other members of the Enterobacteriaceae typically produce black colonies (*Escherichia coli*) or colourless colonies (*Proteus* species).

Different manufacturers use similar substrates to distinguish between α- and β-galalactosidase-producing bacteria, with characteristic coloured colony formation.

Identification of suspect colonies

Every laboratory has an SOP for identification of salmonella and shigella from culture media. The first step is usually to carry out a urea test, as both are urease negative; any urease-positive colonies (*Proteus* species being a prime example) are therefore screened out. Serology tests may then be performed using polyvalent PSO and PSH sera for salmonella, followed by specific O and H sera. The most commonly isolated serotypes are *Salmonella* Enteritidis O9:Hgm and *Salmonella* Typhimurium O4:i. Both these and other serotypes isolated in human infections are strictly serovars of *Salmonella enterica*, as described in *Section 9.3*, but are usually referred to in this simpler form. Similarly, suspected colonies of *Shigella* species are tested against specific antisera for the four genera. Confirmation may be achieved using an API strip: a 10S or 20E. Antibiotic susceptibility testing is always carried out, to give guidance on treatment and for epidemiological purposes.

Campylobacter media and identification of colonies

There are several media available for the culture of campylobacters, all of which contain antibiotics to suppress the growth of faecal flora and enhance the growth of campylobacters. Some of the supplements are named after the people who developed the media, for example Skirrow and Kamali, or Preston, where a considerable amount of developmental work took place. Some of the media require incubation at 42°C, whereas others may be incubated at 37°C. The bacteria are micro-aerophilic and grow preferentially in an atmosphere of 5–6% oxygen, 10% carbon dioxide and 85% nitrogen for 48 hours. Campylobacter-selective agar (Preston) contains blood agar and a mixture of antibiotics, e.g. polymixin B, rifampicin, trimethoprim and cyclohexamide, and incubation is carried out at 42°C. Modified CCDA Preston, on the other hand, is blood-free and contains charcoal and the antibiotics cefoperazone and amphotericin B, with incubation at 37°C.

Identification of the suspect colonies (see the Case study in *Box 9.2*) is performed by an oxidase test (campylobacters are oxidase-positive) and a Gram stain showing the characteristic curved Gram-negative bacteria (see *Figure 9.6*). Antibiotic susceptibilities are performed to give guidance for treatment, which includes ciprofloxacin and erythromycin. Testing for antibiotic susceptibility also enables surveillance of any emerging resistance to ciprofloxacin.

Escherichia coli O157

Isolation and identification of these bacteria is achieved using a modified MacConkey agar plate, with sorbitol substituted for lactose. The bile salts are inhibitory and the sorbitol is present to distinguish sorbitol-negative *E. coli* O157 from other faecal flora and pathogens. Clear sorbitol-negative colonies are then identified using a specific latex test, where latex particles coated with antibodies to O157 react with specific bacterial antigens. The emergence of sorbitol-positive strains has necessitated further testing of cultured bacteria. Isolates are tested for oxidase and all negative colonies are tested with the latex kit, especially in patients under 15 years and over the age of 65 years, for whom the infection is more likely to lead to HUS (haemolytic uraemic

Box 9.2 Case study

A 25-year-old male consults his GP. He has felt unwell for about a week and thought he was going to develop flu as he was feverish, had aching limbs and a headache. However, after a few days he began to have diarrhoea, with 3–5 bowel movements a day, and developed cramping pains in his abdomen. He was concerned when he thought he saw some blood in his stool sample. He had not recently been abroad and did not think he had eaten anything unusual. The GP gave him a specimen pot and the appropriate request form and suggested he take a specimen to the microbiology laboratory at the local hospital.

The specimen was cultured onto selective media for faecal pathogens including a CCDA medium for the isolation of *Campylobacter* species. A wet preparation was prepared and examined microscopically. +++ white cells and + red cells were seen.

The culture plates were examined at 24 hours, with no suspected faecal pathogens isolated on the standard salmonella and shigella agars. After 48 hours of incubation in micro-aerophilic conditions the CCDA plate was inspected. Grey colonies were observed spreading across the plate. A Gram stain was prepared and an oxidase test performed. Gram-negative curved bacteria, resembling seagull shapes, were seen on the Gram stain and the oxidase test was positive.

Questions
1. What is the most likely identity of the bacteria seen on the Gram stain?
2. What are the most likely sources of his infection?
3. Why is it important that antibiotic susceptibility tests are carried out on the isolate?
4. Why were these bacteria not isolated on the routine faecal selective agar?

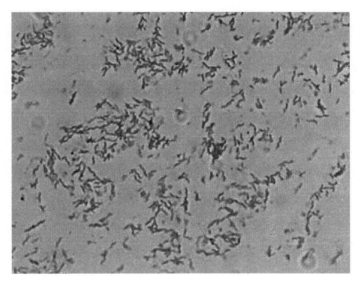

Figure 9.6
Gram stain of *Campylobacter* species, showing the characteristic curved bacteria.

syndrome). Positive isolates are then further identified using an API 20E test. The bacteria have a low infective dose and testing after primary isolation is carried out at containment level 3. Chromogenic agar for the identification of *E. coli* O157 is also available.

Vibrio cholerae *and* V. parahaemolyticus

Culture is only performed if the patient details and travel history suggest it may be a possibility. The faecal sample is inoculated on to TCBS (thiosulphate, citrate, bile salts and sucrose) medium, a selective medium that suppresses faecal flora for at least 24 hours. An alkaline peptone water for enrichment may also be inoculated and subcultured to a TCBS plate after 24 hours. The colonies of *Vibrio cholerae* are yellow and flat, whereas those of *V. parahaemolyticus* and *V. vulnificus* are blue–green. Other bacteria of faecal origin will also grow on the medium with similar, but smaller, colonies and so further testing and identification is essential. *Vibrio* species are oxidase-positive, short fat curved Gram-negative bacilli. They can be further confirmed with specific antisera for 01, 0139 and by the API 20E test. All isolates are tested for antibiotic susceptibility.

All of the bacterial isolates described here are reported to the HPA and local and regional services as appropriate; for example, the Environmental Health Officer and the Consultant in Communicable Disease Control (CCDC) in the UK. The reporting is an essential part of epidemiology and surveillance as well as tracing the sources of infection.

Concentration and examination for faecal parasites

If the patient has travelled to endemic areas and tests for the presence of ova cysts and parasites are requested, a concentration of the faeces is prepared and all the deposit examined under the microscope.

Concentration is achieved either by the following method or the use of commercial concentration kits. This is a matter of choice; the commercial kits are disposable but more expensive if greater numbers are tested routinely. The formol ether method is a cheaper alternative.

- Emulsify a pea-sized piece of faeces into a clean universal bottle containing 7 ml of 10% formalin (one volume of 40% formaldehyde diluted with 9 volumes of distilled water).
- Sieve the contents through a 'tea strainer', pore size approx 425 μm, and collect in a suitable container (sieves should be thoroughly washed for reuse).
- Transfer filtrate into glass or polypropylene container for centrifugation.
- Add 3 ml of ethyl acetate and either vortex for 15 secs or shake for 60 secs.
- Centrifuge at 1500 *g* for 60 secs or 1100 *g* for 2 mins.
- Loosen and remove fatty layer with swab stick before emptying contents of tube, leaving a few drops in the base.
- Resuspend the deposit.
- Place a drop of resuspended deposit on to a microscope slide and apply a coverslip. Iodine may be added if preferred.
- Scan the entire area using low power (10×) objective and medium power (40×) for examining morphological features.

The identification of helminths includes the ova of nematodes, trematodes and cestodes and is made by shape and, importantly, size, measured using the microscope graticule. It is really useful to have a chart available in the immediate vicinity of the microscope that shows both shape and relative size of the ova likely to be seen. All of the concentrated specimen is examined systematically by moving the microscope stage up, across and down until the whole area under the coverslip has been viewed. When viewing a Sellotape slide for *Enterobius vermicularis* it is sometimes difficult to see clearly through the tape layer. Adding a drop of immersion oil under the tape improves the clarity. The eggs appear larger than expected and are relatively easy to identify.

Examples of nematode ova that may be seen include the threadworms, *Ascaris lumbricoides*, hookworms and *Trichuris trichiura*. All of these have distinctive ova that are relatively easy to recognize (see *Figures 9.7–9.10*).

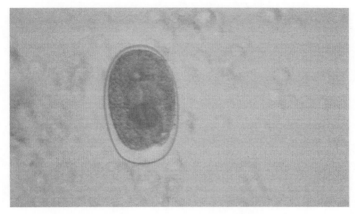

Figure 9.7
Hookworm ovum. Hookworms are nematodes, either New World hookworms (*Necator americanus*) or Old World hookworms (*Ancylostoma duodenale*). The eggs are passed in faeces into the soil and the resulting larvae then penetrate host skin, enter the lungs in the circulation, are coughed up and swallowed. Worms develop in the intestine. Hookworm infection cause anaemia, coughing, wheezing and abdominal pain. The ova measure 65 µm in length.

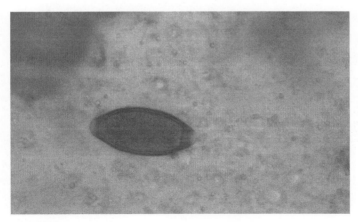

Figure 9.8
Trichuris ovum. Ova of the nematode worm *Trichuris trichiuria*, the whipworm are ingested and the larval form migrates to the caecum. There may be asymptomatic infection or it may lead to bloody diarrhoea, and rectal prolapse in a heavy infection. The ova measure 50 µm in length.

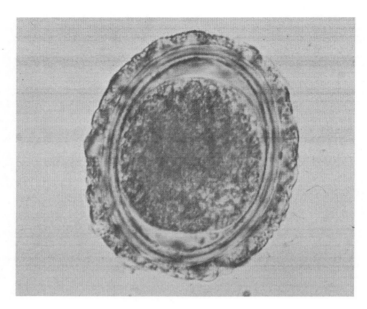

Figure 9.9
Ovum of the nematode *Ascaris lumbricoides*. *Ascaris lumbricoides* are large pink worms. Infection occurs when fertilized eggs are ingested. The larvae migrate in the bloodstream to the lungs. They are coughed up, swallowed and return to form worms in the intestine. They can cause pneumonitis and intestinal obstruction. These ova measure 60 µm in length.

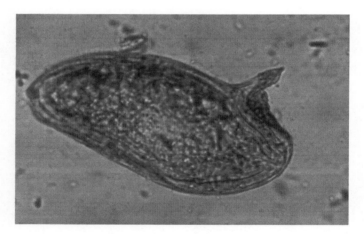

Figure 9.10
Ovum of *Schistosoma mansoni*. Schistosomes are trematodes (flukes). *Schistosoma mansoni* infects the mesenteric veins, and causes intestinal schistosomiasis. These are large ova measuring 150 µm in length.

The trematodes include parasitic flukes found in human infections. Examples of these are the schistosomes *Schistosoma mansoni, S. haematobium* and *S. japonicum,* which would not be missed because of their large size, and also *Fasciola hepatica* and *Clonorchis sinensis.*

Cestode (tapeworm) ova may occasionally be seen in patient specimens or NEQAS samples. Examples include *Taenia solium* and *T. saginata*, tapeworms acquired from pork and beef respectively.

These examples are by no means a comprehensive list of the ova that may be present, but give an idea of the identification process.

The identification of the cause of viral gastroenteritis
Identification of most viruses is best achieved by preparing a faecal sample and viewing under the electron microscope, where the characteristic viral morphology aids identification. Many cases of viral gastrointestinal infection are undiagnosed because of their short duration and self-limiting nature. Norovirus ELISA kits are available and rotavirus is investigated on a seasonal basis using an ELISA method.

9.9   REPORTING AND STORAGE

At each stage of the investigation of the sample, results are entered into the computer until all the tests are complete and a report is generated. The report will list the tests performed on the sample: microscopy, culture, faecal concentration, cryptosporidia stain, etc., and the results (with antibiotic susceptibilities if performed) on a positive culture. Positive cultures of *Salmonella* species and *Shigella* species are sent for confirmation to a reference laboratory. Copies of the reports are sent to relevant communicable disease control personnel if notifiable pathogens are isolated, e.g. salmonellae, shigellae, campylobacters, *Escherichia coli* O157, *Vibrio cholerae* and *V. parahaemolyticus, Giardia lamblia, Cryptosporidium parvum*, ova cysts and parasites.

The samples are stored at +4°C for up to 7 days before being discarded. Negative culture plates are kept for a limited time and positive culture plates for longer, before being discarded.

SUGGESTED FURTHER READING

Brazier, J. (2008) *Clostridium difficile*: from obscurity to superbug. *Br. J. Biomed. Sci.* **65:** 39–45.

Perez, J.M., Cavalli, P., Roure, C., Renac, R., Gille, Y. & Freydière, A.M. (2003) Comparison of four chromogenic media and Hektoen agar for detection and presumptive identification of *Salmonella* strains in human stools. *J. Clin. Microbiol.* **41:** 1130–1134.

Schroeder, G.N. & Hilbi, H. (2008) Molecular pathogenesis of *Shigella* spp: controlling host cell signalling, invasion and death by type III secretion. *Clin. Microbiol. Rev.* **21:** 134–156.

Van Lieshout, L. (2006) Protozoan parasites in the human intestine. *The Biomedical Scientist,* **50:** 608–610.

Vonberg R.-P., Kuijper, E.J., Wilcox, M.H. *et al.* (2008) Infection control methods to limit the spread of *Clostridium difficile*. *Clin. Microbiol. Infect.* **14 (s5):** 2–20.

Wren, M.W.D., Sivapalan, M., Shetty, N.P. & Kinson, R. (2009) Laboratory diagnosis of *Clostridium difficile* infection. An evaluation of tests for faecal toxin, glutamate dehydrogenase, lactoferrin and toxigenic culture in the diagnostic laboratory. *Br. J. Biomed. Sci.* **66:** 1–5.

www.cidrap.umn.edu/cidrap/content/fs/food-disease/causes/noroview.html contains a useful review of norovirus.

SELF-ASSESSMENT QUESTIONS

1. Outline the most common routes of transmission for gastrointestinal infections.
2. Which general characteristics must microorganisms with the ability to cause infection in the GI tract have in common?
3. Explain the methods used to identify *Salmonella* species in the laboratory.
4. Describe how *Shigella* species cause the symptoms of diarrhoea and dysentery in individuals. Which of the species is responsible for severe childhood dysentery in developing countries?
5. In 1996 there was a large outbreak of *Escherichia coli* O157 in Scotland. After the initial infections from the meat source, there was a second wave of infection among people who had not eaten the meat. Suggest a reason for this. What further complications can arise from the infection in certain groups of patients?
6. Describe the life cycle and pathogenesis of *Giardia lamblia*.
7. Why are selective media so important in the isolation of bacterial faecal pathogens? Outline the selective mechanism of one such medium.
8. Discuss the problems associated with an outbreak of norovirus on a cruise ship.
9. The request form accompanying a faecal specimen states that the patient has travelled to India and trekked in Nepal. What additional media and investigations should be included? Give reasons for your choices.
10. Why is it important that laboratories have accurate and timely methods for the diagnosis of *Clostridium difficile* toxin?

Answers to self-assessment questions provided at:
www.scionpublishing.com/medmicro

The diagnosis of infection from wounds, genital and ENT specimens

Learning objectives
After studying this chapter you should confidently be able to:

■ **Outline the principal pathogens likely to be isolated from specimens taken from these body sites**
Wound swabs are taken from a variety of sites of infection, from superficial skin wounds, ulcer swabs and burns to deep post-operative wounds. The range of pathogens is also varied and the significance of the isolation of particular bacteria is related to the site of infection and the presence of normal flora. Any pathogen isolated from a sterile site, e.g. a bile swab or intravenous line, is considered significant. *Staphylococcus aureus*, beta-haemolytic streptococci, coliforms including *Pseudomonas aeruginosa,* and anaerobic organisms are frequent isolates in wound swabs. Coagulase-negative staphylococci from the patient's own skin flora may be the source of infection in an intravenous line. Appropriate culture media to cover the range of potential pathogens are inoculated. The principal pathogens isolated in the general microbiology laboratory from female genital swabs are *Candida* species, Group B streptococci, coliforms, *Trichomonas vaginalis, Gardnerella vaginalis*, and *Neisseria gonorrhoeae. Actinomyces* species may be isolated from intrauterine contraceptive devices (IUCDs). Group A and other beta-haemolytic streptococci are the most frequently isolated bacteria from throat swabs; a wider range of pathogens are isolated from ear swabs, including *Staphyloccus aureus*, beta-haemolytic streptococci, *Streptococcus pneumoniae, Proteus* species, *Pseudomonas aeruginosa*, anaerobic bacteria, yeasts and filamentous fungi.

■ **Describe the laboratory culture of the various specimens and the identification of the isolated pathogens**
A range of culture media are inoculated to ensure the isolation of the most likely pathogens. This will depend on the site of infection and clinical details. After primary isolation further identification tests are performed on significant pathogens and antibiotic susceptibilities carried out to inform treatment choices.

■ **Explain the rationale for the choice of culture media and identification methods used**
Culture media are selected to ensure that the range of pathogens likely to be present at the site of infection are given the optimal conditions to grow and can be differentiated for primary identification. Further tests are performed as outlined in *Chapter 6.*

10.1   SPECIMEN COLLECTION AND RECEPTION

This area of the microbiology laboratory is usually split into distinct sections: one dealing with general wound swabs, pus and bile; a second handling genital specimens; and ear, nose and throat swabs in another. MRSA screening is performed either separately or incorporated into one of the other sections. Many of the specimens are swabs in transport medium. Bacteriological investigations are the principal focus and specimens for chlamydia testing and viral or dermatophyte infections are dealt with in the appropriate section. However, chlamydia testing and screening for syphilis are included in this chapter as they are sexually transmitted infections.

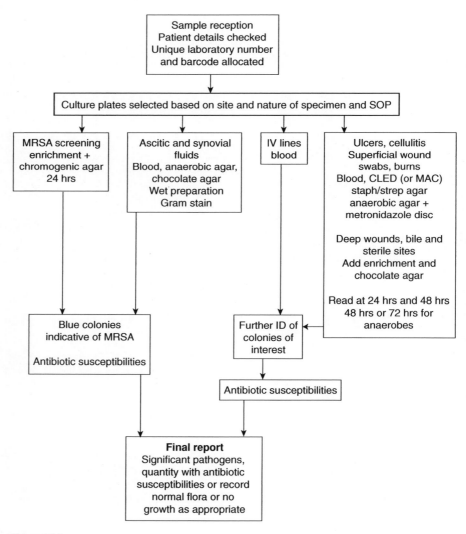

Figure 10.1
Flow chart to describe process of general wound swabs.

A large number of different specimens from body sites are received for investigation. On receipt they are checked for the main points of identification, numbered and entered on to the computer system. The specimens are then transferred to the appropriately labelled racks for each section described above and inoculated on to appropriate culture media depending on the nature of the specimen. These clinical details are guided by the appropriate SOP. Flow diagrams for each of the three sections described are shown in *Figures 10.1–10.3*.

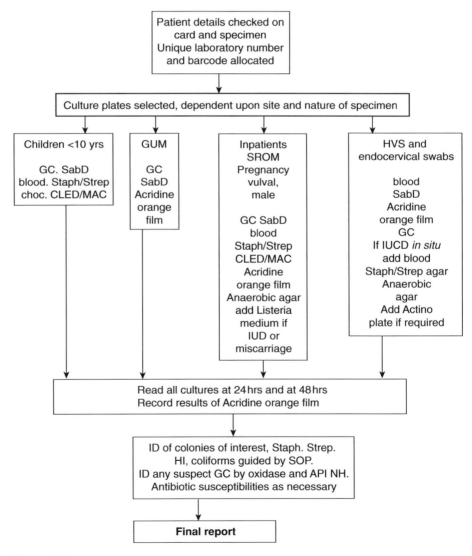

Figure 10.2
Flow chart for processing of genital specimens.

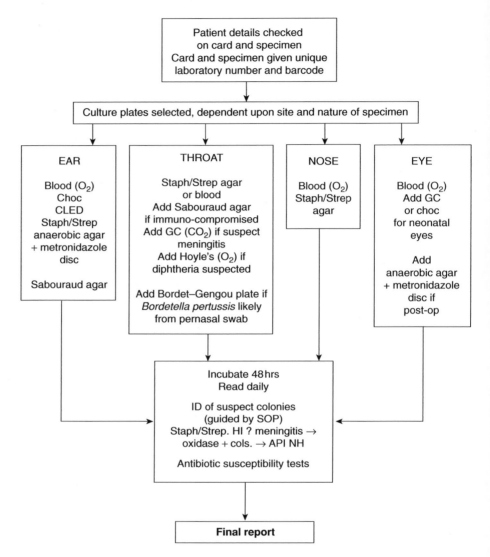

Figure 10.3
Flow chart to describe processing of ENT swabs.

10.2 GENERAL WOUND SWABS

Specimens received in this section include swabs from skin and soft tissue infections (including ulcer swabs, burns, and bites), deep wounds, specimens of bile and pus drained from wounds and abscesses, and fluid from normally sterile areas such as ascitic and joint fluids. The range of pathogens isolated is relatively wide and includes aerobic and anaerobic bacteria and yeasts. The culture media used are selected for the ability to isolate the major pathogens, and extra media are added as necessary for particular specimens.

Skin and soft tissue infections

The skin and soft tissue (see *Figure 10.4*) are composed of several layers: the epidermis, dermis, a subcutaneous layer, and the superficial fascia separating the skin from the muscles. The epidermis is a thin (0.1 mm deep) self-renewing sheet. The keratinocytes at the base of the epidermis divide, differentiate and stratify to produce an outer layer of dead cells called the stratum corneum. These cells are rich in keratin, held together by neutral lipids and are regularly sloughed off the skin surface. Fixed tissue macrophages (the Langerhans cells), lymphocytes and melanocytes are also found in this layer. A basement membrane separates the dermis from the epidermis. The dermis provides a strong supportive structure, being composed of connective tissue, collagen and elastin embedded in a matrix of glycoprotein. The area is well vascularized and restriction of blood flow limits access to nutrients and immune defences and thus predisposes to infection. The subcutaneous layer contains lipid cells and provides heat insulation and calorie reserves, and also acts as a shock absorber. The superficial fascia below separates the skin from the muscles. The area is well protected from exogenous infection by the presence of skin flora on the outer layer, antibiotic peptides, Langerhans cells, lymphocytes and the components of the innate immune system, as well as the continuous shedding of cells. The normal flora of the area have adapted to the pH, salt levels, dryness or presence of sweat, fatty acids and the lower temperature than that of the internal organs.

Potential pathogens arriving on the surface of the skin have to be able to survive these conditions and compete with the resident bacteria for receptor sites and nutrients. If they attach to the outer layers they must be aerobic or facultatively aerobic, or have the capacity for invasion to reach more anaerobic conditions in the deeper layers. To spread within the dermal and subcutaneous layers they need to express additional enzymes and/or toxins to break down the connective tissue and resist the activity of complement and the immune cells. Spread within the fascial

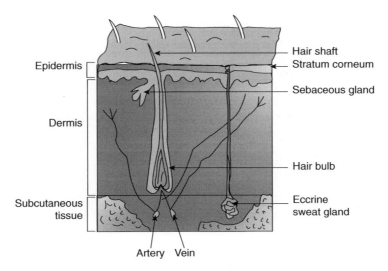

Figure 10.4
The structure of skin, showing the epidermis, dermis and subcutaneous tissue.

layer is fortunately infrequent, involving a small range of anaerobic or facultatively anaerobic bacteria and leading to serious and life-threatening infections.

Bacteria (and fungi, see *Chapter 13*) may be exogenous or from the individual's own flora, and enter the skin through cuts, wounds, trauma, bites (whether insect, human or animal), burns, open ulcers, accompanying foreign bodies and instrumentation, including lines and catheters. They may also arrive at the skin from underlying tissue or the blood circulation. Some patients are predisposed to skin and soft tissue infection:

- diabetics as a result of restricted oxygen supply and blood flow accompanied by peripheral sensory neuropathy
- patients who are immuno-compromised as a result of pre-existing disease and the insertion of catheters, lines and following surgery
- patients with limited mobility have poor circulation and decreased tissue viability which may lead to spontaneous tissue breakdown and tissue that is easily damaged and difficult to heal, predisposing them to the formation of ulcers.

Superficial skin infections

These are characterized by inflammation, failure to heal and sometimes the presence of pus. There are several examples, including erysipelas, which presents as a painful red fluid-filled area of skin, sometimes with small vesicles on the surface. Impetigo appears as red areas on the skin which may result in vesicles or develop into pustules that rupture and crust. Folliculitis is the infection and inflammation of a hair follicle. Paronychia is a superficial infection of the nail fold.

Scalded skin syndrome, where the skin blisters and then peels, is caused by *Staphylococcus aureus* infection where production of exfoliative toxin splits the junctions between the cells. MRSA may colonize or infect skin in hospitalized patients whereas *Staphylococcus aureus* is a common pathogen in the community, with an increasing incidence of strains possessing Panton–Valentine leukocidin (PVL) and scalded skin toxin.

The principal pathogens involved in all these infections, and in insect bites, are *Staphylococcus aureus* and Group A streptococcus. *Pasteurella multocida* is often isolated from dog bites, but any members of the oral flora may be sources of infection. Groups C and G streptococci may also be isolated in cases of erysipelas and impetigo; *Pseuodomonas aeruginosa* and *Candida* species in folliculitis and paronychia may also be caused by yeasts, anaerobic bacteria (folds in the area provide a more anaerobic niche) and *Haemophilus influenzae*. Superficial mycoses (see *Chapter 13*) are further possible causes of infection.

Lyme disease

Lyme disease is caused by the spirochaete bacteria *Borrelia burgdorferi,* transmitted by the bite of an infected tick. The ticks, *Ixodes ricinus*, are associated with mice and deer and the disease is therefore more prevalent in forested areas where deer are known to graze. The early stage of Lyme disease is a characteristic red area called erythema migrans at the site of the tick bite. If undiagnosed the disease can progress to early disseminated Lyme disease, which may include numbness and pain in the legs, Bell's palsy or meningitis. Late Lyme disease includes joint pain, memory loss and chronic muscle pain. It is therefore important to diagnose the condition in the early stage.

However, *Borrelia burgdorferi* is not diagnosed from a skin swab but from a serum sample which is tested for antibodies to the bacteria and if this is positive, confirmatory antibody tests are carried out to ensure that the antibodies are specific for *Borrelia burgdorferi*.

Venous or arterial ulcers

Ulcers involve deeper layers of the skin; the open area becomes colonized with bacteria, which may be commensal skin flora or pathogens that further prevent the healing process. A large majority of swabs received in the laboratory are from chronic venous ulcers and the accompanying clinical details may not indicate whether there are signs of inflammation and infection, making the interpretation of the culture more difficult. Anaerobes may be present and give rise to an unpleasant odour, and the presence of bacteria such as *Staphylococcus aureus*, Group A streptococcus and *Pseudomonas aeruginosa* is more likely to be clinically significant. Diabetic foot ulcers are a serious complication of the disease that can progress to gangrene and the necessity for foot amputation. Infection is caused by a wide variety of aerobic bacteria, including methicillin-sensitive and -resistant *Staphylococcus aureus* and anaerobes such as *Bacteroides fragilis* and *Fusobacterium* species.

Burns

Burns, depending on their severity, can involve any layer of the skin, destroying the skin-related immune defence and rendering the area more prone to exogenous infection and the possibility of sepsis, an important cause of death in burns patients. *Box 10.1* details the microorganisms most likely to be isolated.

Box 10.1 Organisms associated with burns

Staphylococcus aureus
Beta-haemolytic streptococci
Pseudomonads, especially *Pseudomonas aeruginosa*
Acinetobacter species
Bacillus species
Enterobacteriaceae
Filamentous fungi, e.g. *Fusarium* species
Candida albicans and other yeasts
Coagulase-negative staphylococci

Cellulitis

Cellulitis is a spreading infection of the deeper layers of the skin and subcutaneous layer, with symptoms of swollen and inflamed skin. A swab will be of little use in ascertaining the causative organism, especially if the skin is unbroken, and a blood culture is the better option.

Deep wound infections

This includes post-operative wounds, abscesses, infective gangrene and necrotizing fasciitis. *Box 10.2* details the bacteria most commonly isolated from post-operative wounds that drain outside the body.

> **Box 10.2 Organisms associated with post-operative wound infections**
>
> *Staphylococcus aureus* including MRSA
> *Bacteroides* species
> *Clostridium* species
> Enterobacteriaceae
> Pseudomonads
> Beta-haemolytic streptococci
> Enterococci
> *Peptostreptococcus* species

Abscesses

Abscesses are localized areas of infection, full of pus, bacteria and debris. They may arise anywhere in the body and the likely pathogens vary with the site and nature of the abscess. Skin abscesses may present as boils or furuncles, causing pressure on the neighbouring tissue. Their development may be associated with intravenous drug abuse. Abscesses of deeper tissues include dental, liver (bacterial and amoebic), lung, peri-rectal, pilonidal, and prostatic areas. Laboratory investigation is performed on the aspirated contents, which are frequently polymicrobial, representing aerobic and anaerobic bacteria and varying for different anatomical sites. Amoebic liver abscesses involve *Entamoeba histolytica* or hydatid cysts.

Infective gangrene and necrotizing fasciitis

These conditions present as necrotic areas of tissue and require surgical debridement as part of the treatment strategy. Fortunately they are relatively rare infections. Progressive synergistic gangrene can be a post-operative complication caused by mixed aerobic and anaerobic bacteria such as *Staphylococcus aureus* and anaerobic streptococci. *Clostridia* species, particularly *Clostridium perfringens*, may infect a wound and lead to cellulitis, myonecrosis (involving the muscle) or gas gangrene, so called because of the gas that builds up in the tissues. *Clostridium perfringens* has a range of toxins that together create an anaerobic nutrient-rich environment ideal for the growth and spread of the bacteria, but at the same time can cause clinical shock and extensive necrosis in the patient.

If swabs are received from injuries sustained as a result of trauma in salt or fresh water, the presence of water-borne bacteria (for example *Aeromonas* species and *Vibrio* species) should be considered. Occasionally these bacteria cause muscle necrosis similar to that of *Clostridium perfringens*.

Necrotizing fasciitis describes a serious infection of the subcutaneous fat layers, soft tissue and superficial fascia. The infection has the capacity to spread rapidly and may prove fatal in a short time. Type I is caused by a mixed infection of an anaerobe, often *Bacteroides* species, and a facultative aerobe, Enterobacteriaceae or streptococci (not Group A). Type II involves Group A streptococci and *Staphylococcus aureus*, both of which have powerful toxins. Group A streptococcal exotoxins include SPE-A, B and C and streptococcal superantigen (SSA). *Staphylococcus aureus* is a less common cause of necrotizing fasciitis and reported cases have been associated with the enterotoxin gene cluster and Panton–Valentine leukocidin.

Bile and bile swabs

Bile is a normally sterile fluid that may become infected as the result of ascending infection resulting from partial obstruction of the biliary ducts, or as a result of cholecystitis (infection of the gallbladder) often caused by the presence of gallstones.

Ascitic fluid

Ascitic fluid is a watery fluid containing albumin, glucose and electrolytes. The fluid accumulates in the peritoneal cavity in association with several disease processes including malignancies, liver disease and spontaneous bacterial peritonitis. In some diseases no infectious agents are involved. Infections of the fluid, as in bacterial peritonitis, are most commonly associated with enteric organisms such as *Escherichia coli* and streptococci.

Synovial (joint) fluid

Synovial fluid is normally present in healthy joints, but may accumulate in arthritic conditions, trauma and infection. Septic arthritis is associated with *Staphylococcus aureus, Haemophilus influenzae*, Gram-negative bacilli, gonococci and streptococci. Samples of synovial fluid can also be tested on the blood culture machine (described in *Chapter 12*). Joint fluids are also investigated if there is suspicion of infection following prosthetic joint surgery or further revision surgery has taken place.

Intravenous cannulae and lines

When these are removed from the patient they may be sent to the laboratory for culture, either for screening or because the patient has shown signs of inflammation and infection at the site of insertion in the surrounding subcutaneous area. Bacteria from the skin are able to enter the body opportunistically and move along the surface of the line to gain access to deeper tissue. Coagulase-negative staphylococci colonize the tip and produce protective biofilms; other pathogens include *Staphylococcus aureus* and MRSA, Enterobacteriaceae, pseudomonads, enterococci and streptococci.

10.3   LABORATORY INVESTIGATION OF WOUND SWABS

The range of culture media inoculated for the samples and infections described must be able to isolate a variety of aerobic and anaerobic bacteria and any yeasts present (see *Box 10.3*). Blood agar is used, and an anaerobic agar with a metronidazole disc added after inoculation. A medium designed to easily differentiate between staphylococci and streptococci may be included, and either CLED or MacConkey agar to differentiate lactose fermentation. Fastidious anaerobes, *Bacteroides* species and *Prevotella* species are possible pathogens and an agar containing sufficient nutrients to support their growth is included. For deep wounds a liquid enrichment medium such as cooked meat broth may be used. This supports the growth of aerobic and anaerobic organisms at varying levels of oxygen availability within the broth, and may also be used as a room temperature storage medium for stock cultures. The inclusion of chocolate agar encourages the growth of fastidious bacteria such as *Haemophilus* species and a Sabouraud agar is included if *Candida* species or other yeasts are likely pathogens.

A small quantity of ascitic fluid is added to a counting chamber for enumeration of white and red blood cells. The fluids are cultured on blood agar, a fastidious anaerobe

Box 10.3 Case study

A leg ulcer swab is received from an elderly patient. After culture the following bacteria are isolated: coagulase-positive and -negative staphylococci, enterococci, lactose-fermenting coliforms, a beta-haemolytic streptococcus, probably Group A, and a significant growth of mixed anaerobes.

Questions

1. Which culture media would have been inoculated to isolate and differentiate the range of bacteria likely to be present?
2. Which bacteria from those listed are more likely to be significant from a leg ulcer swab?
3. What further tests would be necessary to confirm the presence of the significant organisms?
4. Why is it necessary to treat these pathogens as part of the clinical management of the patient?
5. Outline some of the factors that may have contributed to the formation of the ulcer.

agar and a chocolate agar. A smear is also taken for examination after Gram staining.

Synovial fluids are cultured on the same media as ascitic fluids and additionally have a wet preparation examined for the presence of red and white blood cells and crystals. The presence of specific types of crystals can be indicative of gout or pseudogout, an inflammatory arthritis. Monosodium urate crystals in conjunction with high levels of polymorphs (neutrophils) are found in gout, whereas calcium pyrophosphate crystals and neutrophils are present in pseudogout.

Cannula tips and lines, which should be at least 4 cm in length, are rolled over the media four times so that any adherent bacteria are transferred. Growth of more than 15 bacterial colonies after incubation is considered significant.

MRSA screening swabs from all sites are important specimens because the results affect the movement and isolation of patients. Nose and groin swabs are most frequently used for this purpose. The ideal sensitive, specific, rapid and cost-effective test is elusive and is the constant focus of research in the area. The method used for MRSA screening varies between laboratories. One of the most widely used is the inoculation of specific chromogenic agar and/or enrichment in a 7% salt broth. Chromogenic agar is produced by several media manufacturers and contains a chromogen detecting either α-glucosidase or phosphatase activity, leading to the production of either green or blue colonies after 24 hours. Cefoxitin is incorporated to detect the methicillin resistance. Molecular methods are available using primers to detect the *nuc* gene of *Staphylococcus aureus,* and *mec* or other MRSA-specific genes. For example, one commercial real-time PCR analyser can probe for the *MecA* gene, providing an answer within 4 hours (2 hours' preparation and 2 hours for the PCR programme). This is considerably faster than culture methods but is more expensive, and culture methods are still required for antimicrobial susceptibility testing. Pulsed-field gel electrophoresis (PFGE) analysis enables epidemic strains to be separated and identified. Advanced genomic profiling techniques will be introduced in the near future to enable the source and spread of infection to be identified and tracked, leading to more effective measures to control infection.

All of the media designed to isolate aerobes or facultative anaerobes are incubated for 24 hours at 37°C in air and re-examined at 48 hours. Anaerobic media are incubated at the same temperature in either an anaerobic cabinet or in anaerobic jars for 48 hours. If the wound is deep or the swab is from an abscess, the anaerobic plates are examined daily and incubated for up to 7 days.

When reading the culture plates the site of the specimen and the clinical details are important. The significance of the colonies present must be interpreted in the knowledge of whether the area supports a normal flora and the nature of this, or whether the area investigated is normally sterile and therefore any growth is significant, as described in *Chapter 4*. For example, a chronic ulcer swab may grow Enterobacteriaceae, enterococci and coagulase-negative staphylococci, representative of saprophytic skin bacteria, and thus be considered normal. A culture of any of these bacteria from a specimen of bile would be clinically significant.

Follow-up of interesting colonies is carried out using the standard identification methods for each pathogen, as outlined in *Chapter 6*, and appropriate antibiotic susceptibility tests are performed. Staphylococci are tested for the presence of coagulase and DNAse. If *Staphylococcus aureus* is isolated from a non-resolving infection, the presence of PVL can be determined by a PCR-based method. Beta-haemolytic streptococci are confirmed by Lancefield grouping; significant Gram-negative bacteria are confirmed by lactose fermentation, oxidase test and API testing as appropriate. Anaerobic bacteria will either be reported as mixed anaerobes sensitive to metronidazole or, if present as a pure culture, further identified by biochemical tests. If *Pasteurella* species are suspected from a bite wound, the bacteria can be identified by their characteristic grey growth on blood agar, similar to other coliforms, but they do not grow on MacConkey agar because they cannot grow in the presence of the bile salts. They are oxidase- and indole-positive and, unusually for Gram-negative rods, sensitive to penicillin. Bacteria that are less commonly isolated are also encountered in the wound section and are investigated following set schema, until a presumptive identification is made. The isolates considered significant for a particular specimen type are then reported along with their antibiotic susceptibilities.

10.4 GENITAL SPECIMENS

Specimens received in this work area include high vaginal swabs, endo-cervical swabs, low vaginal and urethral swabs from children, IUCDs, aspirates from cysts and abscesses in the genital area, and specimens of amniotic fluid from cases of intrauterine death. Male specimens include penile swabs and specimens of semen. Screening swabs from the genitourinary clinic are also routinely processed. Chlamydia and syphilis testing is included in this part of the chapter, although the tests would not be carried out in this work area.

Principal pathogens

Significant pathogens isolated from genital specimens may be representative of either sexually transmitted disease (STD) or non-sexually transmitted infection.

Non-sexually transmitted infection

The range of non-sexually transmitted genital infections in females is age and hormone related. Between the menarche (onset of menstruation) and menopause the level of oestrogen keeps the pH of the vagina at a slightly acidic 5.5 and the level of glycogen in the vaginal epithelia encourages the growth of *Lactobacillus* species in the area. The presence of the lactobacilli provides colonization resistance to potential pathogens. Hormonal changes during the menstrual cycle have an effect on the normal flora, the growth of coliforms being more common when the oestrogen levels are lower, with lactobacilli dominating during and after ovulation (luteal phase). Overgrowth of *Candida* species is more likely when oestrogen levels are higher. Group B streptococci may be part of the normal flora and become significant in the final stages of pregnancy as the baby passes through the birth canal. The incidence of neonatal infection and meningitis is low. A study by the HPA in 2002 reported an incidence figure of 0.7 per 1000 live births in the UK, with 67% being early onset disease and 33% late onset disease (7–90 days after birth). Serious disease generally arises as a result of lack of maternal antibodies and infection with serotype III (less commonly with Ia/c and V), which accounts for 90% of strains isolated from neonatal Group B streptococcal meningitis.

The normal vaginal flora may also contain coagulase-negative staphylococci, coliforms, enterococci, diphtheroids and *Bacteroides* species and low levels of *Staphylococcus aureus*. Less common bacteria include *Ureaplasma urealyticum* and *Mycoplasma* species, which may also lead to infection. Post-menopausal women have fewer protective lactobacilli and often have increased levels of coliforms in their normal flora. The clinical details accompanying high vaginal swab specimens often suggest an increased vaginal discharge, itching, or vaginitis as the reason the patient sought clinical advice. Infection can be caused by increased levels of *Staphylococcus aureus*, Group B streptococci, Group A streptococci or anaerobic bacteria.

Candida species are frequent causes of infection, most commonly *Candida albicans*, but other *Candida* species such as *C. krusei*, *C. kefyr*, *C. tropicalis* and *C. glabrata*, which are less responsive to initial treatment, may be the cause of 10–15% of yeast infections. Candidosis, overgrowth of *Candida* species, is associated with high levels of oestrogen, diabetes, pregnancy, obesity and the use of oral contraceptives. Its incidence may be increased following antimicrobial treatment. Although it is not classified as an STD infection, yeasts can be passed between sexual partners, leading to re-infection.

Bacterial vaginosis, caused by a combination of bacteria including *Gardnerella vaginalis*, leads to increased discharge. Bacterial vaginosis was considered harmless until research evidence demonstrated an association with several clinical conditions including increased risk of ectopic pregnancy, pelvic infection and premature births, and an increased risk of acquiring sexually transmitted infections. Children do not have the protection of lactobacilli beyond the first few weeks of life when maternal oestrogen is present, and so infections may be caused by a wide variety of bacteria including staphylococci, streptococci, and *Haemophilus* species.

After removal, IUCDs may be sent for culture if an infection is suspected. Possible pathogens may include *Actinomyces* species such as *A. israelii* or *A. naeslundii*.

The normal flora of the male genital tract consists of skin flora and coliforms. Non-sexually transmitted disease in males can present as inflammation of the glans penis (balanitis) caused by yeasts, Group A or Group B streptococci, *Staphylococcus aureus* or anaerobes. Non-sexually transmitted urethritis can be the result of infection with pseudomonads or Enterobacteriaceae.

Sexually transmitted infection

Sexually transmitted infections (STIs) diagnosed from genital swabs include gonorrhoea and trichomoniasis. The presence of infection with *Neisseria gonorrhoeae* and *Trichomonas vaginalis* can be diagnosed from endocervical, urethral, rectal and pharyngeal swabs and either wet preparations or stained smears, respectively. Other major STDs such as *Chlamydia trachomatis*, genital herpes, HIV and syphilis are diagnosed using molecular or serological methods.

Neisseria gonorrhoeae

Neisseria gonorrhoeae, gonococci, are capable of infecting any mucosal site, leading to symptomatic disease or asymptomatic mucosal infection in males and females of all ages, and also neonatal infection. Disseminated gonococcal infection is a rare complication of the initial infection, and is diagnosed by isolation of the bacteria from blood or sterile fluids. The bacteria are Gram-negative capsulated diplococci, indistinguishable on a Gram film from *Neisseria meningitidis*, and are obligate human pathogens. The outer membrane lacks side chains and is therefore referred to as lipo-oligosaccharide (LOS), rather than LPS (lipopolysaccharide). They are fragile organisms that do not survive outside the body, hence the necessity for them to be passed by intimate contact. The term gonorrhoea means 'flow of the seed' as the connection between sexual activity and the cause of the disease was made long before Neisser discovered the bacterial cause. Gonococci also present a challenge in terms of culture – the transport medium should be able to maintain their viability and the culture medium used has to contain sufficient growth factors to enhance growth and give good colony formation, accompanied by antibiotics to suppress the growth of other bacteria. The fragility of the bacteria can be overcome by examining a Gram stain prepared immediately after the specimen is taken from the patient. Culture plates are inoculated and incubated in the clinic prior to their transport to the laboratory. Gonococci attach to columnar and cuboidal epithelial cells in the endocervix, urethra, ano-rectal area and the pharynx.

Gonococci attach to CEACAM receptors on epithelial cells by pili, type IV fimbriae, and the outer membrane protein Opa (also called P.II). After attachment they invade the epithelium and subepithelium. This stimulates a strong inflammatory response; however, antibodies produced to the bacteria are short-lived in their effectiveness and not protective because of the antigenic variation of the pilin protein. Genetic rearrangement of the protein allows up to a million variations in the antigenic structure. The bacterial capsule further enhances pathogenicity by avoidance of opsonization by complement proteins and phagocytosis by neutrophils. Males infected with urethral gonorrhoea usually present with asymptomatic urethritis, dysuria and purulent discharge. Ano-rectal infection may be asymptomatic or lead to proctitis. Pharyngeal infection may also be asymptomatic in males and females and is detected in specimens from patients with a clinical history of oro-genital exposure.

In females the bacteria can be isolated from the cervix, and from urethral swabs in patients who have had a hysterectomy. Some infections are symptomatic, with increased vaginal discharge, dysuria and itching, while others are silent. The bacteria are able to ascend through the cervix and reach the Fallopian tubes where infection and healing cause scarring (fibrosis) of the tissue. Pelvic inflammatory disease (PID) can also result from the bacteria moving out from the female reproductive organs. Both situations can result in infertility and ectopic pregnancy due to the blocked Fallopian tubes. *Chlamydia trachomatis* is also a major cause of PID, either as a single infection or in conjunction with *Neisseria gonorrhoeae*. Neonates exposed to the bacteria during birth are at risk from the eye infection ophthalmia neonatorum.

Trichomonas vaginalis

This protozoan infection causes vaginitis and presents with symptoms of a frothy cream discharge. It is carried asymptomatically by men and is nearly always acquired by women as a result of sexual contact. The discharge is the symptom that drives women to seek a diagnosis, but asymptomatic carriage in pregnant women can lead to low birth weight and pre-term delivery. The infection can be treated with metronidazole (Flagyl).

Chlamydia trachomatis

Chlamydia trachomatis is the most frequently diagnosed STI in the UK, with around 190 000 new cases diagnosed annually, compared with around 17 000 cases of gonorrhoea and 2700 cases of syphilis in 2010. The disease is most prevalent among younger people aged between 15 and 24 years, the age range targeted by the national chlamydia screening programme, launched in 2003. *Chlamydia trachomatis* is an important infection to diagnose because it is asymptomatic in up to 70% of females and 50% of males. Undiagnosed infection can lead to complications in both sexes; urethritis and epididymitis in men, and more serious consequences in women. The infection can ascend through the uterus and infect the Fallopian tubes, increasing the risk of ectopic pregnancy and infertility. Release of the elementary bodies into the peritoneal cavity can lead to pelvic inflammatory disease, as described above in relation to gonococcal infection. Chronic infection can be the cause of arthritis in both sexes. Any STI also increases the risk of infection with HIV because the infection attracts immune cells to the area, and it is the immune cells that become infected with HIV.

Once diagnosed, *Chlamydia trachomatis* is easy to treat with antibiotics, such as doxycycline or azithromycin, which are able to combat intracellular infections. Pelvic inflammatory disease is treated with a combination of drugs including doxycycline, metronidazole and ceftriaxone.

Syphilis

The spirochaete *Treponema pallidum* has eluded all attempts to be grown on an *in vitro* culture medium and of necessity is diagnosed from serological markers. The bacteria can be visualized directly from a primary lesion, but the opportunity to view such specimens is rare. Syphilis has a long history, so much so that entire textbooks have been written on the subject. Fortunately the disease is now treatable and the prevalence in the UK is relatively low; there were 2700 newly diagnosed cases in 2010. The disease has three stages – the primary chancre, an ulcer-like lesion, appears a few days after infection, heals and the spirochaetes spread. Secondary syphilis manifests itself two to ten weeks after the initial infection with a rash accompanied by general malaise, which can be difficult to diagnose without confirmatory serological evidence. Tertiary disease in untreated patients can become evident after up to 30 years of latency, and again can mimic other conditions such as dementia and other neurological problems. Tertiary disease can affect any area of the body – heart, eyes, brain, nerves, bones, liver or joints. All pregnant women in the UK are tested for syphilis antibodies as part of their antenatal screening.

HIV

The diagnosis of HIV infection is described in *Chapter 3*.

10.5   LABORATORY DIAGNOSIS

Standard operating procedures are, as always, essential for guiding the most appropriate culture plates to be inoculated from specific specimens. Patient details, age, source of specimen (genitourinary clinic, GP or hospital ward) and clinical details further influence this choice (see *Figure 10.2*).

Vaginal swabs

For high vaginal swabs, possible pathogens are isolated on blood agar and either a Sabouraud or chromogenic agar for isolating and identifying yeasts. A Granada plate can also be inoculated to identify Group B streptococci. Enterococci are not normally significant and their presence can be determined by the addition of a penicillin disc to the blood agar plate. Enterococci are resistant to penicillin and so if there is a zone of susceptibility, further testing can be performed on the susceptible bacteria, such as Lancefield grouping. A smear can also be prepared from the swab for staining with acridine orange to identify *Trichomonas vaginalis*. This will also indicate the presence of yeasts, neutrophils and clue cells (see *Figure 10.5*). Some laboratories prefer to examine unstained wet preparations for the presence of *Trichomonas vaginalis* (see *Figure 10.6*). *Trichomonas vaginalis* can also be cultured in *Trichomonas* culture medium for 48 hours at 35–37°C. Motile trichomonads can be visualized at low magnification on the inverted light microscope. The plates are kept sealed during incubation and reading. If the patient is post-menopausal an anaerobic plate is included, as bacterial vaginosis is more likely. Bacterial vaginosis is a mixed infection of anaerobic and aerobic bacteria that characteristically attach to epithelial cells. The presence of these cells covered in bacteria, some of them characteristically curved *Mobiluncus* species, together with the presence of anaerobes and a lack of lactobacilli on the blood plate, are all factors leading to a suggestion of bacterial vaginosis.

Urethral and low vaginal swabs, male urethral swabs

Urethral and low vaginal swabs from children may contain significant coliforms or *Haemophilus influenzae* and require the addition of CLED or MacConkey agar,

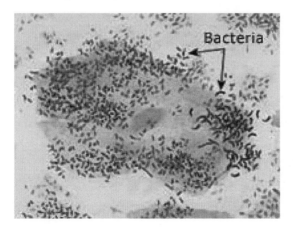

Figure 10.5
Clue cells, suggestive of bacterial vaginosis.

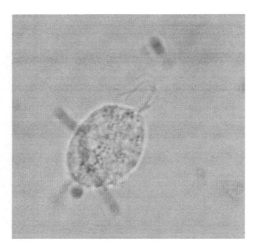

Figure 10.6
Trichomonas vaginalis in a wet preparation from a vaginal swab.

and also chocolate agar. Male urethral specimens are also inoculated on to CLED or MacConkey agar in addition to blood agar. Staphylococci, streptococci, coliforms and *Haemophilus influenzae* are identified by standard confirmation tests.

Endocervical swabs

Endocervical swabs with relevant clinical details and all specimens from the genitourinary (GUM) clinic are cultured for *Neisseria gonorrhoeae* using a specially formulated culture medium. There are several commercially available media such as New York City agar, Thayer–Martin and 'special chocolate'. They all contain antibiotics. VCAT is a common combination including vancomycin, colistin, amphotericin B and trimethoprim to suppress the growth of susceptible organisms. Growth of gonococci is enhanced by growth supplements such as vitox or polyvitox. An ideal gonococci culture medium should produce pure growth of creamy colonies after incubation at 37°C in an atmosphere of CO_2. The colonies are confirmed as *Neisseria gonorrhoeae* by Gram stain and a positive oxidase test, followed by an API NH and/or Gonochek test. *Neisseria meningitidis* and *N. gonorrhoeae* are distinguishable by their sugar reactions: **m**eningococci ferment **m**altose and **g**lucose, but **g**onococci, **g**lucose only. Susceptibility tests are performed to guide appropriate treatment, such as cefixime or ciprofloxacin.

Gonorrhoea can also be diagnosed using a nucleic acid amplification test where specific primers for a sequence of the genome are used to identify and amplify gonococcal DNA. An automated system is described below in the diagnosis of *Chlamydia trachomatis*. Automated amplification systems can also be used to identify both *Neisseria gonorrhoeae* and *Chlamydia trachomatis* from a single specimen.

Amniotic fluid

Specimens from amniotic fluid in cases of stillbirth require additional culture to detect the presence of *Listeria monocytogenes*. The incidence of infection in pregnancy is fortunately low, but carries a risk of miscarriage, premature delivery and neonatal infection. The selective culture medium contains inhibitory factors, including lithium chloride, acriflavine and antibiotics that are effective in inhibiting Gram-negative bacteria. *Listeria monocytogenes*, a Gram-positive rod, is identified by black colonies produced by the hydrolysis of aesculin and the formation of black phenolic iron compounds.

Intrauterine contraceptive devices
IUCDs are added to nutrient broth and a series of dilutions made. The initial dilution is then inoculated on to blood, chocolate and either CLED or MacConkey agar, and incubated aerobically for up to 48 hours. The remaining dilutions are inoculated on to blood or anaerobic agar, or specific *Actinomyces* agar, and incubated for 10 days to allow for growth and for characteristic colony formations of *Actinomyces* species to develop. Identification is then confirmed by colony appearance and further identification if necessary. *Actinomyces* are branching Gram-positive rods.

Testing for Chlamydia trachomatis
Testing for *Chlamydia trachomatis* must be sensitive, specific, cost-effective and capable of detecting low levels of infection in clinical samples. Molecular nucleic acid amplification tests are the preferred option. An example of an automated system is the BD VIPER, using strand displacement amplification to visualize the amplified product (described in *Section 6.8*). A hairpin probe specific for a sequence of the *Chlamydia trachomatis* genome anneals to the single-stranded DNA and is nicked by a restriction endonuclease to separate the fluorophore and the quencher, allowing a signal to be emitted. Both urine and swab samples can be tested on the system.

Syphilis testing
Syphilis testing is performed on serum samples, in a separate section of the laboratory. The most frequently used test is an ELISA technique, enabling large numbers of samples to be screened simultaneously. The test uses syphilis antigen as the solid phase to bind with antibodies specific for *Treponema pallidum*. Patients who have been infected with the bacteria and have been successfully treated will still have detectable levels of antibody in their serum. Positive samples would be sent to a reference laboratory for further testing.

10.6   EAR, NOSE AND THROAT SPECIMENS

The upper respiratory tract (URT) is a frequent site of infection (see *Figure 10.7*), as it is in close communication with the environment and aerosol-borne pathogens. The infections are generally mild and often viral in origin; for example, rhinoviruses and coronaviruses, which give rise to cold symptoms, cause recurrent infections but do not spread beyond the nasal area as the viruses survive better at the slightly lower temperature found there. The lining of the nose and throat provides a warm moist environment for colonization of bacteria and viruses. Infections of the eyes and ears are less frequent in healthy adults; children are more prone to ear infections because the ear canal is wider. The eyes are protected by the presence of lacrimal (tear) fluid bathing the conjunctiva; the fluid contains antibacterial substances including lysozyme. The ear is protected by the presence both of normal flora on the skin surfaces and of earwax, which provides a physical barrier, and by the narrow ear canal. The nasal and

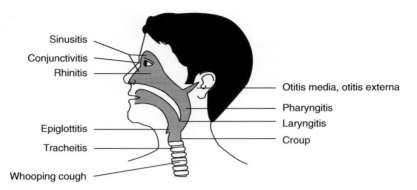

Figure 10.7
Structures and infections associated with the ENT area.

pharyngeal areas also support normal flora on their epithelial surfaces and are covered in mucus containing antibacterial peptides and secretory IgA.

Eyes

Infections of the eye include conjunctivitis, blepharitis, keratitis (inflammation of the cornea) and infection of the eyelid.

Neonatal eye infections may be the result of contact with pathogenic bacteria in the birth canal or exogenous pathogens in the first weeks of life. The most frequent causes of ophthalmia neonatorum are *Neisseria gonorrhoeae* or *Chlamydia trachomatis*. *Treponema pallidum* is also a rare cause of keratitis leading to blindness and is part of the congenital syphilis syndrome. *Staphylococcus aureus* infections (often known as 'sticky eyes') are more likely to occur 5–10 days after birth. *S. aureus* is the major pathogen isolated in cases of blepharitis and styes (folliculitis).

Endogenous infections caused by constituents of the normal skin flora, as well as by *Haemophilus influenzae*, staphylococcal and *Streptococcus pneumoniae* infections, occur sporadically at any age. *Pseudomonas aeruginosa* enters the eye through trauma, contamination of contact lenses or fluid with the bacteria in tap water, post-operatively, or through the use of infected eye creams or drops. For this reason, eye drops are always stored at +4°C and both drops and creams have a strictly limited expiry date after opening. Conjunctivitis can also occur as a symptom of Weil's disease, caused by *Leptospira* species.

Acanthamoeba infections are rare causes of reusable contact lens contamination.

Nose and throat infections

Infections of the nasopharynx and oropharynx (pharyngitis) are common and frequently the result of viral infection. *Staphylococcus aureus* can colonize the nasal epithelium, leading to carriage and a source of endogenous infection. Nasal swabs are included in screening procedures for *S. aureus* and MRSA. Screening for the presence of yeasts is important in immuno-suppressed patients.

Whooping cough, caused by *Bordetella pertussis* or *B. parapertussis* infection, is a rare occurrence in non-immunized individuals and, if suspected, a pernasal swab is taken for investigation.

One symptom of pharyngitis and tonsillitis, a painful throat (especially when swallowing), is frequently caused by viruses or bacteria, notably Group A streptococci (*Streptococcus pyogenes*). Other β-haemolytic streptococci, Groups C or G, are sometimes implicated and *Fusobacterium necrophorum* infection can be the cause of pharyngitis and tonsillitis. *Staphylococcus aureus* may be carried asymptomatically, as may small numbers of *Neisseria meningitidis*, commensal *Neisseria* species and *Streptococcus pneumoniae*. The oropharynx is an extragenital site for *Neisseria gonorrhoeae* infection.

Widespread childhood immunization has rendered *Corynebacterium diphtheriae* infections in the UK extremely unlikely; however, travel to endemic areas increases the risk of toxigenic or non-toxigenic infection and must be considered if the clinical details are suggestive of exposure. Similarly, Hib vaccination has dramatically reduced the number of cases of epiglottitis.

Respiratory syncytial virus (RSV)

RSV is a negative single-stranded RNA paramyxovirus. More than 50% of infants are likely to have been exposed to the virus during their first year of life. The majority will experience mild respiratory symptoms or be infected asymptomatically. However, those more seriously affected will develop bronchiolitis or viral pneumonia and require diagnosis and treatment. The infection rates peak in December and January, and may be the cause of respiratory problems in older children and adults.

The virus attaches to and gains entry to the cytoplasm of respiratory epithelial cells via the F protein on the viral surface. The F protein also causes cell membranes on neighbouring cells to merge, forming syncytia. The infection is spread by direct contact, as the virus does not survive in the environment for long.

The virus can be diagnosed from naso-pharyngeal aspirate (NPA) by a single-use solid phase ELISA. Alternatively, diagnosis can be made by molecular methods using a reverse transcriptase PCR-based amplification method.

The antiviral drug ribavirin can be given as an aerosol in the treatment of RSV. Ribavirin acts as a nucleoside and interferes with the metabolism of viral RNA. Children at risk from RSV because of chronic lung conditions can be given prophylactic monthly injections during the high risk season of a monoclonal antibody to RSV called palivizumab.

Ear infections

Clinical details are important when ear swabs are sent for investigation. Infections of the ear may involve the outer auditory canal (otitis externa), are either acute or chronic, and have similar causes to skin and soft tissue infections elsewhere. *Staphylococcus aureus*, Group A streptococci and fungi are frequent isolates. *Pseudomonas aeruginosa* is another common cause and is often called 'swimmer's ear'. Antibiotic treatment can be administered as a topical antibiotic cream. Polymicrobial infections include mixed anaerobic bacteria.

Otitis media is a more serious condition, causing acute illness, and involves the presence of fluid in the middle ear following the upward movement of oropharyngeal flora along the Eustachian tube. Infections are more common in children and may lead to hearing loss if not diagnosed and appropriately treated with oral antibiotics. *Streptococcus pneumoniae* and *Haemophilus influenzae* are the principal pathogens; others include *Staphylococcus aureus*, Group A streptococci and *Moraxella catarrhalis*.

10.7   LABORATORY DIAGNOSIS

Eye swabs

The principal bacterial pathogens isolated from eye swabs grow on either blood or chocolate agar, and are incubated in CO_2 and read at 24 and 48 hours. Eye swabs are the most common specimens received; occasionally an eye clinic or ward will request that the plates are sent to them for direct inoculation from corneal scrapes. If *Chlamydia trachomatis* infection if suspected, an appropriate swab sample is submitted for testing as described earlier. The presence of acanthamoeba can be detected by adding washings from the contact lens to a nutrient agar plate seeded with *Escherichia coli*. After prolonged incubation of 7–10 days, the effect of the ingestion of the bacteria by the amoebae can be observed by viewing the culture plate microscopically. More sensitive molecular amplification methods are also available.

After incubation of the blood and chocolate agars, suspect colonies are further identified by, for example:

- sensitivity to optochin for *Streptococcus pneumoniae* (also distinguishes optochin-resistant viridans streptococci)
- X and V plates for *Haemophilus influenzae*
- coagulase and DNAse tests for staphylococci
- an oxidase test for *Pseudomonas aeruginosa*.

Antibiotic susceptibility tests for the different pathogens are then performed.

Throat swabs

Blood agar is a good isolation medium for most of the suspect pathogens, with the addition of chocolate for enhanced isolation of *Neisseria* species. A specialized medium for isolating *Neisseria gonorrhoeae* is added if oro-pharyngeal infection is suspected. A CNA agar plate (blood agar with staph/strep supplement added) is often the medium of choice; however, two blood agar plates may be inoculated and incubated aerobically and anaerobically, or alternatively a single blood plate may be incubated anaerobically. A bacitracin disc can be added to the blood plate – Group A streptococci are sensitive to the antibiotic. A Sabouraud dextrose agar is included if the clinical details suggest that a candida infection is a possibility. Similarly a Hoyle's tellurite medium is inoculated if *Corynebacterium diphtheriae* is clinically indicated.

Identification tests on presumptive colonies from the blood and chocolate agar, in addition to those described for isolates from the eye, include:

- Lancefield grouping for β-haemolytic streptococci
- oxidase and species identification for *Neisseria* species
- Gram stain for fusobacteria.

Characteristic black colonies suggestive of *Corynebacterium diphtheriae* growing on the tellurite agar are identified by their Gram stain morphology – Gram-positive rods often form 'V' shapes or Chinese letter formations and this can be confirmed by a commercial identification system such as API Coryne.

Pernasal swabs, for suspected *Bordetella pertussis* and *B. parapertussis* infections, are transported in charcoal medium, and cultured on to a special Bordet–Gengou agar, a blood agar with charcoal and containing cephalexin. After incubation the characteristic pearl-like colonies are identified by Gram stain (they are Gram-negative coccobacilli) and the oxidase test. *B. pertussis* is oxidase-positive and *B. parapertussis* oxidase-negative. Confirmatory testing is effected by the use of specific antisera to the two species.

Ear infections

The range of pathogens isolated from ear swabs means that a greater number of culture media are required to cover the suspect organisms and also to give a better presumptive identification from primary culture. Blood agar is used or a CNA staph/strep agar. Chocolate agar is included for more fastidious bacteria and either a CLED or MacConkey agar to distinguish lactose-fermenting coliforms from *Pseudomonas aeruginosa*. All of these culture media are incubated in CO_2 and read at 24 and 48 hours. The possibility of anaerobic infection warrants the inclusion of an agar for this purpose, whether this is a fastidious anaerobic agar or another anaerobic agar. Yeast and filamentous fungi are selected using a Sabouraud agar. After incubation suspect colonies are confirmed as described above.

10.8   ANTIBIOTIC SUSCEPTIBILITY TESTING

The choice of antibiotics for given pathogens in wound, genital and ENT swabs is guided by several factors, including the age of the patient, whether or not they are pregnant, the site of infection, and the properties of the pathogen in terms of intrinsic resistance, including the potential to produce enzymes such as β-lactamases and extended spectrum β-lactamases. Each hospital trust has an antibiotic prescribing policy outlining the recommended drugs for particular clinical symptoms and bacterial isolates. Initial therapy for an unknown infectious cause is empirical and includes a broad-spectrum antibiotic and one covering anaerobic bacteria. When the causative agent is known, specific testing can be performed. The antibiotics tested reflect current prescribing policy, epidemiological data and the pharmacokinetics of the individual drug that make it suitable for a given clinical situation. If the infection is deep within the body, the drug must be able to reach the area at a plasma concentration around the MIC to be effective.

SUGGESTED FURTHER READING

Abdurahman, S. (2007) *In vitro* interaction between methicillin-resistant *S. aureus* and various types of honey. *The Biomedical Scientist,* **51**: 908–909.

Abu-Sabaah, A.H. & Ghazi, H.O. (2006) Better diagnosis and treatment of throat infections caused by group A b-haemolytic streptococci. *Br. J. Biomed. Sci.* **63**: 155–158.

Appelbaum, P.C. (2006) MRSA – the tip of the iceberg. *Clin. Microbiol. Infect.*
12: 3–10.

Church, D., Elsayed, S., Reid, O., Winston, B. & Lindsay, R. (2006) Burn wound
infections. *Clin. Microbiol. Rev.* **19:** 403–434.

Davies, A., Thng, C. & Morgan, E. (2007) Laboratory testing in resistant
Trichomonas vaginalis infection. *The Biomedical Scientist,* **51:** 733–735.

Lagacé-Wiens, P.R.S., Alfa, M.J., Manickam, K. & Harding, G.K.M. (2008)
Reductions in workload and reporting time by use of methicillin-resistant
Staphylococcus aureus screening with MRSA*Select* medium compared to
mannitol-salt medium supplemented with oxacillin. *J. Clin. Microbiol.* **46:**
1174–1177.

Miller, L.G., Perdreau-Remington, F., Rieg, G. *et al.* (2005) Necrotizing fasciitis
caused by community-associated methicillin-resistant *Staphylococcus aureus*
in Los Angeles. *N. Engl. J. Med.* **352:** 1445–1453.

Morgan, W.R., Caldwell, M.D., Brady, J. *et al.* (2007) Necrotizing fasciitis due to
a methicillin-sensitive *Staphylococcus aureus* isolate harboring an enterotoxin
gene cluster. *J. Clin. Microbiol.* **45:** 668–671.

Naber, C.K. (2008) Future strategies for treating *Staphylococcus aureus*
bloodstream infections. *Clin. Microbiol. Infect.* **14:** 26–34.

Wishart, K., Goldsmith, C.E., Loughrey, A., McClurg, B. & Moore, J.E. (2008)
Methicillin-resistant *Staphylococcus aureus*: a microbiological update. *The
Biomedical Scientist,* **52:** 39–41.

SELF-ASSESSMENT QUESTIONS

1. Why is the skin a potentially challenging area for exogenous bacteria to infect? How do bacteria either overcome these natural defences or gain access to the skin and soft tissues?

2. What is necrotizing fasciitis and which major pathogens are most likely to be involved?

3. A swab is received from a patient with a deep post-operative wound. Which culture plates would need to be inoculated and why?

4. Why is it important to know the age of the patient and some clinical details when a genital specimen is received from a female patient?

5. How is *Neisseria gonorrhoeae* cultured and identified from clinical specimens?

6. Which factors will influence the significance of culturing Group B streptococci from female genital specimens?

7. Which pathogenic bacteria are most commonly isolated from eye infections?

8. Why is it important for the clinical details accompanying an ear swab to distinguish between otitis externa and otitis media?

9. What is the most probable bacterial pathogen to be isolated from a patient with acute tonsillitis / pharyngitis? How would this be cultured and identified?

10. Why is it necessary to inoculate a greater number of culture media for an ear swab than a throat swab?

Answers to self-assessment questions provided at:
www.scionpublishing.com/medmicro

Lower respiratory tract infections

Learning objectives

After studying this chapter you should confidently be able to:

■ **Describe the structures and defence mechanisms of the upper and lower respiratory tract**
Hairs and ciliated mucous membranes in the upper respiratory tract trap particles and bacteria. The tonsils, which are lymphoid tissue, protect the sinuses and middle ear and are important because infections can quickly spread through these systems. In the lower respiratory tract the pleura, a double-layered mucous membrane, encloses the lungs and a ciliated membrane lines the lower respiratory tract; particles trapped in these ciliated membranes are moved from the lower respiratory tract to the throat by a 'muco-ciliary escalator' where they can be expelled or swallowed. Additional defence is provided by mucosal defence mechanisms and macrophages, neutrophils and lymphocytes.

■ **Outline host predisposition for lower respiratory infection and describe the range of infections**
Some people are more predisposed to lower respiratory tract infection because of pre-existing lung disease, lifestyle, occupational or travel exposure to pathogens and immuno-suppression related to disease or medical procedures. The range of infections includes bronchitis, both acute and chronic, bronchiolitis, pneumonia and lung abscesses.

■ **Discuss the principal pathogens implicated in disease of this area**
The principal bacterial pathogens include *Streptococcus pneumoniae*, *Haemophilus influenzae*, *Mycobacterium tuberculosis*, *Moraxella catarrhalis*, *Mycoplasma pneumoniae*, *Pseudomonas aeruginosa*, *Staphylococcus aureus* and MRSA, and less commonly *Chlamydia pneumoniae*, *Legionella pneumophila* and *Coxiella burnetii*. Viruses associated with lower respiratory tract infection include flu, respiratory syncytial virus and cytomegalovirus. *Aspergillus* species, *Cryptococcus* species and *Pneumocystis jirovecii* can cause fungal infections in the area.

■ **Discuss the diagnosis of lower respiratory tract pathogens from clinical specimens**
The specimens received are usually sputum, broncho-alveolar lavage (BAL) and pleural effusions. Tuberculosis can be diagnosed from all these specimens and also from urine, pus swabs or lymph nodes. Before the culture media are inoculated, either for routine or TB culture, sputum samples are treated to break up the mucus and release trapped bacteria, and other fluids are centrifuged. Samples for TB testing are also decontaminated to remove normal flora prior to culture. Culture isolates are identified using standard confirmatory tests and tested against appropriate antibiotics to guide therapy. Isolates of TB are sent to reference laboratories for confirmation and susceptibility testing. Non-cultural methods to identify other significant pathogens include serology and molecular identification methods based on the amplification of target sequences of DNA.

Respiratory tract infections can arise in both the upper and the lower respiratory tract. Infections of the upper respiratory tract involve the ears, eyes, nose and pharynx and associated structures, such as the sinuses, naso-lacrimal and Eustachian tubes, which generally empty into the upper throat. Infections of the lower respiratory tract involve the bronchial tubes (bronchitis and bronchiolitis) and the lobes of the lung (pneumonia, abscesses and chronic airway disease). *Figure 11.1* shows the structure of the respiratory tract.

Upper respiratory tract infections are common, as the system is continuously exposed to the environment and organisms suspended in the air. However, they are usually mild but have a major economic burden in terms of time lost from work and visits to general practitioners. Many are self-limiting, such as the common cold and other respiratory viruses, and do not require laboratory diagnosis. Upper respiratory tract infections include infections of the ears, eyes, nose and throat, and their diagnosis from appropriate swab samples was discussed in *Chapter 10*. The specimens described in this chapter are processed in a Category 3 containment area, as there is always the possibility of a specimen being infected with tuberculosis.

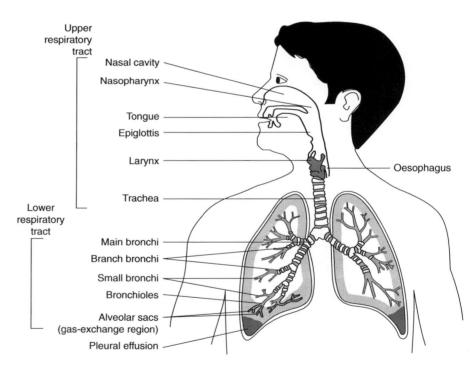

Figure 11.1
Structure of the respiratory tract.

11.1 SPECIMEN COLLECTION AND TRANSPORT

The main specimens sent to clinical microbiology laboratories for diagnosis of respiratory tract infections are nose, throat and ear swabs for upper respiratory tract infections (see *Chapter 10*) and sputum, bronchial washings (lavage) and pleural effusions for lower respiratory tract infections. Bronchial washings are collected through a suction tube placed in the bronchial tree with the aid of a bronchoscope. Saline is introduced into the bronchial tree to help release some of the thick bronchial mucus. Broncho-alveolar lavage (BAL) is a more invasive form of bronchial washing and involves using an endoscope to introduce 50 ml of saline into the lower bronchial tree. The aspirated saline contains material from the alveolar spaces.

Because most of the pathogens can be transmitted in aerosol form and there is an increased possibility that specimens may contain *Mycobacterium tuberculosis*, respiratory specimens are dealt with at containment level 3 for health and safety purposes. The type and colour of the sputum or effusion specimen has to be noted because sometimes a sputum specimen may arrive which consists of saliva only; these specimens should be repeated as they are representative of the oral flora rather than the infected area in the lower respiratory tract.

On arrival at the laboratory, in common with other specimens, the samples and request cards are checked for their points of identification, given a unique laboratory number and entered on to the computer system. Details are again checked in the respiratory section in containment level 3 and a description of the specimen entered on to the computer. Appropriate personal protective equipment as required for working in a containment area is worn, and personnel must have evidence of immunity to tuberculosis.

Lower respiratory tract infections caused by non-culturable bacteria, viruses and fungi are also described in this chapter, although they are not directly diagnosed from sputum or pleural effusions but from serum samples, which are not treated under Category 3 conditions.

11.2 SOURCES AND SYMPTOMS OF INFECTION

Respiratory infections can be bacterial, viral, fungal or parasitic in origin. They are transmitted by aerosols from person to person, by aspiration of the patient's own normal flora into the lung, zoonotic transmission from animals and birds or from an environmental source, where fungal elements are inhaled. They can be community-acquired: person to person, via occupational exposure to aerosols, animals and fungi, or by travel exposure to endemic pathogens and by being predisposed to community-acquired infection as a result of pre-existing chronic airway disease. Immuno-compromised patients are at risk from hospital-acquired respiratory infections as a result of HIV positivity (these patients are equally at risk in the community), organ transplantation, ventilator assisted breathing and loss of consciousness.

Defences

The upper respiratory tract has several defences against pathogens:

- It has hairs and ciliated mucous membranes to trap particles and bacteria.
- The tonsils are two oval lymph glands at the junction of the nose and throat that form part of a ring of tissue, called Waldeyer's ring, encircling the back of the throat. In early life the tonsils are at their largest, diminishing in size with age, and they aid the development of antibodies to airborne pathogens. This

explains why children are prone to infection in this area as they encounter new pathogens and induce inflammation in the area of tonsillar tissue.

As the nose and throat are connected to the sinuses and middle ear, infections can spread through these systems, particularly in children as their Eustachian tube is wider. The nasal sinuses are four air-filled cavities sited within the bones of the face. They each connect to the nasal cavity via an opening called the ostium and can become infected.

The lower respiratory tract includes the larynx, trachea, bronchial tubes and alveoli (the air sacs making up the lung tissue). These structures are protected by the presence of the normal flora and by two main types of mucous membranes:

- a ciliated membrane which lines the lower respiratory tract. Particles trapped in the ciliated membranes are removed from the lower respiratory tract to the throat by a 'muco-ciliary escalator' where they can be expelled or swallowed. In common with other mucous membranes, further protection is provided by the presence of secretory IgA antibodies, defensins and lactoferrin and in the lungs by alveolar macrophages, neutrophils and lymphocytes.
- the pleura, a double-layered membrane enclosing the lungs.

The presence of the normal flora of the respiratory tract provides colonization resistance along the mucosal surfaces, by occupying receptor sites and thus inhibiting the attachment of pathogens. The most common organisms found as part of the upper respiratory tract flora are Gram-positive cocci, viridans streptococci, beta-haemolytic streptococci (other than *Streptococcus pyogenes*), *Staphylococci* species, anaerobic bacteria, non-pathogenic *Neisseria* species, diphtheroids, *Haemophilus* species and yeasts.

Members of the normal flora can sometimes become endogenous pathogens if they gain access to different areas of the tract or if they overgrow because of altered conditions in the micro-environment (see *Chapter 4*). In contrast, the lower respiratory tract is relatively sterile as a result of the effectiveness of the mucus-based entrapping systems. These are designed to prevent potential pathogens from reaching the lung, and remove those that do; these two processes protect the delicate gaseous exchange processes in the lung. If the area becomes infected and inflamed, pathogens are able to cross the cell barriers separating the alveoli and the blood vessels and enter the bloodstream.

Host predisposition

Some respiratory pathogens will always cause infection in non-immune individuals, whereas others target the immuno-compromised, such as hospital inpatients and people with pre-existing respiratory disorders and impaired defences. Examples of these categories and associated pathogens are shown in *Table 11.1*.

Infectious diseases of the lower respiratory tract

The main lower respiratory tract diseases caused by infection are:

- bronchitis
- bronchiolitis
- pneumonia
- lung abscesses.

Table 11.1 Lower respiratory pathogens associated with different categories of susceptible patients

Community-acquired	Occupation-associated, zoonotic and environmental	Chronic lung disease, smokers, alcoholics	Cystic fibrosis	Hospital-acquired	Immuno-compromised, including HIV positive
Streptococcus pneumoniae	Aerosols containing *Legionella pneumophila*	*Streptococcus pneumoniae*	*Staphylococcus aureus*	*Staphylococcus aureus* and MRSA	*Pneumocystis jirovecii*
Haemophilus influenzae	*Coxiella burnetii*	*Haemophilus influenzae*	*Haemophilus influenzae*	CMV (organ transplant)	*Mycobacterium tuberculosis, Mycobacterium avium-intracellulare* and other environmental mycobacteria of low pathogenicity
Mycobacterium tuberculosis	*Brucella* species	*Mycobacterium tuberculosis*	*Pseudomonas aeruginosa*	*Streptococcus pneumoniae*	*Cryptococcus* species
Mycoplasma pneumoniae	*Bacillus anthracis*	*Pseudomonas aeruginosa*	*Burkholderia cepacia*	*Klebsiella pneumoniae*	*Aspergillus* species
Flu and other respiratory viruses, e.g. RSV	*Chlamydia psittaci*	*Klebsiella pneumoniae*	*Aspergillus* species	*Serratia marcescens* and other Gram-negative bacilli	
Chlamydia pneumoniae	Fungal pathogens, *Aspergillus* species	*Staphylococcus aureus*		Aspiration pneumonia: Enterobacteriaceae, mixed anaerobes of oral origin, *Pseudomonas aeruginosa*	
Staphylococcus aureus with Panton–Valentine leukocidin	Allergic reactions leading to chronic lung disease – ornithosis and farmer's lung	*Moraxella catarrhalis* *Neisseria meningitidis*			

Bronchitis

Bronchitis describes an inflammatory infection of the tracheo-bronchial tree. The condition may be an acute illness or a chronic condition. The main symptom of acute bronchitis is a hacking cough, which may bring up purulent mucus. Other symptoms include tightness of the chest, breathlessness and wheezing because of the congestion and impaired air exchange, and classical symptoms of infection: fever or chills, headaches, aches and pains. A sore throat and blocked nose are also sometimes present. Acute bronchitis can be caused by flu and other respiratory viruses, *Mycoplasma pneumoniae, Streptococcus pneumoniae* and *Haemophilus influenzae*.

Chronic bronchitis is characterized by a sputum-producing cough that lasts for more than two successive years. Chronic bronchitis is a syndrome, where infection is one component along with cigarette smoking and occupational exposure to dust and fumes. Bacterial infection can be the cause of acute exacerbations of chronic bronchitis and often involves *Streptococcus pneumoniae* and *Haemophilus influenzae*. *Moraxella catarrhalis*, a commensal bacteria known to colonize the upper respiratory tract, can also cause infection in patients with chronic lung conditions. If chronic bronchitis also involves obstruction to the airflow, this is called chronic obstructive bronchitis.

Bronchiolitis

This childhood disease arises when the small airways in the lungs, the bronchioles, become infected and inflamed and this again leads to a build-up of mucus; it commonly affects babies less than 2 years old. Bronchiolitis is often undiagnosed as the symptoms are similar to those of a common cold, but if the symptoms become severe the child may experience difficulty in breathing because of necrosis of the bronchiolar epithelial cells. Respiratory syncytial virus is the main pathogen, implicated in 75% of cases; the remaining number are also viral in origin.

Pneumonia

Pneumonia is an inflammation of the lungs (one or both), usually caused by an infection, and is the most serious of the three diseases and the most common cause of infection-related death. Typical pneumonia refers to patients with cough, fever and chest pain and can be community- or hospital-acquired. Atypical pneumonia is more insidious than typical pneumonia and the symptoms include fever and cough, but also headache and myalgia (muscle pain). Pneumonias can also be sub-classified into community-acquired (CAP) where the patient has not recently visited a hospital, and hospital-acquired where the patient has spent at least 48 hours in hospital prior to infection.

Clinical characteristics are used to define pneumonias as either acute (duration of less than 3 weeks) or chronic. Acute pneumonias are also divided into bacterial bronchopneumonias (such as that caused by *Streptococcus pneumoniae*), atypical pneumonias (e.g. the interstitial pneumonitis caused by infection with *Mycoplasma pneumoniae*, *Chlamydia pneumoniae* or *Legionella pneumophila* or viruses) and aspiration pneumonia syndromes. Most infections caused by *Chlamydia pneumoniae* are asymptomatic but they can cause severe disease which is not clinically distinguishable from diseases caused by *Mycoplasma pneumoniae*. Chlamydiae are Gram-negative bacteria that are obligate intracellular parasites lacking the mechanisms for producing metabolic energy, whereas mycoplasmas are bacteria lacking in cell walls.

Aspiration pneumonia can either be acquired in the community, where it accounts for 15% of CAP, or in the hospital environment. Empyema, abscesses, acute respiratory failure and lung injury follow inhalation of the stomach contents or oropharyngeal secretions. *Streptococcus pneumoniae*, *Haemophilus influenzae*, *Staphylococcus aureus*, *Streptococcus anginosus* (*milleri*) group and peptostreptococci are associated with community-acquired infection, whereas nosocomial infection is associated with oral anaerobes, peptostreptococci, Enterobacteriaceae, *Pseudomonas aeruginosa* and MRSA. Risk factors for aspiration pneumonia include alcohol abuse, general anaesthesia, seizures, strokes and head injury. Ventilator-associated pneumonia, a variant of hospital-acquired pneumonia, occurs after at least 48 hours of intubation and mechanical ventilation. When a patient is on a ventilator, air is delivered directly to the lower respiratory tract and bypasses the defences of the upper respiratory tract.

X-rays are also useful in the diagnosis of pneumonia as they are able to distinguish between the following types:

- lobar pneumonia, affecting one or more lobes of the lung, which are rendered solid by the build-up of inflammatory exudates
- bronchopneumonia, where the X-ray shows a more diffuse and patchy consolidation of the lungs
- interstitial pneumonia, where the tissue separating the alveoli, the interstitium, is infected
- lung abscesses, also known as necrotizing pneumonia, where a specific area of lung tissue is affected, leading to cavitation and destruction.

Mycobacterial (TB), fungal, or mixed bacterial infections can lead to chronic pneumonia. Allergic hypersensitivity reactions to mouldy hay (farmer's lung) and bird feathers or droppings cause chronic pneumonia-like illnesses. These are diagnosed by testing the patient's serum for antibodies to the relevant antigen responsible for the chronic allergic reaction.

Lung abscesses. These can occur as a complication of pneumonia, leading to necrotizing pneumonia, as a result of damage to the lung tissue. They can also be caused by:

- aspiration of fluid from the stomach or mouth, particularly in unconscious patients, alcoholics and epileptics
- an infected blood clot (embolus) lodging in the lung, and leading to abscess formation
- a bronchial carcinoma causing compression of the lung tissue.

The most common pathogens associated with necrotizing pneumonia and lung abscesses are *Klebsiella pneumoniae, Staphylococcus aureus, Pseudomonas aeruginosa* and mixed infections of oral streptococci and anaerobes.

11.3 THE PRINCIPAL PATHOGENS

A wide range of pathogens are known to be implicated in lower respiratory disease, as shown in *Table 11.1*.

Streptococcus pneumoniae (pneumococci)

Streptococcus pneumoniae is the main causative agent for lobar pneumonia in humans and is responsible for 60% of cases of community-acquired pneumonia. The bacteria enter the body by the nasal–oral route in aerosols / droplets and attach to the oro-pharyngeal epithelial tissue. Bacterial choline-binding protein A assists in initial adhesion to a poly-immunoglobulin receptor and to platelet-activating factor (PAF). Transient colonization of the pharynx helps the spread of the disease. The disease presents as a rapid onset of fever (41°C) and shaking chills; these symptoms may be post-viral, as the virus infection damages the mucosal cells and facilitates attachment of the pneumococci. Patients usually have a productive cough and blood in the sputum. The organisms have dense capsules surrounding them and this is their principal virulence determinant, protecting them from phagocytosis by inhibiting the deposition of C3b (an opsonic complement component) on the bacterial surface, which in turn impairs the immune response to *S. pneumoniae*. *S. pneumoniae* also undergo autolysis and this releases pro-inflammatory cell wall fragments. The toxin pneumolysin is also released. Worldwide, *S. pneumoniae* is the most common cause of community-acquired pneumonia (see *Box 11.1*).

Box 11.1 Vaccination for *Streptococcus pneumoniae*

There are now two effective vaccines for the prevention of severe pneumococcal disease. The pneumococcal polysaccharide vaccine (PPV), Pneumovax, containing 23 serotypes known to cause 90% of disease, was introduced in the UK in 1992 and given to everyone over the age of 65 years or at clinical risk of disease. This includes everyone with chronic heart, liver or kidney disease and the immuno-suppressed. Anyone who has lost their spleen is also eligible because the immune response to pneumococci involves cells within the spleen. In 2006 a childhood vaccine, the pneumococcal conjugated vaccine (PCV) Prevenar, was included in the childhood vaccination schedule and covered seven serotypes. This has now been replaced by an improved Prevenar covering 13 serotypes.

Haemophilus influenzae (HI)

Haemophilus influenzae accounts for about 5% of all pneumonias in the UK. In the pre-vaccine era, *H. influenzae* type B (Hib), an invasive capsulated strain, accounted for a significant number of childhood bacterial pneumonias between the ages of 4 months and 4 years. Since the introduction of the Hib vaccine in 1992 (see *Box 11.2*) the incidence of serious invasive disease has fallen dramatically. *Haemophilus influenzae* is still frequently identified in the yellow–green sputum produced during

---

Box 11.2 The success of vaccination for *Haemophilus influenzae* type B (Hib)

Prior to the introduction of the Hib vaccine in 1992 there were around 900 cases of invasive *Haemophilus influenzae* type B infection, an incidence of 34 cases per 100 000, in children under five years old, reported annually to the Health Protection Agency. The peak age for infection was 10–11 months. Invasive Hib disease includes meningitis with or without bacteraemia, epiglottitis, septic arthritis, osteomyelitis and cellulitis, often with lasting effects such as intellectual problems, seizures or deafness. Although a vaccine made from purified capsular polysaccharide had been introduced in the 1970s it was ineffective in producing an adequate response in children less than 18 months old and so missed the peak age for serious infections. The polysaccharide vaccine was then conjugated to a protein carrier, making it more effective in young children, and included in the UK vaccination schedule in 1992. A dramatic decline in serious disease was noted in the following years, to fewer than 50 cases in the under-5s in 1995. From 1999 there was an overall small gradual increase and a booster campaign was introduced in 2003. Currently the vaccine is incorporated in the Pediacel vaccine, administered at 2, 3 and 4 months of age. This combined vaccine contains diphtheria, tetanus, acellular pertussis, inactivated polio and Hib. At 13 months Hib is given in one injection (Menitorix) combined with meningitis C.

Infections with non-Hib strains are associated principally with respiratory infections in susceptible individuals; for example, those with pre-existing respiratory disease such as chronic bronchitis.

Data taken from www.hpa.org.uk.

exacerbation of adult chronic bronchitis and may be the cause of pneumonia in chronic bronchitis sufferers and emphysema patients.

Moraxella catarrhalis

Moraxella catarrhalis is a member of a group of non-motile, non-fermentative and oxidase-positive small Gram-negative bacilli that are generally associated with upper respiratory tract infections, but can occasionally cause pneumonia in susceptible individuals. Rare cases of pneumonia have been caused by *Pasteurella* species (more commonly associated in humans with wound infections from cats and dogs, but the cause of 'snuffles' in rabbits) and *Neisseria meningitidis,* causing a mild form of bronchopneumonia in patients with underlying pulmonary disease.

Mycobacterium tuberculosis

Tuberculosis is caused by *Mycobacterium tuberculosis* and less frequently by the mycobacterium complex members *M. bovis* and *M. africanum. Mycobacterium tuberculosis* is a Gram-positive acid-fast bacillus transmitted via the respiratory tract. Small droplets or aerosols containing the bacteria are inhaled and reach the alveoli, where they grow. The host immune response is to recruit large numbers of macrophages to the area, where they attempt to engulf the bacteria. The bacteria are able to survive within these cells and more macrophages aggregate around the bacteria in an attempt to kill them. The severity of the disease caused by the infection depends on the number of mycobacteria inhaled and the immunity of the host. In the majority of cases exposure and initial infection will result in the bacteria being walled off in a calcified nodule, called a tubercle, where they can remain dormant for many years. However, the patient is harbouring latent TB which can be reactivated. If the infection is not controlled at an early stage the bacteria can multiply in the lungs, causing the classic symptoms of a cough, with night sweats and loss of weight. Tubercle bacilli are spread as the patient coughs and can be transmitted to other susceptible people. This is a problem particularly in crowded and socially deprived populations. Reactivation can be triggered by co-factors such as exposure to coal dust and industrial pollutants over a number of years, declining immunity with age and, importantly, infection with HIV. During the initial infection bacteria may have travelled to other body sites such as the bladder or bones before they are controlled, and thus reactivation can occur in these sites distant from the initial respiratory infection. Co-infection with HIV, which attacks and infects the key cells of the immune system, weakens the immune surveillance responsible for the control of the latent TB, and renders the patient more susceptible not only to *Mycobacterium tuberculosis* but also to normally low pathogenic environmental mycobacteria such as *Mycobacterium avium-intracellulare.*

Tuberculosis was endemic in the UK until the middle of the twentieth century (see *Box 11.3*), before the introduction of the BCG (bacille Calmette–Guérin) vaccination and effective drug regimes. There were only around 8600 cases of confirmed TB in the UK in 2010, a slight drop on the previous year when there were 9000 cases, the highest number in 30 years. Of these, 1.2% were multi drug resistant. TB remains endemic in many areas of the world and with easy world travel, population movements, inappropriate and inadequate drug use, coupled with HIV and poverty, TB is recognized as a global problem and is monitored by a worldwide surveillance

---

Box 11.3 Current vaccination strategy for tuberculosis in the UK

The BCG vaccination was, until 2005, a feature of all teenagers' lives in the UK. The tuberculin test, also known as the Heaf test, was given first, and everyone found to be non-immune, i.e. with no reaction to the purified protein derivative of TB, was subsequently given the BCG injection. The BCG (bacille Calmette–Guérin) consists of a live attenuated strain (a Danish strain 1331) of *Mycobacterium bovis* and remains effective in 70–80% of people against the most severe forms of TB. However, there is considerable investment in research to develop a safe and effective replacement vaccine for worldwide use. Following the NHS and Department of Health national action plan, *'Stopping TB in England'*, published by the Chief Medical Officer in 2004, the Joint Committee on Vaccination and Immunisation reviewed the data of disease incidence and recommended bringing an end to the national school-based programme. Disease surveillance data showed that new cases of TB were mainly in high-risk areas and in high-risk groups, or in patients who were born in countries where the level of TB is high. The revised BCG immunization programme targets individuals most at risk from being infected with the disease and the vaccine is administered earlier. The following data are summarized from the Department of Health 'Green Book', *Immunisation against infectious disease*, published in June 2010. The following groups should be offered BCG:

- All infants living in areas of the UK where the annual incidence of TB is 40/100 000 or greater (offered the BCG in the first year of life)
- Infants whose parents or grandparents were born in a country with an annual TB incidence of 40/100 000 or higher
- Previously unvaccinated people who have recently arrived from high prevalence countries
- Schoolchildren are screened for risk factors, e.g. those with parents or grandparents from high incidence countries are tested and vaccinated as appropriate
- Those at occupational risk – health care workers, veterinary staff, prison staff, staff of hostels for the homeless and refugees
- Contacts of known cases
- Individuals who intend to live or work in countries with a high prevalence of TB.

In common with other countries the Mantoux test has replaced the Heaf test in the UK as the skin test initially used to measure any previous immune response to TB, and can be used in children over 6 years old. A tiny amount, 0.1 ml, of purified protein derivative (PPD), containing seven strains of *Mycobacterium tuberculosis*, is injected under the skin and viewed after 48–72 hours. If the area of inflammation is less than 6 mm, the BCG is given. If it is between 6 and 15 mm the patient is considered immune, and if the area is greater than 15 mm they are referred to a clinician as this is indicative of active disease.

---

and control system coordinated by the World Health Organization. World-wide surveillance monitors the prevalence of both drug sensitive and multi-drug-resistant TB.

Staphylococcus aureus with Panton–Valentine leukocidin (PVL)

The incidence of community-acquired pneumonia with *Staphylococcus aureus* as the causative organism has been low, but recently cases of severe haemorrhagic necrotizing pneumonia in previously healthy young adults, caused by strains producing the extracellular toxin PVL, have increased. The production of PVL occurs in both methicillin-sensitive and -resistant strains and is produced in addition to haemolysins, leading to toxin activity against a range of cells. The PVL-producing strains have an affinity for the basement membrane in the lung ciliary epithelial cells, which is exposed after viral infection. The bacteria multiply rapidly, destroying the neutrophils present and releasing inflammatory mediators, which leads to destruction of the lung tissue.

Further causes of community-acquired pneumonia

Mycoplasma pneumoniae is responsible for 20% of community-acquired pneumonias. This is often called 'walking pneumonia' because it is considered to be a mild form of pneumonia, as most patients do not require hospital treatment, and it occurs in epidemics every 4–5 years. *Chlamydia pneumoniae* and respiratory syncytial virus are further causes of community-acquired pneumonia. *Legionella pneumophila* is the causative organism of an environmentally acquired atypical pneumonia, where these Gram-negative bacteria are transmitted by aerosols from infected water, often the cooling tanks of air conditioning systems and showerheads. The bacteria are intracellular in habit and live in biofilms or within amoeba. Inside the human host they maintain an intracellular life within alveolar macrophages, release toxins and cause destruction to the lung tissue.

Some occupations, such as those of farmer and veterinary surgeon, are at more risk of some of the rare causes of pneumonia. For example, those in contact with birds may develop *Chlamydia psittaci* pneumonia. *Coxiella burnetii*, a small coccobacillus, is an obligate intracellular pathogen, forming spores that are environmentally stable; it causes Q (query) fever, a rare zoonotic infection in the UK, transmitted from cattle, sheep and goats. Farmer's lung, an allergic pneumonia, is the result of exposure to spores of the thermophilic *Actinomycetes* species of fungi (see *Chapter 13*).

Further rare causes of lower respiratory tract disease are the larvae of *Ascaris lumbricoides,* hookworms, *Strongyloides stercoralis* and the lung fluke *Paragonimus westermani,* acquired in endemic countries. Also at risk are travellers to areas such as the south-western USA where the fungal pathogens *Histoplasma capsulatum* and *Coccidioides immitis* are endemic (see *Chapter 13*).

Patients with cystic fibrosis suffer repeated and chronic lower respiratory infections because of the abnormal physical conditions prevailing in their lungs. The genetic abnormality affects the sodium chloride balance, resulting in high salt levels, excess mucus, poorly active defensin activity and the presence of neutrophils. In younger patients *Staphylococcus aureus* and *Haemophilus influenzae* are common infections, replaced by chronic infection by *Pseudomonas aeruginosa* as they grow older. *Aspergillus* species and *Burkholderia cepacia* infections are also a problem.

Hospital-acquired pneumonia

The majority of cases of hospital-acquired pneumonia are related to various Gram-negative bacilli (more than 50%) and *Staphylococcus aureus* (20%) and can cause a severe, necrotizing pneumonia. In the intensive care unit, distributions are generally more balanced, with *Staphylococcus aureus, Pseudomonas aeruginosa, Klebsiella pneumoniae* and *Enterobacter* species responsible for about 20% of infections each. In hospital-acquired pneumonia viruses cause 10–20% of infections, with the main agents being influenza and respiratory syncytial virus and, in the immuno-compromised host, cytomegalovirus. These patients usually have an underlying illness and while in hospital may be exposed to multiply drug-resistant bacteria, so the disease has a higher morbidity and mortality rate than community-acquired pneumonia (see also *Box 11.4* and *Box 11.5*).

Box 11.4 Case study

G. was a 93-year-old man living in a nursing home. He suffered from emphysema, a chronic obstructive pulmonary disease, and vascular dementia. He suffered occasional chest infections, successfully treated with oral antibiotics. He had been vaccinated some years earlier with Pneumovax (although the effect of the vaccine on a weakened immune system with pre-existing respiratory problems may have been diminished) and received annual flu vaccinations. During a particularly cold spell in the winter he developed breathing difficulties and was in obvious distress, with some blueness around the lips (because of the shortage of oxygen). His GP referred him to the local hospital where he was given oxygen in the A&E department and sent for a chest X-ray. The X-ray showed an area of consolidation in the right lung and a diagnosis of pneumonia was made. He was started on intravenous augmentin. Despite the antibiotic treatment his condition deteriorated and he died five days later.

Questions
1. What was the most likely cause of his pneumonia?
2. Which other respiratory pathogens could have caused the disease?
3. Outline the predisposing factors in this case.
4. How would these bacterial pathogens be cultured and identified if a specimen of sputum had been taken?

Box 11.5 Case study

F. is a retired coal miner. Recently he has noticed that his cough has worsened and that he has lost some weight. He feels generally unwell and visits his GP. He is referred to the chest clinic at the local hospital, where he is examined, has a chest X-ray and a sample of sputum is taken. Several nodules and a 'shadow' are seen on the chest X-ray. The routine sputum culture grows no significant pathogens. He is asked to submit three more sputum samples to test for TB and within a few days his doctor calls him and tells him that the initial tests suggest TB, and that confirmation of this will follow in due course. He is started on a course of antibiotics.

Questions
1. Why was the initial sputum culture negative?
2. Why was F asked to submit three specimens of sputum for TB testing?
3. Is this likely to be a new case of TB or a reactivation of a past infection? If it is a reactivation, suggest reasons why this patient has become symptomatic.
4. Outline the recommended treatment for TB. Why is it important that F completes the full course of treatment and has regular check-ups?
5. The laboratory report identifying TB was sent to the GP after a short time. At which point in the laboratory diagnosis does this suggest that the bacteria were diagnosed?

Severely immuno-compromised patients are additionally at risk from infection by the fungal pathogens *Pneumocystis jirovecii, Cryptococcus* and *Aspergillus* species (see *Chapter 13*).

11.4   LABORATORY DIAGNOSIS

Gram films can be a useful first step in the microbiology investigation, especially in a normally sterile specimen, whether to determine the presence and type of any bacteria present and the level of pus cells, or to give a quick indication of the potential pathogen. Gram stains can provide a rapid diagnosis for some major respiratory infections, for example, *Streptococcus pneumoniae* (a Gram-positive diplococcus) or *Haemophilus influenzae* (a small Gram-negative rod). A description of the macroscopic appearance of the specimen is recorded before culture. A film is also prepared prior to culture for specimens investigated for TB and stained using either Ziehl–Neelsen (ZN) or phenyl auramine.

Culture

Sputum specimens are generally thick and contain large amounts of mucus in which bacteria are trapped. Because there is a risk that the bacteria would not have the opportunity to benefit from the culture medium and grow in untreated sputum, the specimens are first mixed with an equal quantity of a reducing agent, dithiothreitol (available as a commercial product such as Mucolyse or Sputasol), that breaks down the disulphide bonds in the mucus protein, for 10–20 minutes. A small quantity (10 µl) of sputum is then diluted in 5 ml of distilled water prior to inoculation on to the culture medium. Specimens of BAL and pleural effusions are centrifuged for 10 minutes in order to concentrate them; the deposit is re-suspended in a small quantity of the supernatant, and cultured.

The specimens are usually cultured on blood agar, chocolate agar and a selective medium such as MacConkey agar to distinguish between some of the Gram-negative bacilli, and observed at 24 and 48 hours. Sabouraud agar is added if there is thought to be the possibility of fungal pathogens. These media will allow the growth of the principal microbial pathogens, *Streptococcus pneumoniae*, *Haemophilus influenzae*, *Klebsiella pneumoniae and Pseudomonas aeruginosa*. Sputum from cystic fibrosis patients will be further cultured on to specialist media for the growth of *Staphylococcus aureus* and *Burkholderia cepacia* and fungal pathogens.

Isolation and provisional identification

Streptococcus pneumoniae colonies are partially α-haemolytic, through the production of hydrogen peroxide. The colonial appearance varies from highly mucoid to drier colonies with an indentation in the centre which resemble a piece in the game of draughts. The bacteria can be distinguished from other α-haemolytic commensal and viridans streptococci by the optochin sensitivity test. A disc containing ethylhydrocupreine hydrochloride, a surface active agent, is placed on the culture plate prior to incubation. *Streptococcus pneumoniae* are lysed by the chemical and so a clear zone is apparent around the disc.

Haemophilus influenzae grow better on the chocolate agar (see *Chapter 6*) as the bacteria are able to obtain haemin and NAD from the lysed blood. The identity of the bacteria is confirmed by the X and V test (see *Chapter 6*) on simple culture media that contain neither growth factor. *Haemophilus influenzae* grow around the XV disc only, whereas *H. parainfluenzae* grow around the XV and V discs.

Klebsiella pneumoniae are lactose-fermenting, capsulated bacteria that appear very mucoid on the culture media. *Pseudomonas aeruginosa* appear as either capsulated colonies, with or without mucoid alginate, or non-capsulated drier-looking colonies. They are non-lactose fermenting, oxidase positive and have a characteristic metallic sweet odour. On selective media for *Burkholderia cepacia* the bacteria form colonies

1–2 mm in diameter and the medium turns pink. The medium is quite selective but there is still some growth of other *Pseudomonas*-related bacteria. Any isolates of *Staphylococcus aureus* are confirmed by coagulase and DNA. If PVL-producing bacteria are suspected because of the clinical condition, the isolate would be sent to a reference laboratory to test for the presence of the toxin using a PCR-based amplification method.

If none of the more common bacterial pathogens are isolated from the clinical sample further investigations are carried out as requested; these may include culture for tuberculosis, culture and/or serology for atypical bacterial pathogens such as *Legionella pneumophila* or latex agglutination tests for *Mycoplasma pneumoniae*, molecular techniques for viruses, fungal culture or microscopic examination for parasitic worms.

Legionella pneumophila are fastidious aerobic poorly staining Gram-negative rods. Legionellae grow slowly (3 days) on complex media such as buffered charcoal–yeast extract, often containing antibiotics to suppress normal flora. Legionellae usually infect immuno-suppressed or elderly people, following inhalation from contaminated air conditioning systems or water supplies. Isolation from sputum samples is difficult and bacteria can be isolated from bronchial washings or lung tissue. Less invasive diagnostic techniques include the detection of legionella antigens in blood or urine or by detecting antibodies in the patient's serum by an indirect fluorescence antibody technique (see *Section 5.3* and *Figure 5.9*). Interestingly, although the bacteria are fastidious to culture they will survive well if kept in distilled water before they are sent to the reference laboratory for full identification.

If the patient's symptoms suggest TB, specimens of sputum, bronchial washings, pleural aspirate, urine, lymph nodes or pus swabs can be cultured. Specimens of BAL are always routinely cultured for TB. To maximize the chance of diagnosing the disease, three consecutive samples of urine and sputum are requested, as the bacteria may only be present in each sample in low numbers. TB testing of urine is best performed on early morning urine samples which are centrifuged to concentrate any bacteria present, prior to decontamination. Specimens taken from body sites known to contain normal flora will first have to be decontaminated, most commonly by the Petroff method. Because mycobacteria are slow-growing bacteria, the specimen needs to be free of faster-growing bacteria that would interfere with TB culture methods. Sputum samples must be treated with a reducing agent, as described earlier.

For decontamination, 3 ml of 4% sodium hydroxide is added to the specimen in a glass universal bottle and left at room temperature for 20 minutes. The bottles are then filled with distilled water to dilute the sodium hydroxide and neutralize the pH (acidified water can be used) and the specimens centrifuged at a speed of 3000 rpm for 10 minutes. After discarding the supernatant, the resuspended deposit can be inoculated either on to solid agar slopes of Lowenstein–Jensen media, one containing pyruvate and the other glycerol, or inoculated into a liquid medium (Middlebrook's) and placed in an automatic monitoring machine. The Middlebrook's method has been shown to be more sensitive and specific. The technology used operates on a continuous monitoring system identical to the automated blood culture machine described in *Chapter 12*. However, the bottles are not agitated as in the blood culture machine. On conventional solid culture media the slopes are incubated at 30°C and checked for growth weekly. Bacterial growth can take up to 10 weeks. Using a liquid culture method, detection is reduced to between 2 and 4 weeks. Isolates of TB are identified further and antibiotic susceptibility tested in a reference laboratory. However, because there is a time delay of several weeks before the susceptibility tests are available, treatment is started.

A film is made of the deposit before culture to give an indication of the presence of mycobacteria and also if suspicious colonies are seen on solid culture or the machine flags positive on an automated system. The film is stained either by the ZN method or using a fluorescent stain such as phenyl auramine (both described in *Chapter 5*).

Non-cultural methods

Mycoplasma pneumoniae has no cell wall and cannot be Gram stained. The bacteria can be cultured on specialized media containing fetal calf serum and this is usually carried out in reference laboratories. In routine laboratories the bacteria can be diagnosed indirectly by testing the patient serum for specific antibodies. If a specimen of serum is taken early in the disease process and then another 10–14 days later, a rising titre of antibodies can be demonstrated, indicative of a current ongoing infection. In the particle agglutination test a series of dilutions of the patient serum is prepared and mixed with latex particles coated with antigen. Agglutination occurs and is dependent on the level of antibodies present. NAAT methods, such as real-time PCR, are also used to detect the DNA of these bacteria. Real-time PCR is also used in the diagnosis of *Chlamydia pneumoniae* (see *Section 6.8*).

Chlamydia psittaci and *Coxiella burnetii* can be diagnosed by serological methods, which detect rising levels of antibodies, or more commonly by a real-time PCR method that amplifies specific gene sequences of these bacteria and uses fluorescent signals to visualize the product. Molecular methods are also used for the fungal pathogens *Histoplasma capsulatum* and *Coccidioides immitis* and for respiratory viruses.

Sputum samples are examined for parasitic ova if *Ascaris lumbricoides*, hookworms and *Strongyloides stercoralis*, or *Paragonimus westermani* infection is suspected.

Pneumocystis jirovecii is identified from BAL specimens by using a fluorescent antibody test to detect the presence of oocysts in the fluid, or by the use of molecular techniques. Cryptococcus species can be diagnosed by antigen testing of BAL.

11.5   ANTIBIOTIC THERAPY

All significant isolates must be tested against a range of antibiotics suitable for treatment of the lower respiratory tract. These would include amoxicillin, erythromycin, cefuroxime, tetracycline, augmentin, and ciprofloxacin. Cases of pneumonia are often treated with intravenous antibiotics, gentamicin, ciprofloxacin and imipenem, vancomycin, clindamycin and flucloxacillin. Rifampicin with erythromycin are suitable for *Legionella* infections. Viral and fungal infections are treated with appropriate antimicrobial therapy, as described in *Chapter 3* and *Chapter 13*, respectively. Tuberculosis is treated with a combination of three or four drugs over an extended period of time to ensure that the slow-growing bacteria are killed and do not develop antibiotic resistance. The drugs used are rifampicin, isoniazid, pyrazinamide and ethambutol and these can be administered before a positive culture result. After the initial phase of two months, treatment is continued with isoniazid and rifampicin for a further four months.

SUGGESTED FURTHER READING

Carroll, K.C. (2002) Laboratory diagnosis of lower respiratory tract infections: controversy and conundrums. *J. Clin. Microbiol.* **40**: 3115–3120.

Christ-Crain, M. & Muller, B. (2007) Biomarkers in respiratory tract infections: diagnostic guides to antibiotic prescription, prognostic markers and mediators. *E. Resp. J.* **30**: 556–573.

Lacoma, A., Prat, C., Andreo, F. *et al.* (2009) Biomarkers in the management of COPD. *E. Resp. Rev.* **18**: 96–104.

McGrath, B., Rutledge, F. & Broadfield, E. (2008) Necrotising pneumonia, *Staphylococcus aureus* and Panton-Valentine leukocidin. *Journal of the Intensive Care Society,* **9**: 170–172.

Mizgerd, J.P. (2008) Acute lower respiratory tract infection. *N. Engl. J. Med.* **358**: 716–727.

Musher, D.M. (2003) How contagious are common respiratory tract infections? *N. Engl. J. Med.* **348**: 1256–1266.

Tuberculosis update, March 2011. Available from www.hpa.org.uk

SELF-ASSESSMENT QUESTIONS

1. Outline the defence mechanisms of the respiratory tract that prevent microorganisms reaching the delicate tissues of the lower respiratory tract.
2. Some pathogens will always cause infection in non-immune hosts. Other hosts are rendered susceptible to a wider range of infections. Discuss the reasons for this.
3. Which principal bacterial pathogens could be isolated by culturing a sputum sample on routine culture media, blood and chocolate agars?
4. Why is it important to ensure that a specimen labelled as sputum is not just a pot of saliva? Three specimens of sputum are requested for the investigation of TB; what is the reason for this?
5. Why is it necessary to request blood specimens rather than sputum if the initial culture results are negative?

Answers to self-assessment questions provided at:
www.scionpublishing.com/medmicro

The laboratory identification of infection from blood cultures and cerebrospinal fluid

Learning objectives
After studying this chapter you should confidently be able to:

■ **Discuss the causes of, and principal pathogens involved in bacteraemia and septicaemia**
Bacteraemia and septicaemia describe the presence of microorganisms in the blood, ranging in significance from transient bacteraemia in healthy individuals to life-threatening septic shock. Microorganisms can gain entry to the bloodstream from an infected site, the focus of infection, and then multiply. Bacteraemia from community-acquired infections is likely to be caused by *Streptococcus pneumoniae*, *Neisseria meningitidis* or *Escherichia coli*. Infective endocarditis, where infected heart valves shed microorganisms into the blood, is often caused by constituents of the patient's own flora. *Staphylococcus aureus*, MRSA, coagulase-negative staphylococci and yeasts are the principal pathogens isolated from hospitalized patients. Immuno-compromised patients are at risk from all the pathogens mentioned.

■ **Explain the symptoms and the pathogens most likely to cause infection of the central nervous system**
Infections of the central nervous system (CNS) are rare but serious events resulting from microorganisms crossing the blood–brain barrier into the meninges and the brain parenchyma. The symptoms of inflammation and infection are exaggerated because of the rigidity of the skull and the pressure on the brain tissue. The area is anatomically well protected but is a hidden area and has fewer defence mechanisms. Infections of the CNS include meningitis, encephalitis and brain abscesses. Symptoms include headaches, stiff neck, vomiting, and altered vision as a result of the raised intracranial pressure. The symptoms of a brain abscess vary depending on the area of brain affected. The pathogens involved in CNS infection can be bacterial, viral, fungal or amoebic, or caused by toxins. In the UK the principal bacterial pathogens isolated in cases of meningitis are pneumococci and meningococci in children and young adults, whereas Group B streptococci and *Escherichia coli* are more commonly associated with neonatal meningitis. Anaerobic streptococci and staphylococci cause brain abscesses but are rarely the cause of meningitis. Viral meningitis is most likely to be caused by enteroviruses in children, whereas herpes simplex virus (HSV) is more common in adults. *Cryptococcus neoformans* is an important cause of meningitis in patients suffering from AIDS.

■ **Outline the laboratory methods routinely used to diagnose infection occurring in these sterile sites**
Bacteraemia is diagnosed by inoculating a sample of the patient's blood into liquid culture media: one anaerobic and one aerobic bottle. The samples are then incubated at 37°C with constant agitation, often in an automated system where they are constantly monitored for several days. Any bottle showing as positive on the system is subcultured on to a range of culture media and incubated. A Gram stain is also performed and direct antibiotic sensitivity testing can be carried out, depending on the results of the Gram stain. Confirmatory testing is then carried out on the cultured bacteria. For the diagnosis of CNS infection a specimen of cerebrospinal fluid (CSF) is examined microscopically for the presence, number and differentiation of cells and bacteria and cultured on to suitable culture media, with confirmatory testing as appropriate. Specimens can also be tested for the presence of viruses if the results are suggestive of viral meningitis.

12.1   SPECIMEN COLLECTION AND TRANSPORT

This chapter examines the causes, symptoms and laboratory diagnosis of infection in two very important sterile sites: the blood and the CNS. The range of pathogens likely to be isolated from blood is more varied than from the more protected area of the brain and spinal cord. A flow diagram for blood cultures is shown in *Figure 12.1*.

Blood cultures

Blood is taken from the patient by venepuncture, taking care not to contaminate the sample with skin flora. The blood culture bottles are then inoculated and, following sterile protocols, placed in the appropriate bag accompanying the request card and sent to the laboratory. They are then numbered, entered on to the computer system and loaded on to the machine as soon as possible. Two samples are recommended for most patients, as this enhances the detection rate.

The volume of blood added to the bottles is important, and a ratio of blood to broth of 1:15 is recommended; this is usually 10 ml of blood per bottle. Aerobic and anaerobic bottles are supplied for adults, giving a volume of 20 ml per set of cultures, whereas for children one paediatric bottle is inoculated with a smaller volume of 1–5 ml blood, depending on the age of the child. The medium used is dependent on the manufacturer of the equipment and varies in terms of supplements, antimicrobial-neutralizing reagents, anticoagulants and headspace atmospheres. For this reason, some systems require venting of the aerobic bottle with a sterile needle before it is incubated.

Cerebrospinal fluid (CSF)

Specimens of CSF are taken from between the lower lumbar vertebrae beyond the extent of the spinal cord. After insertion of the needle the fluid is collected into three sterile containers, appropriately numbered and labelled, packaged with the request card and sent off to the laboratory marked as an urgent specimen. CSF specimens should be processed as quickly as possible (within 2 hours of collection) to avoid

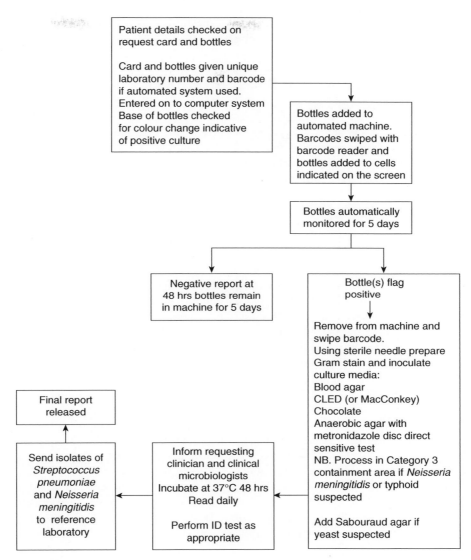

Patient details checked on
request card and bottles

Card and bottles given unique
laboratory number and barcode
if automated system used.
Entered on to computer system
Base of bottles checked
for colour change indicative
of positive culture

Bottles added to
automated machine.
Barcodes swiped with
barcode reader and
bottles added to cells
indicated on the screen

Bottles automatically
monitored for 5 days

Negative report at
48 hrs bottles remain
in machine for 5 days

Bottle(s) flag
positive

Remove from machine and
swipe barcode.
Using sterile needle prepare
Gram stain and inoculate
culture media:
Blood agar
CLED (or MacConkey)
Chocolate
Anaerobic agar with
metronidazole disc direct
sensitive test
NB. Process in Category 3
containment area if *Neisseria
meningitidis* or typhoid
suspected

Add Sabouraud agar if
yeast suspected

Inform requesting
clinician and clinical
microbiologists
Incubate at 37°C 48 hrs
Read daily

Perform ID test as
appropriate

Send isolates of
*Streptococcus
pneumoniae*
and *Neisseria
meningitidis*
to reference
laboratory

Final report
released

Figure 12.1
Flow diagram for blood culture.

deterioration of any cells present. The minimal acceptable volume is 1 ml, although as
large a volume as possible is required for the investigation of possible mycobacterial
meningitis. Glucose and protein levels, and examination for xanthochromia by
spectrophotometry, are usually carried out in the clinical biochemistry department on
one of the specimens. Cell counts and culture in microbiology are usually performed
on the third or final sample taken. Xanthochromia is the term for yellow pigment in
the CSF, indicating the presence of bilirubin from the breakdown of haemoglobin,
and is useful in the diagnosis of brain haemorrhages. Blood cultures should also
be taken, as should an EDTA (ethylenediaminetetraacetic acid, an anticoagulant)

specimen of blood. This is for diagnosis by a nucleic acid amplification technique if bacterial meningitis is suspected.

12.2   SOURCES AND SYMPTOMS OF BACTERAEMIA

Definitions

Bacteraemia, sepsis, septicaemia and septic shock are all terms used to describe the presence of microorganisms in the blood with varying severity of disease. Bacteraemia literally means the presence of bacteria in the bloodstream, whether transient, intermittent or continuous.

Transient bacteraemia

Transient bacteraemia occurs in healthy individuals every time commensal bacteria enter the bloodstream as a result of gums bleeding during teeth cleaning, entry of faecal bacteria during defecation, entry from minor skin infections, from squeezing spots, or the use of contaminated needles by intravenous drug abusers. Patients suffering from renal infections may also have transient bacteraemia. The small numbers of bacteria involved and the combination of host defence mechanisms in the blood, coupled with the ability or not of the bacteria to survive in the bloodstream, ensure that the immune system successfully clears the bacteria with no effect upon the host. The presence of an abscess in the abdominal cavity leaking bacteria into the bloodstream can lead to intermittent bacteraemia and this is also true of the early stages of pneumococcal pneumonia.

Continuous bacteraemia

Continuous bacteraemia suggests that a combination of sheer numbers of bacteria or very virulent organisms have overwhelmed the immune system. The patient is symptomatic and this condition is often described as septicaemia. When there is clinical evidence of infection as well as a response to infection, demonstrated by fever and increased heart rate (tachycardia), the condition is described as sepsis. When there are severe symptoms of sepsis and altered perfusion of any organ this is described as sepsis syndrome. This, accompanied by hypotension which may lead to multi-organ failure, is called septic shock.

Defences

The normal defence systems of the blood include the complement cascade system (see *Chapter 4*) where low levels of circulating proteins sensitive to the presence of bacteria deposit C3b on to the cell wall and initiate the alternative pathway, and mannose-binding lectins (MBL) attach to mannose and initiate the cascade via the MBL pathway. Neutrophils are attracted by the presence of the bacteria and the opsonization by the C3b. Acute phase proteins are released from the liver and with the cytokine response raise the body temperature; activated neutrophils engulf and kill the bacteria. The adaptive immune response is alerted by uptake and presentation of bacterial antigen on the surface of macrophages to specific lymphocytes, with the production of IgM antibodies and later IgG. Immunoglobulins raised to past infections of the same bacteria may also be present. The blood also contains further non-specific defences in the form of lysosyme and iron-binding proteins. Any defect in aspects of the immune system will compromise the normal clearance mechanisms and predispose the patient to bloodstream infection. This will therefore include all immuno-compromised patients, whether through pre-existing disease, instrumentation, surgery or treatment.

Sepsis syndrome and septic shock are the body's reaction to toxic components of the bacteria. This is often the result of overwhelming infection with Gram-negative bacteria. When the bacteria die they release large quantities of lipopolysaccharide (LPS). When LPS is released in steady amounts the immune system reacts to its presence by the production of acute phase proteins and cytokines, resulting in raised temperature and myalgia. This is an innate immune response involving migration of neutrophils, activation of the complement, coagulation, and arachadonic acid cascades, leading to a specific immune response and clearance of the infection. If LPS is released in large quantities the immune system reacts to the increased levels of lipid A and the resultant immune response may lead to hypovolaemia, leaky blood vessels and multi-organ failure. When LPS is released it is bound to LPS-binding protein which is up-regulated in response to its presence, and which then attaches to the CD14 receptor on macrophages. The sequence of events is shown in *Figure 12.2*.

Microorganisms other than bacteria may also be the cause of symptomatic septicaemia, for example *Candida* species may lead to fungaemia in susceptible patients. Viraemia may also accompany systemic viral infection and is detected in the blood by serological or molecular methods for significant infections: levels of HIV RNA, hepatitis C RNA and hepatitis B antigenaemia. Organ transplant patients are at risk from overwhelming viral infections as a result of immunosuppression.

Sources and foci of infection

Bacteraemia may develop from an infected site in previously healthy individuals, hospitalized patients and those who are immuno-compromised. Bacteraemia and septicaemia arise in a variety of situations, from a particular focus of infection, which may be community or hospital-acquired. This could result from invasive procedures or treatments, leading to immune suppression. The causative organisms may be pathogens or constituents of the patient's own normal flora that have gained access to the blood via surgical sites or instrumentation. *Escherichia coli* and coagulase-negative staphylococci are the most frequent isolates from blood cultures.

Bacteraemia arising from community-acquired infections

Community-acquired pneumonia caused by *Streptococcus pneumoniae* in previously healthy individuals may lead to bacteraemia, as the pneumococci are well adapted to survival in the bloodstream. Five to six thousand cases of invasive pneumococcal disease (septicaemia, pneumonia and meningitis) are reported to the HPA annually. *Neisseria meningitidis* is associated with meningococcal septicaemia, with or without the symptoms of meningitis. The symptoms are life-threatening and require immediate treatment. The characteristic rash, purpura fulminans, is the manifestation of dysfunctional clotting mechanisms and loss of thrombo-resistance in the vascular endothelium in response to the release of endotoxin. Ultimately this may lead to disseminated intravascular coagulation and septic shock. Untreated gonorrhoea may

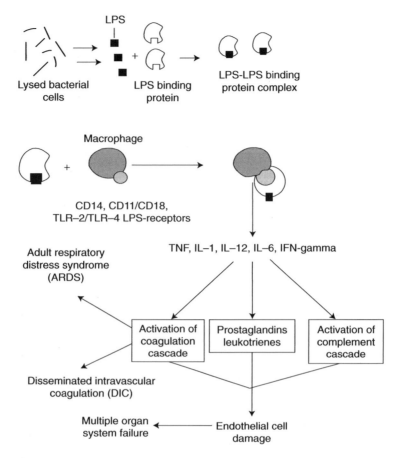

Figure 12.2
The development of septic shock.

cause bacteraemia in a minority of patients, with symptoms of polyarthritis and myalgia.

The principal causes of community-acquired bacteraemia are summarized in *Table 12.1*. Vaccination programmes have changed the profile of childhood bacteraemia; *Haemophilus influenzae* type B (Hib) is rare and the introduction of the pneumococcal vaccine and that for meningitis C also has a positive effect on infections caused by the serotypes included in the vaccines. The most commonly isolated pathogens at present are *Streptococcus pneumoniae*, *Neisseria meningitidis*, *Staphylococcus aureus* and *Escherichia coli*. Over 25 000 cases of *E. coli* septicaemia were reported in 2009. Neonatal infection is most commonly caused by Group B streptococci, *Escherichia coli*, coagulase-negative staphylococci and *Candida* species.

Infective endocarditis
Infective endocarditis, infection of the heart endocardium, may affect the native heart valve, most commonly the mitral valve, or prosthetic valves. The most frequently

Table 12.1 Causes of bloodstream infection in different patient populations

Community-acquired	Hospital-acquired	Immuno-compromised – in addition to those in other columns
Escherichia coli	Coagulase-negative staphylococci	Non-fermentative Gram-negative rods
Streptococcus pneumoniae	*Escherichia coli*	*Listeria monocytogenes*
Staphylococcus aureus	*Staphylococcus aureus* including MRSA	*Corynebacterium* species
Other Enterobacteriaceae	Other Enterobacteriaceae (*Proteus* species, *Providentia, Enterobacter, Klebsiella, Citrobacter, Serratia* species)	*Candida* species and other fungi
Neisseria meningitidis	*Pseudomonas aeruginosa*	*Mycobacterium* species
β-haemolytic streptococci	Enterococci including glycopeptide-resistant strains	Viruses
Fusobacteria (rare, causing necrobacillosis, Lemierre's syndrome)	Anaerobes	*Cronobacter* infections in neonatal units
	Streptococcus pneumoniae	
	Yeasts	
	Acinetobacter species	

isolated bacteria are from the patient's own flora including oral streptococci, staphylococci, enterococci and *Streptococcus bovis*. Infection of prosthetic valves is usually with coagulase-negative staphylococci, *Staphylococcus aureus,* Gram-negative rods, streptococci and enterococci, *Candida* and *Aspergillus* species and corynebacteria. Patients with endocarditis shed bacteria into the blood from the infected valve.

Bacteraemia in hospital patients

A number of factors put hospitalized patients at risk from bacteraemia, including the number of invasive treatments, instrumentation, length of stay in hospital and the age of the patient. The profile of microorganisms isolated reflects the nature of hospital-acquired infection and includes opportunistic organisms such as coagulase-negative staphylococci and yeasts, originating from the patient's own flora (see *Table 12.1*).

Since April 2001 there has been mandatory surveillance of all *Staphylococcus aureus* (including MRSA) septicaemia in all the NHS trusts in England. The data are collected by the HPA on behalf of the Department of Health and the figures are updated regularly on the HPA website. Mandatory surveillance extends to septicaemias caused by glycopeptide-resistant enterococci (see *Box 12.1*).

Bacteraemia in immuno-compromised patients

Patients who are immuno-compromised because of hereditary defects of the immune system or neutropenia following treatment, patients with AIDS or malignancy,

---

Box 12.1 Mandatory surveillance of bloodstream infections caused by *Staphylococcus aureus* and glycopeptide-resistant enterococci

Healthcare-acquired infections are of great concern as they not only cause significant morbidity and mortality to patients, but prolong their stay in hospital, with all the associated additional costs of treatment. Bloodstream infections represent 6% of all healthcare-associated infections and are often related to intravenous devices and following surgery. Colonization with the causative organism, for example methicillin-resistant *Staphylococcus aureus* (MRSA), is also a risk factor, as is advancing age (over 75 years).

Mandatory reporting of MRSA bloodstream infections has been in place since 2001 and since 2005 also includes patient data. The reports are categorized as 'trust apportioned' if the patients are inpatients, day patients, emergency assessment, and the specimen was taken in the acute trust four or more days after admission. All other patients are categorized as 'non-trust apportioned'. The data are analysed every quarter and compared with previous quarters, as well as with the baseline quarterly average figures for MRSA bacteraemia in England for 2003–2004 of 1925 cases. The figures for England for October to December 2010 (330 reports) represent a decrease of 82.9%. The figures are also expressed as cases per 100 000 bed days; these latest figures represent 1.6/100 000 bed days compared with 3.9/100 000 bed days in the same quarter of 2008.

The incidence of glycopeptide-resistant (vancomycin, teicoplanin) enterococci bacteraemia has also been subject to mandatory reporting since 2003 when the annual incidence was 620. The figures for 2009 had fallen to 559 cases.

The advantage of mandatory surveillance of these serious infections by hospital trusts is to raise awareness of the rates of serious healthcare-acquired infection and effective infection control, and to provide epidemiological data to contribute to a better evidence base for recognizing risk factors.

The data for MRSA were taken from HPA Quarterly Analyses, mandatory MRSA bacteraemia and *Clostridium difficile* infection in England (up to October 2010). London HPA, March 2011. Available at www.hpa.org.uk.

---

and those who have undergone transplantation, are susceptible to all of the microorganisms listed in *Table 12.1* as well as to low pathogenicity microorganisms which may be considered contaminants in healthier patients.

12.3   LABORATORY DIAGNOSIS

Considering the numbers of cases of bacteraemia / septicaemia diagnosed each year (around 15 000 for *Staphylococcus aureus* and slightly more for *Escherichia coli* in the UK) the rapid detection, isolation and identification of microorganisms from blood cultures are of paramount importance. Ideally the system used must be able to detect small numbers of organisms as quickly as possible, and therefore the quality of the culture media used is important. Contamination of cultures must be minimal and the effect of antimicrobial substances either from treatment or from the blood itself must be neutralized. Various systems are available, both automated and manual.

Manual systems at their most simple involve the inoculation of the patient's blood into liquid culture medium, incubation and then subculture on to agar plates at regular intervals. More recent manual systems indicate growth of microorganisms by positive pressure – the growth is indicated by the displacement of blood / culture medium into a separate chamber (see *Figure 12.3*). Many laboratories now have fully automated continuous monitoring systems, of which there are several commercially

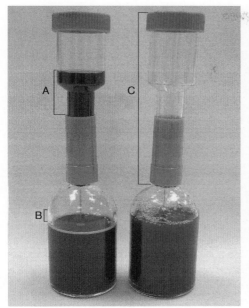

Oxoid Signal blood culture system

A. This is the signal produced by the production of gas by the organism. This area between the top of the locking sleeve and the meniscus of the media is the measurement area.

B. This is a visual sign of the displacement of the media into the device. The production of gas displaces the media by positive pressure up the needle.

C. This is the signal device. The needle of the device pierces the rubber bung, creating a seal, and protudes into the media. The locking sleeve holds it upright onto the bottle. The device, bottle, and media complete the system.

Figure 12.3
Oxoid signal bottle.

available. The modular design of these machines enables laboratories to select the most appropriate size and then 'add on' if necessary (see *Figure 12.4*).

Each automated system supplies compatible bottles containing liquid culture medium to which the correct volume of patient's blood is added. The bottles have a sensor incorporated into the base of the bottle, resulting in a colour change when the bottle has significant growth in it. All bottles must be checked for positivity prior to introduction into the machine and subcultured immediately if found to be positive. The bottles are incubated at 37°C with continuous agitation for a period of 3–5 days. Detection of microbial growth depends on colorimetric technology and tracks the carbon dioxide produced by growing organisms. The presence of carbon dioxide is detected and measured every 10 minutes by reflected light, via photodiodes and LEDs. The algorithmic data are analysed and a curve of the reflected signal can be viewed on the system software.

When a specimen flags as a positive, an audible alarm sounds and the bottles are removed. A specialized sterile needle is inserted into the bottle to allow a specimen to be taken for subculture on to a range of solid culture media designed to grow and isolate relevant pathogens: blood agar, CLED, chocolate and an anaerobic agar with a metronidazole disc added. A Gram stain is also prepared from the positive culture.

Culture media

A range of media are chosen to isolate the most likely pathogens:

■ blood is a good, non-selective agar for most pathogens, staphylococci, streptococci and coliforms

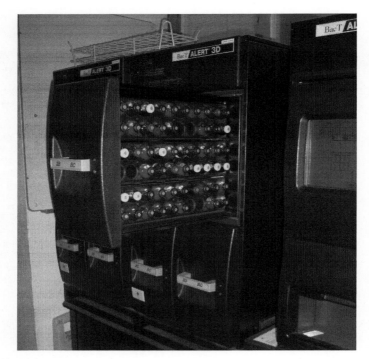

Figure 12.4
Automated blood culture machine. Additional drawers, similar to the one shown in this
photograph, can be physically added on to the machine and interfaced with the computer system.

■ chocolate agar contains haemolysed blood-releasing X and V factors for
   Haemophilus species and other fastidious organisms such as *Neisseria meningitidis*
■ CLED, MacConkey or chromogenic agar for the differentiation of lactose and
   non-lactose fermenting bacteria
■ anaerobic agar for the isolation of anaerobic bacteria.

The appearance of the bacteria or yeasts seen on the Gram stain also guides the
choice of additional media. If a yeast infection is suspected, a Sabouraud agar is
added. If streptococci are seen, an optochin disc can be added to the blood agar
plate to identify the presence of *Streptococcus pneumoniae*. If the Gram stain
contains Gram-positive cocci suggestive of staphylococci, a tube coagulase test can
be performed directly from the positive blood culture to give an early indication of
the presence of *Staphylococcus aureus*: 1 ml of rabbit plasma is added to 2 ml distilled
water and two or three drops of the blood culture are added and incubated at 37°C
for 4 hours; if a clot has formed in this time the result is positive (*Staphylococcus
aureus* is used as a positive control).

Blood and chocolate agars are incubated at 37°C aerobically in 5% carbon dioxide,
or anaerobically in a specialized cabinet or jar. Direct sensitivity tests, using antibiotics
covering the likely identity of the organism suggested by the Gram stain, are carried
out at the same time. If *Neisseria meningitidis* septicaemia is suspected from the
Gram stain, an EDTA specimen of blood is requested and tested using a PCR method

for the presence of the bacteria, detecting the presence of the *ctrA* gene, which codes for a capsular transport protein. Positive blood cultures with clinical details or Gram stain appearance suggestive of either *Neisseria meningitidis* or typhoid are processed at containment level 3, for health and safety reasons.

Further identification tests performed after primary culture

Further identification tests are carried out from the primary culture plates, and follow the guidance for confirmation of, for example, staphylococci, streptococci, coliforms, *Haemophilus* species and *Neisseria* species (see *Chapter 6*). Because the isolation of organisms causing bacteraemia is so important, the identification is often taken a stage further, including biochemical test strips to identify bacteria to species level. Automated methods, including the Vitek 2, or analysis by MALDI-TOF are also used for identification of blood culture isolates. If a focus of infection is suspected where a pathogen has already been isolated, confirming the exact profile of both isolates is of clinical interest; for example, a catheter-related coliform infection or a staphylococcal infection originating from a cannula site. The confirmation of the presence of MRSA or ESBL-producing bacteria is also important. Antibiotic susceptibility testing is performed on all significant isolates, guided by the identity of the organism and the local antimicrobial prescribing policy.

Significance of isolates

Not all isolates are significant; coagulase-negative staphylococcus from one bottle may reflect skin contamination, especially if the patient is asymptomatic and diphtheroids are most likely to be contaminants – these are decisions made at a clinical level. False positives, where no organisms are seen either on the Gram stain or on the culture plates, may be the result of high white cell counts in the blood giving off detectable levels of carbon dioxide, or of the inoculation of too large a volume of blood. If the bottle flags as positive and bacteria are seen in the Gram stain, but there is no growth on the culture plates, this may indicate the presence of *Streptococcus pneumoniae* that have undergone autolysis and are non-viable. If *S. pneumoniae* is the likely pathogen, direct antigen testing could be performed (using for example Binax Now) and/or some of the blood culture sample can be added to a new bottle and returned to the machine in the hope of recovering viable organisms. Alternatively, the absence of growth on the media selected may indicate a more fastidious organism requiring special growth conditions.

Reporting and storage

Isolates of *Streptococcus pneumoniae* and *Neisseria meningitidis* are sent to reference laboratories for further typing for epidemiological purposes and all isolates are notified to the HPA for inclusion in voluntary and mandatory surveillance schemes. Significant isolates are also retained locally and stored at −70°C.

When blood culture bottles become positive the requesting clinician is telephoned and the consultant microbiologist informed. Positive culture results along with the isolate's antibiotic susceptibilities are entered on to the computer system and reported according to current laboratory practice. Negative bottles are removed from the machine after 5 days but are reported as 'blood culture negative' after 48 hours.

12.4   INFECTIONS OF THE CENTRAL NERVOUS SYSTEM

Infections of the central nervous system include meningitis, encephalitis and brain abscesses.

The brain and spinal cord are suspended in CSF and surrounded by three layers of meninges, the pia mater and the arachnoid mater, together called the leptomeninges, and the dura mater or pachymeninges. To be anatomically correct, infection of the brain parenchyma is called encephalitis, infection of the meninges is meningitis, and infection of the spinal cord tissue is myelitis. However, all of the areas may be infected at the same time (see *Figure 12.5*).

Infections occur relatively infrequently but have extremely serious consequences; untreated bacterial meningitis is fatal in 70% of cases, a figure reduced to less than 10% with antibiotic treatment. Childhood CNS infections can, however, leave their victims with severe neurological impairment.

Defences

The anatomical area is distinctive in that it is well protected and isolated by the skull and blood–brain barrier, but at the same time highly vulnerable to significant damage. Because of the rigidity of the skull, minor swelling and inflammation are magnified, causing significant damage and pressure. Possible involvement of the brain tissue causes further complications and systemic effects.

In normal circumstances the blood–brain barrier, a membrane consisting of endothelial cells with tight junctions, inhibits the passage of microorganisms and toxic substances into the brain. The membrane is permeable to oxygen, carbon dioxide and

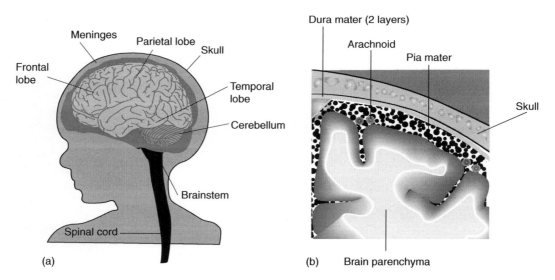

Figure 12.5
Structure of the brain and spinal cord, showing the meningeal area. The brain and spinal cord are suspended in cerebrospinal fluid and surrounded by three layers of meninges; the pia mater and arachnoid (together they form the leptomeninges) and the dura mater (the pachymeninges). Infection of the brain and meninges cause severe symptoms because they are enclosed within the skull.

lipid-soluble molecules such as steroid hormones, alcohol, amphetamines and heavy metals. The passage of antibodies and cellular defence components is impeded and only certain antibiotics are able to pass through. If the tight junctions are relaxed during acute infection the passage of antibiotic substances is increased.

Despite being well protected anatomically, the CNS is a relatively hidden area with fewer defence mechanisms. Complement levels are low because of partial inactivation by the CSF and also because of poor penetration of the blood. Furthermore, phagocytosis and lysis of bacteria does not occur to the same extent in the brain, meninges and CSF. The microglial cells do provide some immunosurveillance and have many surface markers in common with circulating blood monocytes. The Virchow–Robin spaces, which are the perivascular sheaths surrounding blood vessels as they enter the brain, have a lymph-like system containing macrophages and lymphocytes, should infection arise.

Sources of infection

Meningitis and encephalitis can be caused by bacterial, viral or fungal pathogens. Infectious agents enter the area via the blood circulation, or by the neural route in the case of viruses such as rabies and HSV. One common place of entry via the blood is thought to be the choroid plexus, where the CSF is formed. The area is highly vascular and organisms present in the blood are able to penetrate the blood–brain barrier. The microorganisms carried in the blood can originate from the pharyngeal area or from any other focus of infection; they are usually capsulated and capable of evading phagocytosis and complement activity. *Figure 12.6* shows a flow diagram for CSF specimens.

Brain abscesses may develop as the result of a local chronic infection, for example of the middle ear or sinuses, a previous acute infection such as meningitis or as a complication of congenital heart disease. Any situation that results in a decrease in blood supply or infarction to areas of the brain can result in encephalomalacia, which is softening of the tissue following cell death. Bacteria transiently carried in the blood then lodge in the tissue and form an abscess. This may happen following trauma to the brain or a meningitis infection, and in children with congenital heart disease. The symptoms vary according to the area of the brain affected; an abscess in the temporal lobe affects vision and speech, whereas one in the frontal lobe affects memory and intellectual performance and causes drowsiness. Medical imaging techniques are used in the diagnosis and the treatment involves drainage of the abscess.

Principal pathogens

Bacteria

Many pathogens may be involved in CNS infection and the bacteria most frequently isolated in meningitis differ from those causing brain abscesses: anaerobic streptococci and staphylococci cause brain abscesses, but rarely meningitis. Pneumococci and meningococci are frequent pathogens in children and young adults, whereas Group B streptococci and neuropathogenic strains of *Escherichia coli* are more commonly associated with neonatal meningitis. All of these bacteria are capsulated, which enhances their virulence in terms of antiphagocytic activity and inhibition of complement activation. There are many different types of *E. coli* but it is the K1 strain that possesses a polysaccharide capsule rich in sialic acid that

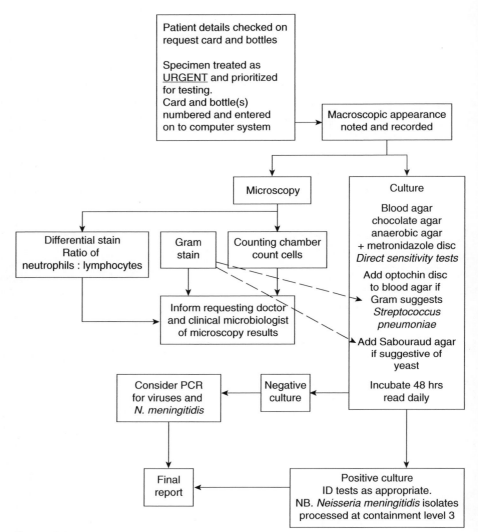

Figure 12.6
Flow diagram for CSF specimens.

is particularly neuropathogenic. Mycobacteria, capsulated *Haemophilus influenzae*, and *Listeria* species are also possible pathogens in susceptible patients. Ventriculo-peritoneal shunts in patients with hydrocephalus are also prone to infection from their own normal flora, in addition to staphylococci, corynebacteria, coliforms and *Pseudomonas aeruginosa*. In cases of neonatal meningitis and septicaemia, an infection with another member of the Enterobacteriaceae should be considered, Cronobacters, formerly known as *Enterobacter sakazakii*, were designated a genus of their own in 2007. Infection has been associated with powdered formula milk and can lead to a fatal meningitis as a result of gross destruction of brain tissue. Specifically designed chromogenic agar enables differentiation of these bacteria from other members of the Enterobacteriaceae. The bacteria can also be detected in food products, using either cultural or molecular methods (see *Chapter 14*).

Neisseria meningitidis

Group B *Neisseria meningitidis* is the most frequent pathogen isolated in cases of meningitis and meningococcal disease (meningitis and septicaemia) in the UK, with around 1000 cases reported to the HPA in 2007–2008 and a similar number in 2008–2009; the disease is most common in the very young and in young adults between 15 and 19 years old (see *Box 12.2*). There were no reported cases of Group A and about 30 each of groups C, W135 and Y over the same period.

Group A disease is associated with drier, hotter climates and a vaccination is available for travellers to endemic areas. Annual figures for pneumococcal meningitis are considerably less than for meningococcal meningitis. The figures for Group C meningitis have fallen dramatically since the introduction of the vaccine in 1999 and continue to decline. The incidence of Group B meningitis rises in the winter months, when viral infections such as flu are also at their peak.

Box 12.2 Case study

A 19-year-old male has a history of headaches and unusual behaviour over a period of several weeks. He is admitted to hospital for investigations and a lumbar puncture is performed. The specimen of CSF is sent to the microbiology laboratory for microscopy and culture. The white cell count is >500 cells/ml, the majority of which are neutrophils. Gram-positive cocci are seen on the Gram stain preparation. Culture of the CSF yields a pure culture of streptococci which are Lancefield Group F. The patient undergoes a brain scan and the presence of a large abscess is revealed, which is subsequently drained and treated.

Questions

1. Which culture media are routinely inoculated for the culture of CSF?
2. Why is the diagnosis of meningitis less likely after the culture result of Group F streptococci?
3. The patient's symptoms could also have been indicative of viral meningitis. What differences would have been seen in the white cell differential preparation? Why is this?
4. Which predisposing factors may have led to the development of the abscess?
5. If the patient had presented with a non-blanching rash in addition to the headaches and stiff neck, what would be the likely diagnosis and pathogen involved?

The epidemiology and pathogenesis of *N. meningitidis* are interesting because up to 10% of people carry the bacteria as part of their normal throat flora. The figure rises to about one-quarter of 15–19 year olds, but very few develop invasive disease. People who have a congenital deficiency in the late components of the complement cascade are known to be more susceptible, but it is still not fully understood why the disease occurs sporadically in normal healthy individuals. Viral infections (particularly in the winter months when the incidence of meningococcal disease is at its height), which cause damage to the epithelial cells, may be a factor in the invasiveness of meningococci. Dry dusty air may also affect the mucous membrane, predisposing the individual to infection, and passive smoking may also be contributory. The bacteria are passed in respiratory secretions and require close contact for spread, as they do not survive long outside the human host. Specific antibodies raised against the strains carried as part of the normal flora are an important feature, whereas the acquisition of a different strain may lead to disease.

To be able to cause disease in the CNS the bacteria have to move from the pharyngeal area across the epithelium and endothelium, into the blood vessels and then across the blood–brain barrier to reach the CSF. The expression of virulence factors is carefully controlled; the capsule is a prerequisite for survival in the blood but is probably not expressed when the bacteria cross the epithelial layer. Specific adhesins must be expressed for attachment to the endothelial cells, thought to be mediated by one of the outer membrane proteins, Opc. Opc binds first to serum proteins such as vitronectin, which then attaches to vitronectin receptors on the endothelial cell. This attachment is enhanced by the expression of pili but inhibited by capsule expression. The production of IgA protease, factors to inhibit the ciliary beat and surface antigen expression are additional virulence factors. The capsule of Group B is non-immunogenic because it has similarities with components of host cell neural adhesion molecules, and as yet no effective vaccine has been developed.

Viruses

Viral meningitis or encephalitis is most likely to be caused by enteroviruses in children, whereas HSV is more common in adults. Varicella-zoster virus is also responsible for some cases of encephalitis. Polio virus, an enterovirus, shows tropism for motor neurons of the spinal cord and medulla, whereas mumps virus affects the ependyma of the fetus. The reason for this is the distribution of receptors used by the viruses and, in the case of polio virus, differences in blood flow. Polio virus affects the anterior horn cells of the spinal cord, often on the side of the dominant hand, which may be the result of increased blood flow. Arboviruses (arthropod-borne viruses) are common in certain geographical areas, for example Japanese encephalitis and St Louis encephalitis.

Fungi and amoebae

The amoeba *Naegleria fowleri* is also a rare cause of meningoencephalitis thought to be acquired by trauma to the cribiform plate after diving into infected water. *Cryptococcus neoformans* is an important cause of meningitis in AIDS patients.

Table 12.2 CSF levels of glucose, protein and cell counts in meningitis

	Total white cell count x 10^6/l	Predominant white cell type	Protein levels (mg/l)	Glucose levels (mmol/l)
Normal	<10		<450	4
Bacterial	Markedly raised 100–10 000	Neutrophils	Raised, e.g. 850	Reduced, e.g. 0.2
Viral	Raised 10–1000	Lymphocytes	Normal	Normal
TB	Raised 50–1000	Monocytes / lymphocytes	Raised, e.g. 1500	Reduced, e.g. 1.0

Toxins and immune-mediated disease

CNS infection may also be the result of toxin- and immune-mediated disease. *Clostridium botulinum*, *Clostridium tetani* toxin, and Guillain–Barré syndrome, a polyneuropathy, are rare sequelae of *Campylobacter jejuni* with serotype O19, and may also follow infection with mycoplasmas and EBV.

Pathogenesis of meningitis

Breaching of the blood–brain barrier, leading to the presence of infectious agents in the area, causes damage to the host cells. The resulting inflammatory immune response causes further damage and symptomatic disease. Host cells are damaged by the release of bacterial toxins, by lytic viral replication, or by intracellular growth of bacteria or fungi. The inflammatory response increases capillary permeability, allowing infiltration of fluid, neutrophils and macrophages. The activity of the neutrophils in phagocytosing and killing bacteria involves toxic molecules and, when the cells lyse, the released enzymes digest cells and tissue in the immediate area. The extent of inflammation varies, depending on the type of bacteria and the immune state of the patient. Pus produced as a result of dead neutrophils builds up in the subarachnoid spaces and may spread over the brain, cerebellum and spinal cord, causing raised CSF pressure; the raised intracranial pressure induces vomiting and headaches. Pressure on the optic nerve may cause altered vision. Viral meningitis (meningoencephalitis), or aseptic meningitis, is a milder disease with low to moderate inflammation and a lymphocytic response, and presents with severe headaches and stiff neck.

12.5 LABORATORY DIAGNOSIS

The macroscopic appearance of the CSF is always recorded. A normal CSF appears clear and colourless, whereas a sample from a severe case of bacterial meningitis will appear milky. If the lumbar puncture has involved a small blood vessel, the appearance will be bloody, as will the sample from a patient with a subarachnoid haemorrhage.

Cell counts

Cell counts are performed using a counting chamber. The CSF is carefully added to the chamber with a fine pipette or sterile capillary tube, taking care not to overfill the area, as this will lead to a false count. Some laboratories add a stain such as methylene blue or crystal violet to the sample at this point to enable white cell differentiation at the same time as the total count. If stain is added then the dilution factor must be taken into account. Similarly if the specimen is heavily blood-stained it may require dilution with saline to obtain a total white and red cell count. Turk's solution (a white cell diluting and differentiating fluid containing acetic acid, water and crystal violet), which lyses the red cells, can be added to the CSF to clear the specimen of red cells and stain the nuclei of the white cells.

The counting chamber is left for 5 minutes to allow the cells to settle and then viewed first at low magnification to locate the position of the squares and then at 40×. At this point five large squares containing 16 smaller squares are counted to give the total number of cells per ml (see *Chapter 6* and *Figure 6.6*).

White cell counts below 10 cells/ml are considered normal, and above that figure the count is considered raised. White cell counts in the order of thousands are seen in cases of bacterial meningitis.

Gram stain and differential count

A sample of the CSF is concentrated by cytocentrifugation for 5–10 minutes at a speed of 800–1200 *g*. The supernatent is transferred to another tube and the cells gently resuspended in the remaining fluid. A Gram stain and a differential stain are then prepared from the deposit. In this instance the slide is not heat dried as this distorts the cells; the slide is instead left to air dry and can be fixed in alcohol. If the differential count has already been satisfactorily performed on the counting chamber, or if the Gram stain is preferred for this purpose, the differential stain is unnecessary. The Gram stain is carefully scanned for the presence of bacteria, which may appear inside the neutrophils or remain extracellular. To increase the chances of visualizing bacteria in the specimen, the Gram preparation can be enhanced, after the initial drop has dried, by adding another drop on top until a thicker smear is achieved. If the presence of *Cryptococcus neoformans* is suspected, a slide is prepared and stained with Indian ink or nigrosin and covered with a coverslip; this enables the distinct capsule surrounding the yeast to be seen.

The ratio of neutrophils to lymphocytes is an important factor in distinguishing bacterial and viral infection. A bacterial infection usually attracts neutrophils to the area and this is also true for the more inaccessible area around the meninges. The exception to this is a mycobacterial infection where the response is monocytic. This reflects the response if mycobacteria are present in the lungs, where macrophages are attracted in large numbers in an attempt to engulf the bacteria. If the meningitis is viral, the response is lymphocytic as in other areas of the body. The ratio of neutrophils to lymphocytes can easily be assessed by counting at least 100 white cells in either the differential or Gram stain.

Glucose and protein levels

The glucose and protein results are also relevant at this stage. Glucose levels are low in a bacterial infection because the bacteria use it for growth, whereas the levels are normal in a viral infection.

Culture of CSF specimens

The use of blood agar, chocolate agar, and anaerobic culture media should identify the major pathogens likely to be causing the infection. An optochin disc is added to the blood plate if the Gram stain is suggestive of *Streptococcus pneumoniae*. If bacteria have been noted in the Gram stain, direct sensitivity tests can be performed on the CSF for the relevant group of bacteria, e.g. Gram-positive cocci, Gram-negative diplococci and Gram-negative rods. Third generation cephalosporins, ceftriaxone and cefotaxime are commonly used to treat bacterial meningitis. If there is any suspicion of mycobacteria on the Gram stain or from the clinical details, then appropriate culture can be performed from the spun deposit: the inoculation of slopes or the relevant liquid culture medium for an automated process.

The blood and chocolate plates are examined at 24 hours and the anaerobic plate after 48 hours. The culture results are reported after 48 hours but many laboratories further incubate for a total of 5 days to ensure the isolation of any slow-growing organisms. Identification tests are performed relevant to the bacteria cultured; appropriate API identification for most pathogens and PCR testing if indicated. Automated methods, including the Vitek 2, or analysis by MALDI-TOF are also used if available. If *Neisseria meningitidis* is suspected, further tests are carried out at containment level 3. If the patient has been treated with antibiotics before the CSF was taken, the culture result may be negative. If meningococcal meningitis is suspected, the EDTA blood specimen can be tested for the presence of meningococcal DNA.

A viral infection can be suspected for a number of reasons, such as a raised white cell count (predominantly lymphocytic), clinical details, or lack of bacteria seen on the Gram stain or grown in culture. The specimen of CSF is then sent for identification by PCR of any virus present. The presence of bacteria in the CSF may occasionally be caused by leakage from a brain abscess and is more likely to have a growth of mixed bacterial flora or facultative anaerobic bacteria such as Group F streptococci, all bacteria which are less likely to be the cause of meningitis.

If the isolate is bacterial, antibiotic susceptibility testing is performed. The antibiotics chosen must be able to cross the blood–brain barrier and penetrate the CSF in an active form and in high concentrations without causing toxicity. β-lactam antibiotics such as cefotaxime or ceftriaxone can be used and, although they normally have poor penetration, entry is enhanced because of the inflammatory process.

Reporting and storage

Initial cell counts and Gram stain results are telephoned to the requesting clinician. All results, whether positive or negative, are entered into the laboratory information system and reported according to current laboratory practice.

After all the tests have been completed, CSF specimens are stored in the cold room for up to 2 months and then discarded.

SUGGESTED FURTHER READING

Goldmeyer, J., Li, H., McCormac, M. *et al.* (2008) Identification of *Staphylococcus aureus* and determination of methicillin resistance directly from positive blood cultures by isothermal amplification and a disposable detection device. *J. Clin. Microbiol.* **46:** 1534–1536.

Hall, K.K. & Lyman, J.A. (2006) Updated review of blood culture contamination. *Clin. Microbiol. Rev.* **19:** 788–802.

Hill, E. E., Herijgers, P., Herregods, M.-C. & Peetermans, W.E. (2006) Evolving trends in infective endocarditis. *Clin. Microbiol. Infect.* **12:** 5–12.

Jones, D., Maxwell, S. & Coulthwaite L. (2011) Rapid identification and susceptibility testing of positive blood cultures. *The Biomedical Scientist,* **55:** 14–15.

Lingwood, M., Abba, M., Pillay, D. & Burrows, K. (2006) Link between inoculum size and blood culture positivity rates. *The Biomedical Scientist* **50:** 422–423.

Pathan, N., Faust, S.N. & Levin, M. (2003) Pathophysiology of meningococcal meningitis and septicaemia. *Arch. Dis. Child.* **88:** 601–607.

Riedel, S., Bourbeau, P., Swartz, B. *et al.* (2008) Timing of specimen collection for blood cultures from febrile patients with bacteraemia. *J. Clin. Microbiol.* **46**: 1381–1385.

HPA Quarterly Analyses, Mandatory MRSA bacteraemia and *Clostridium difficile* infection in England (up to October 2010). London HPA, March 2011. Available at www.hpa.org.uk.

SELF-ASSESSMENT QUESTIONS

1. Outline the role of LPS in the development of sepsis and septic shock.
2. Why is it important for patients with prosthetic heart valves to maintain good oral hygiene?
3. What is the principle of automated blood culture machines?
4. Why is it important to have clinical input when interpreting the results of blood cultures?
5. Outline the tests necessary to identify Gram-positive cocci seen on a Gram stain from a blood culture.
6. Infections of the central nervous system are relatively rare but have serious consequences – why is this?
7. How do pathogenic microorganisms gain access to the central nervous system?
8. Distinguish between meningococcaemia and meningitis caused by *Neisseria meningitidis*.
9. A CSF sample contains 1000 white cells per cubic mm, the majority of which are lymphocytes. Protein and glucose levels are normal. What are the most likely pathogens and how would they be identified?
10. How have childhood vaccination patterns affected the epidemiology of meningitis in the UK in recent years?

Answers to self-assessment questions provided at:
www.scionpublishing.com/medmicro

Mycology

Learning objectives
After studying this chapter you should confidently be able to:

■ **Explain the terminology used to describe fungal infections**
Diseases caused by fungi are called mycoses. The fungal pathogens may be divided into two groups, the filamentous mycelium-forming fungi (moulds) and the yeasts. Mycoses are described according to the area they infect: superficial, cutaneous, subcutaneous or systemic (involving the invasion of several internal organs). Superficial infections of the epidermis and stratified corneum of the skin are often caused by filamentous fungi called dermatophytes. These skin infections are described as tinea (ringworm). Yeasts are single eukaryotic cells that generally divide by budding; they are the cause of opportunistic infection which ranges from mild to life-threatening disease. Fungal pathogens may also be dimorphic, showing both yeast and mycelial forms.

■ **Outline the different types of fungi and yeasts causing mycoses in humans**
Superficial mycoses, affecting the outermost layers of hair and skin, are often cosmetic and caused by *Piedraia hortae*, *Trichosporon beigelii* or the yeast-like *Malassezia furfur*. Dermatophyte infections involve the genera *Trychophyton*, *Epidermophyton* and *Microsporum*. Subcutaneous mycoses are rare diseases often acquired through trauma; an example is *Sporothrix schenckii*, a dimorphic fungus causing sporotrichosis. Systemic mycoses include the dimorphic fungi *Histoplasma capsulatum, Coccidioides immitis, Aspergillus* species, and yeasts such as *Candida* species and *Cryptococcus neoformans*. Pneumonia in severely immuno-deficient hosts can be caused by *Pneumocystis jirovecii*.

■ **Discuss the symptoms of the more common mycoses**
Dermatophyte infections affect hair, nails and skin, causing hair loss, thickened nails and ringworm lesions. Tinea versicolor is a skin condition where pigmentation of the skin is varied, caused by *Malassezia furfur*. Overgrowth of yeast can lead to thrush and also systemic infections. Capsulated yeasts such as *Cryptococcus neoformans* cause pneumonia and systemic disease in the immuno-compromised. Sporotrichosis is a chronic infection resembling an ulcerated bacterial skin infection, and is difficult to treat. Systemic mycoses involve the invasion of major internal organs, lungs, liver and the central nervous system.

■ **Describe the laboratory diagnosis of fungal infections**
Laboratory diagnosis relies on both microscopy and culture on special media. Immunological techniques are also used to measure levels of antibodies and precipitins produced in response to the initial infection (e.g. *Aspergillus* infections). Microscopy is useful to visualize fungal elements directly from patient specimens and give an initial indication of infection prior to culture. It is often sufficient to diagnose *Malassezia furfur* from skin scrapings and clinical details. Specialized culture media are used for fungal and yeast identification. Specimens are inoculated on to one medium containing cycloheximide and one without. Dermatophytes can grow in the presence of cycloheximide, whereas non-dermatophytes cannot. Microscopy of the fungal growth is

then performed and identification made on the appearance of the hyphae and conidia in conjunction with the colour of the growth of the surface and underside of the colony. Chromogenic agar is often used to distinguish between different yeasts, whereas specialized media are necessary for the growth of *Cryptococcus neoformans*. Molecular techniques are used in the diagnosis of the severe systemic infections such as *Histoplasma capsulatum* and *Coccidioides immitis*.

13.1   SPECIMEN COLLECTION AND RECEPTION

Fungal pathogens, yeasts and moulds are isolated from several different specimens sent to the microbiology laboratory. For example, a Sabouraud medium is included in the investigation of genital, ENT and wound swabs in addition to all patients who are immuno-compromised. A specimen of CSF or a blood culture may also be positive for fungal pathogens. Specimens sent for specific culture for fungal infections include hair, skin and nail clippings, where the symptoms are suggestive of a mycosis. They are generally processed in a discrete area of the laboratory reserved for the purpose. Specimens for mycology are sent to the laboratory in appropriate sterile specimen containers, which may be pots or cassettes solely for hair and skin scrapings, and on receipt are checked for the four points of identification, given a laboratory number and entered on to the computer before transfer to the mycology section (see *Figure 13.1*).

13.2   SOURCES AND SYMPTOMS

Fungi are eukaryotic cells belonging to the kingdom Eumycota, with a nuclear membrane and membrane-bound organelles similar to human cells. There are important differences in their structures, such as the presence of ergosterols in the cell membrane, rather than the cholesterol found in mammalian cells, and these provide targets for selective toxicity when developing treatment strategies. Fungi are abundant in nature where they perform an essential role as saprophytes, breaking down dead material. Over 100 000 fungi are recognized but only a few of these are of clinical importance. Many are used in commercial processes: yeasts for brewing, the ripening of cheeses by *Penicillium roqueforti* and *P. camemberti*, and the production of antibiotics. They also have destructive activities when they spoil food products and damage fabrics. Human hosts come into contact with potentially infectious fungi from the environment, from person to person spread, and from endogenous infection from yeasts present in the normal human flora.

The fungi involved in human infections may be divided into two groups, the filamentous fungi (moulds) and yeasts. The diseases they cause range from the superficially cosmetic to life-threatening systemic infections. The immune status of the host is also an important factor, as immuno-compromised patients are much more susceptible to opportunistic fungal infections. The isolation of opportunistic pathogens from a patient sample can no longer be dismissed as insignificant without knowledge of the clinical status. Fungal infections are also a problem for the elderly, diabetics, chronic alcoholics and a risk for patients with cystic fibrosis.

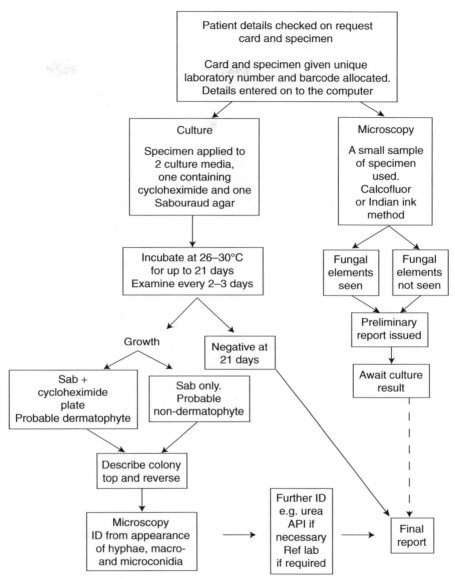

Figure 13.1
Flow diagram to show investigation of fungal infection from hair, skin and nails.

Filamentous moulds

The filamentous moulds (see *Figure 13.2*) grow as hyphae, long filaments that criss-cross and form a mat-like structure called a mycelium. The hyphae may either be co-enocytic (continuous without cross walls but with multiple nuclei) or septate (divided into sections). These features are helpful when trying to identify fungal growth microscopically. When grown on culture media they will also develop aerial hyphae and spores called conidia. These are described by size as either macroconidia

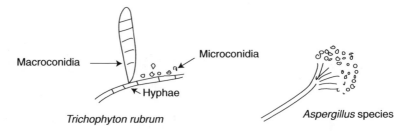

Figure 13.2
Basic filamentous moulds, *Trichophyton rubrum* and *Aspergillus* species.

or microconidia. The shape and position of the conidia are also used to identify fungal pathogens under the microscope. The appearance of the colonies growing on the agar plate provides the starting point for identification. They are much slower growing than bacteria and produce dusty colonies that are often brightly coloured. The growth on the surface of the agar may also be a different colour from the underside of the plate.

Filamentous moulds shed numerous spores called arthrospores into the air, both in the environment and when growing on culture media. They can therefore cause contamination to other cultures in the laboratory, and may be inhaled by anyone in the vicinity. *Aspergillus niger* is a prime example, as the black growth contaminates everything in the area and may also lead to an allergic reaction in susceptible individuals. For a vulnerable patient such as a child with cystic fibrosis, the inhalation of the spores into a compromised lung environment may be the start of a chronic infection.

Yeasts

Yeasts are single eukaryotic cells with rigid cell walls. They generally divide by budding, in which blastospores and daughter cells are formed. *Candida*, *Saccharomyces* and *Cryptococcus* species are examples of yeasts. *Candida* species are present as part of the normal flora and grow on culture media such as blood agar from skin or vaginal swabs. The colonies are often larger than bacterial colonies and on a Gram stain large ovoid Gram-positive cells are seen. They are opportunistic pathogens, taking the chance to overgrow when the host defences are compromised (patients on intensive care units have to be checked regularly for yeast infections), or as a result of treatment, from chemotherapy to a course of antibiotics where the normal prokaryotes are killed and the eukaryotic yeast survive. Some yeasts produce a polysaccharide capsule, for example *Cryptococcus neoformans* (see *Figure 13.3*), and this enhances the organism's pathogenicity.

Dimorphic fungi

Nothing is ever straightforward in microbiology – there are always exceptions to the general rules and behaviour, and this is certainly true of fungal pathogens. Many important fungi can behave as moulds or yeasts, displaying both yeast and mycelial forms. Some will form hyphae at environmental temperatures but change to yeast cells in the body, the switch being induced by changes in temperature and the nature

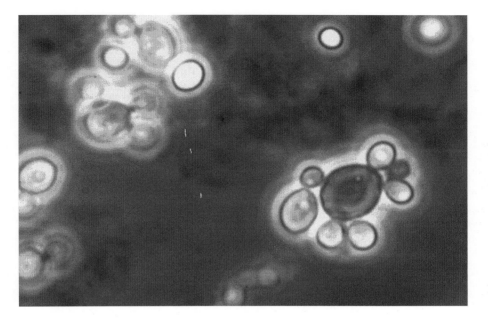

Figure 13.3
Cryptococcus neoformans negatively stained with nigrosin to demonstrate presence of capsules.

of existence from free-living to parasite. *Coccidioides immitis* and *Histoplasma capsulatum* are both inhaled as arthrospores and then adopt yeast-like forms when they become parasitic in the tissue; both are the cause of serious systemic diseases. *Candida albicans* behaves in the reverse fashion, behaving as a yeast on surface mucosa but forming mycelia when it becomes more invasive and pathogenic. Filamentous moulds such as *Aspergillus* species, however, always behave as moulds and *Cryptococcus neoformans* remain as yeasts.

13.3 PATHOGENS CAUSING MYCOSES

Infections caused by fungal pathogens are called mycoses and may be superficial, cutaneous, subcutaneous or systemic, depending on the nature of the pathogen and the immune state of the host. Mycoses (see *Figure 13.4*) may affect most areas of the body including the skin and mucous membranes, and may cause systemic infections involving major organs.

Superficial and cutaneous mycoses

The term superficial mycosis is used solely to describe infections of the outermost layers of hair and skin. The infections are generally mild, with little or no involvement of an inflammatory response, are easily diagnosed and respond well to treatment. They are often cosmetic, affecting the hair, skin and nails. Black and white piedra caused by *Piedraia hortae* and *Trichosporon beigelii* affect the hairs of the scalp and beard. Infection with a yeast-like organism called *Malassezia furfur* causes changes in the pigment of hairless skin called pityriasis versicolor.

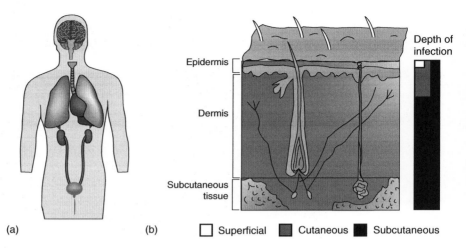

Epidermis

Dermis

Subcutaneous
tissue

Depth of
infection

(a)   (b)   □ Superficial   ■ Cutaneous   ■ Subcutaneous

Figure 13.4
Skin structure showing different levels of mycosis. (a) shows the major organs that can be infected by systemic mycoses and (b) shows the different levels of mycotic infections of the skin.

Dermatophyte infections

The superficial and cutaneous mycoses include infections of the epidermis and stratified corneum, invading only superficial keratinized tissue of the skin, hair and nails. These infections are caused by filamentous fungi known as dermatophytes. They are spread by direct contact, allowing transfer of arthrospores, and are the cause of athlete's foot and ringworm. The characteristic skin lesion is called a ringworm because as the infection moves out from a central point it provokes an inflammatory response (a delayed hypersensitivity reaction) in the form of a raised red scaly area that resembles a circular worm under the skin. The centre of the lesion contains no viable fungi, rather similar to the fairy ring formation of mushrooms growing in the wild. The terminology used to describe dermatophyte infections can sometimes be confusing; the clinical term for these infections is *tinea*, the Latin word for worm, and the request form accompanying a specimen for mycology will perhaps give the diagnosis as tinea pedis, fungal infection of the foot, or tinea capitis for an infection on the head, using Latin nomenclature for the areas of the body (see *Figure 13.5*). There are also many colloquial descriptions, such as athlete's foot and jock itch.

The dermatophytes comprise three genera, *Epidermophyton*, *Microsporum* and *Trichophyton*. The source of dermatophyte infection may be anthrophilic, from person to person; zoophilic, where an animal is the source; or geophilic, where infection comes from the environment. Athlete's foot is frequently caused by *Trichophyton rubrum* caught from an anthrophilic source when the arthrospores are shed from skin in a communal shower. *Trichophyton verrucosum*, however, is caught from cattle. *Microsporum canis* causes infections of the scalp and skin, particularly in children, and is acquired from infected cats and dogs.

Subcutaneous mycoses

Subcutaneous mycoses are rare diseases that affect the dermis and subcutaneous tissue and cause more serious infections; they are often acquired through trauma.

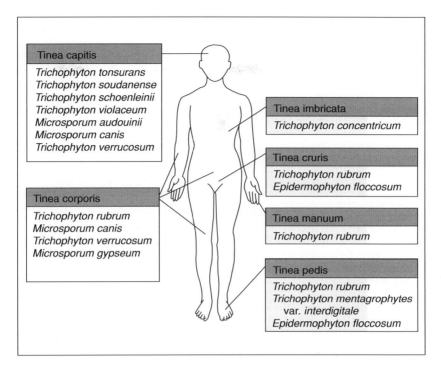

Figure 13.5
Location of dermatophyte infections and likely infecting organisms.

They can be difficult to treat and may require surgery to excise the infection and even amputation in some cases. Laboratory diagnosis is important because the lesions can mimic bacterial infections. *Sporothrix schenckii* causes sporotrichosis, a chronic infection characterized by lesions affecting the skin, subcutaneous layers, local lymph nodes and, systemically, affecting the skeletal system. The fungi are dimorphic, demonstrating mycelial growth, with hyphae and conidia at lower temperatures and forming budding cells at 35–37°C. The disease is rare in Europe but does occur in the USA and is associated with chronic alcoholism and occupationally with farm workers, gardeners and florists.

Systemic mycoses

Systemic mycoses, as their name suggests, involve the invasion of major internal organs. They may be caused by primary pathogens, capable of causing infection in healthy hosts, or opportunistic pathogens (mostly of low pathogenicity), capable of causing disease in immuno-compromised hosts. *Histoplasma capsulatum* and *Coccidioides immitis* are primary pathogens, whereas *Aspergillus*, *Candida* and *Cryptococcus neoformans* are opportunists.

The primary pathogens, *Histoplasma capsulatum*, *Coccidioides immitis*, *Blastomyces dermatidis* and *Paracoccidioides brasiliensis*, are all dimorphic fungi, inhaled from the environment in arid or semi-arid environments in North, Central and South America. They are unlikely pathogens to be encountered in the UK unless there is a relevant travel history. The Ohio and Mississippi river valleys of the mid-western USA are known as the 'histo belt', and the disease also occurs in Africa. *Coccidioides immitis* is also known as San Joaquin River Valley fever. Once the arthrospores of these pathogens have entered the lung they change into the yeast phase and form spherules, which may develop into pneumonia and also cause micro-abscesses and granulomas. A significant number of infections are asymptomatic and the outcome is dependent on the initial infecting dose and the ability of the host immune system to clear the pathogen.

In the UK the systemic mycoses encountered in the laboratory are more likely to be opportunistic in nature, affecting hosts with lowered resistance (see *Table 13.1*). Susceptible individuals would therefore include intensive care patients, those who are HIV positive, patients undergoing chemotherapy or treatment with broad-spectrum antibiotics, those with cystic fibrosis, organ and bone marrow transplants, burns, long-term catheters, malignancies and any condition where the functioning neutrophil count is lowered.

Table 13.1 Systemic mycoses caused by opportunistic fungi

Disease	Fungal pathogen	Predisposing factors	Organ involvement
Candidiasis	*Candida albicans*	Immunosuppression, broad-spectrum antibiotics, instrumentation Diabetes Specific T cell defects Intravenous drug abuse	Mucosal areas, GI tract, blood and other organs Chronic mucocutaneous candidiasis Endocarditis
Aspergillosis	*Aspergillus* species, *fumigatus* and others	Immunosuppression, chemotherapy, etc. Cystic fibrosis	Lungs and other organs
Cryptococcosis	*Cryptococcus neoformans*	Immunosuppression, none if large inoculum	Lungs, CNS
Others, including zygomycosis	Zygomycetes genera *Mucor, Rhizopus* and *Absidia*, and other infrequent fungi	Diabetes, burns, immunosuppression	Lungs, sinuses, CNS, soft tissue

13.4   LABORATORY DIAGNOSIS

The routine laboratory diagnosis of fungal infections relies on microscopy and culture on selective media, although molecular-based amplification techniques and mass spectrometry methods are being developed. Immunological techniques are used for detecting *Aspergillus* precipitins in suspected cases of farmer's lung and allergic aspergillosis, where the patient has a hypersensitivity reaction to the fungal spores. Molecular amplification methods are also available for the diagnosis of some of the more dangerous pathogens, such as *Histoplasma capsulatum* and *Coccidioides immitis.* MALDI-TOF mass spectrometry can also be used to differentiate different species of yeast isolates (the method is described in *Section 6.8*).

Microscopy

Microscopy techniques allow the visualization of fungal elements directly from the patient specimen and also detailed observation of hyphae, macro- and microconidia after culture. The characteristics of the cultures, colour and texture, along with the microscopic features usually lead to a satisfactory identification. This is true of specimens sent primarily for fungal culture (hair, skin and nails in particular), whereas yeast may be cultured from many other types of specimens and would only need microscopy if there was any doubt over their identity as *Candida* species.

The initial preparation for microscopy involves adding a small quantity of the sample to a drop of 10% potassium hydroxide and Indian ink on a slide. Alternatively a fluorescent stain such as calcofluor may be used. The potassium hydroxide is necessary to soften hard samples such as nail clippings and also acts as a clearing agent for most organic substances, allowing the fungal elements to be seen easily; a drop may also be used with the calcofluor for the same purpose. Calcofluor binds to the β1–3 and β1–4 polysaccharides present in fungal cell walls, cellulose and chitin, and fluoresces when exposed to UV radiation. If Indian ink is used, the fungal elements stain blue; if stained with calcofluor they are brilliant blue in colour. In most cases, the fungal elements seen are small segments of hyphae or mycelium across the cells. An initial report may then be produced, with identification after culture to follow. The method for microscopic examination after culture is described in the section covering fungal culture.

The causative agent of pityriasis (tinea) versicolor, *Malassezia furfur,* forms part of the normal flora of the majority of adults. It may also be the cause of pneumonia and catheter-associated sepsis in patients receiving intravenous lipids over a long period. The organism has a requirement for lipids and will grow on a lipid-supplemented medium. For this reason the findings of the characteristic microscopic appearance coupled with the clinical details are often sufficient.

Fungal culture

Culture of yeasts from clinical specimens

The choice of culture medium again depends on the type of specimen received, as samples specifically for fungal culture are treated differently from swabs in other sections of the laboratory. One of the standard culture media for general purpose identification of yeasts and fungi is Sabouraud agar or a specific chromogenic agar. Sabouraud dextrose agar contains mycological peptone and glucose and *Candida* species grow characteristic creamy colonies. The knowledge that *Candida albicans* form pseudohyphae when incubated in rabbit serum for a few hours may also be used to distinguish their presence. The hyphae and yeast cells are also clearly seen in Gram stain samples taken from vaginal swabs (see *Figure 13.6*) and in acridine orange stained smears (see *Chapter 10*).

With the rise of serious *Candida* species bloodstream infections it is often important to distinguish between the species, as the more common *Candida albicans* is sensitive to treatment with azole compounds, whereas some of the other species are resistant. Chromogenic media can distinguish between five major species of

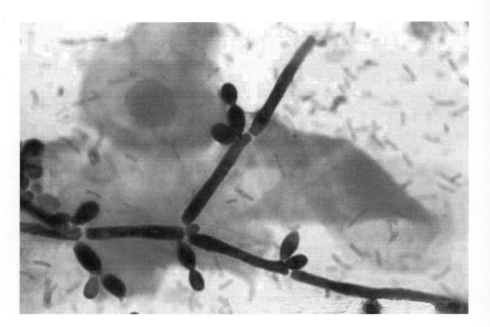

Figure 13.6
Gram stain of yeast in vaginal sample.

Candida by detection of hexoaminidase (X-NAG) and alkaline phosphatase (BCIP) activity. On this medium *Candida albicans* and *C. dubliniensis* are identified as green colonies, *C. krusei* colonies are dry and pink–brown and those of *C. glabrata, C. kefyr, C. parapsilosis* and *C. lusitaniae* appear as beige, brown or yellow. This is also advantageous for identifying non-*C. albicans* infections of the genitourinary tract that have been unresponsive to treatment with fluconazole (Diflucan) and also for patients in intensive care who need to be screened on a regular basis (see *Box 13.1*).

Culture differentiation of dermatophytes and non-dermatophytes
All specimens received specifically for fungal culture are cultured on to two separate types of agar, one containing cycloheximide (also known as actidione), for example dermasel agar or dermatophyte test medium (Sabouraud dextrose plus cycloheximide), and one without, Sabouraud. Non-dermatophytes cannot grow in the presence of cycloheximide and this provides a good basis for identification, along with the microscopy and the colony growth description. The specimens are cut up into small pieces, which is particularly advantageous with large segments of nail clippings, and applied to the surface of the agar. Four pieces of nail can be pushed into the top of the agar; hair and skin scrapings are firmly applied to the surface.

Dermatophytes are slow-growing and may take up to 3 weeks to produce good colony growth, whereas non-dermatophytes grow at a much faster rate. All culture plates are incubated at 30°C or at room temperature if no suitable incubator is available. The plates are then examined every 2 or 3 days for growth.

If there are colonies growing on both plates, with and without cycloheximide, the growth is likely to be a dermatophyte of the genera *Epidermophyton, Microsporum*

Box 13.1 Case study

A 73-year-old female patient is undergoing treatment for leukaemia and is neutropaenic as a result of the chemotherapy. She has an intravenous catheter for administration of the drugs. At the time of her most recent treatment she had a raised temperature and was feeling unwell. The intravenous catheter was replaced and the tip sent to the microbiology laboratory for culture. Blood cultures were also taken.

Characteristic colonies of yeast were isolated from the culture plates inoculated from the tip. The blood culture flagged as positive on day 2 of incubation and large ovoid cells were observed on the Gram stain. Colonies of yeast were visible on the culture plates after incubation. When the isolates were subcultured on to chromogenic agar, blue colonies were present. When the isolates were incubated into rabbit plasma, germ tubes were observed.

Questions
1. From the description and the further tests performed, what is the most likely identity of this pathogen?
2. Explain why this patient has several risk factors for local and bloodstream infections.
3. Suggest an appropriate antifungal treatment for the infection.
4. Topical yeast infections occur in various body sites. Outline some of the more common manifestations.
5. Outline some further causes of opportunistic yeast infections in susceptible patients.

---

or *Trichophyton.* The clinical details also provide clues to the identity of the isolate; if the diagnosis suggests athlete's foot (tinea pedis), the most likely organisms are *Trichophyton rubrum* and *T. mentagrophytes* (see *Figure 13.5*).

The colonies are observed and the colour of the upper surface and the reverse are recorded. Most colonies are fluffy and downy on the surface and are often distinctively and brightly coloured. A culture preparation for microscopy is then prepared using Sellotape. The sticky side of the tape is pressed on to the surface of the colony and then on to a microscope slide, on to which a drop of lactophenol cotton blue or 0.1% acid fuchsin has been placed. The slide is viewed on medium (40×) magnification under a light microscope and should demonstrate hyphae, macro- and microconidia (see *Figure 13.7*).

Non-dermatophytes

Non-dermatophytes are faster-growing and produce colonies only on the agar without cycloheximide. They are examined macroscopically and microscopically in the same way. Some of them may be considered contaminants and indeed this is sometimes true; equally they may be the cause of opportunistic infection in

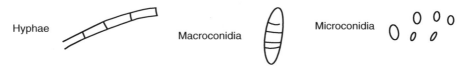

Figure 13.7
Identifying markers: hyphae, macroconidia and microconidia.

susceptible patients. Examples include *Aspergillus* species, isolates from the skin and other body sites. *Acremonium* and *Fusarium* species may be contaminants but also cause eye infections; *Scopulariopsis brevicaulis* similarly may cause toenail infections. All of these grow rapidly within 3 days and have distinctive microscopic features.

Laboratory diagnosis of systemic mycoses

Aspergillus *species*
Aspergillus species cause allergic reactions and serious aspergillomas (fungus balls) in the lungs, which may lead to disseminated disease in neutropaenic patients. Serological tests are useful in aiding the diagnosis because titres of antibody are high in cases of farmer's lung and 10–20% of asthmatics react to *Aspergillus fumigatus* with elevated levels of IgE. Highly specific molecular techniques, such as the PCR–ELISA targeting of the *Aspergillus* mitochondrial gene, are useful for diagnosing invasive pulmonary aspergillosis in bronchial lavage specimens from neutropaenic patients. The culture of bronchial lavage and sputum specimens is less reliable.

Cryptococcus neoformans
Cryptococcus neoformans is a capsulated yeast, and is the cause of cryptococcosis, a subacute or chronic infection of the lungs and central nervous system, most commonly seen in immuno-compromised patients. The yeasts are found in large quantities in bird droppings (most commonly from pigeons), in soil contaminated with droppings, and also in rotten fruit and vegetables. They may cause disease in healthy individuals if inhaled in large enough quantities, although the organisms are most frequently associated with meningitis in AIDS patients, and with cancer patients on chemotherapy. The virulence factors are the presence of the capsule, a phenol oxidase enzyme enabling enhanced survival in the presence of the immune system, and the ability to grow at 37°C; they also appear to be trophic for the central nervous system. Other members of the genus, of which there are 37 in total, are unable to grow at this temperature.

In cases of meningitis, the yeasts are visible in the CSF specimen and cultured on cornmeal Tween 80 agar incubated at 25°C for 72 hours. The colonies are fast-growing and slightly pink or yellow in colour. The yeasts are urease-positive, will grow in the presence of cycloheximide and produce brown colonies if grown on birdseed agar. This is because the activity of the phenol oxidase enzyme results in the production of melanin. The capsules can be seen as clear areas around the cells if the sample is stained with Indian ink. Capsule production is enhanced if the yeasts are grown in a 1% peptone solution.

Recovery, after treatment with an appropriate antifungal drug such as fluconazole or amphotericin B with 5-fluorocytosine, is dependent on the clinical state of the patient, and the prognosis is poor if the patient is severely immuno-compromised.

Pneumocystis jirovecii
Until the late 1980s *Pneumocystis* was thought to be protozoan but has been reclassified as a unicellular fungus on the basis of the nucleic acid composition of its ribosomal RNA and mitochondrial DNA. The organism was first discovered in 1909

by Carlos Chagas and first isolated from humans by Dr Otto Jirovec. The original organism known to cause human interstitial pneumonia was called *Pneumocystis carinii* in common with similar animal pathogens. Recognition that the fungi causing human disease were genetically different from those isolated in animals led to the name change to *P. jirovecii*. *Pneumocystis* is found in the lungs of healthy people, and most children have been exposed to the organism; however, it only causes disease when the immune system is impaired. Interstitial pneumonia caused by the fungus was recognized in central and eastern Europe during the Second World War among premature babies and malnourished children.

The fungus is inhaled as a cyst and multiplies in the alveoli of the lung. Both cyst and trophozoite forms of the fungus exist and can be seen in infected specimens. The presence of the fungi induces an infiltration of mononuclear cells, which, in immuno-compromised patients, are unable to clear the infection, and the area fills with exudate. As a result of the infection, desquamation of alveolar cells takes place and the permeability of the capillary membrane increases. Pulmonary oedema develops and further lung damage leads to the appearance of cysts, blebs or cavities in the lung and may cause a pneumothorax (collapsed lung). The symptoms develop slowly over a period of weeks or months and include a cough, fever, rapid breathing and shortness of breath.

Pneumocystis pneumonia, known as PCP (*Pneumocystis carinii* pneumonia, from when the organism was named *carinii*), is associated with patients who are severely immuno-compromised. This group includes post-transplant patients, patients undergoing chemotherapy and particularly in those with advanced HIV infection. With the advent of better treatment strategies (for example HAART for HIV) the number of cases has decreased in countries where this treatment is available. The disease remains highly prevalent in HIV-positive children in Africa.

Laboratory diagnosis is carried out on a broncho-alveolar lavage (BAL) specimen, either by fluorescent antibody tests, where a fluorescent labelled antibody is added to a smear of the BAL, incubated and washed and then viewed under a fluorescence microscope, or by histological stains such as Giemsa, DifQuik or silver stains to visualize the cysts and trophozoites.

Fungal treatment is ineffective, whereas treatment with the antibiotic cotrimoxazole (sulphamethoxazole and trimethoprim) or intravenous pentamidine, an anti-protozoal drug, is successful. The mortality rate in HIV-negative patients remains high, between 30 and 50%.

Candida fungaemia
Candida fungaemia is diagnosed by a blood culture specimen followed by microscopy and culture once the bottles have flagged positive on the system.

Further laboratory identification tests for yeasts and moulds
Most common dermatophyte, non-dermatophyte and yeast infections are diagnosed by the tests described above and do not need further analysis. Occasionally it may be necessary to distinguish between genera by the urease reaction and this can be performed by culturing the specimen on a Christensen's urea medium. A urease-positive reaction will cause a pH change as ammonia is formed and this is detected by a pH indicator incorporated into the medium. API strips are also available for identification. If antifungal susceptibility testing is required, the specimens are sent

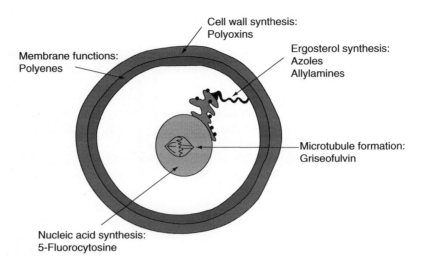

Figure 13.8
Target sites for antifungal therapy.

to the reference laboratory, where antibody levels are tested for *Aspergillus* species, *Candida* species, farmer's lung, avian antigens and antigens of *Aspergillus*, *Candida* and *Cryptococcus* species. E test strips are available for some of the antifungal agents.

13.5   TREATMENT

Antifungal treatments are much more difficult to develop than antibacterial agents because there are fewer targets for selective toxicity. The targets are ergosterol in the membrane, RNA synthesis and prevention of nutrients reaching the fungal cells.

Cutaneous mycoses are treated with topical creams or orally with griseofulvin; this is used for skin and nail infections, is slow-acting and therefore has to be taken over a longer period of time. The drug accumulates in the stratum corneum, forms a barrier to prevent further penetration and starves the cells of nutrients. Terbinafine is also used. Candida infections are treated with nystatin for oral thrush and fluconazole for vaginal infections.

More serious and systemic fungal infections need to be treated with more powerful drugs such as amphotericin B, a polyene (containing large numbers of double bonds) antimycotic. Amphotericin B binds to sterols and has a greater affinity for ergosterol than cholesterol but still has toxicity for human cells. Intravenous treatment with the drug leads to cell leakage and death. It is active against *Aspergillus*, *Candida*, *Cryptococcus* and *Trichosporon* species in immuno-compromised hosts. Resistance is rare but the drug has unpleasant side-effects, including damage to the renal tubules. The azole drugs are more frequent drugs of choice and are given orally. They are synthetic compounds that inhibit ergosterol synthesis with reduced toxicity to the host. Fluconazole, ketoconazole and itraconazole are prescribed for systemic candida and cryptococcal infections. High serum concentrations are achieved because the drugs have low protein binding. Resistance has, however, been seen in HIV patients suffering from candida and cryptococcal infections. *Cryptococcus neoformans* infections are also treated with 5-fluorocytosine (flucytosine). The active compound 5-fluorouracil disrupts protein synthesis and inhibits fungal DNA synthesis as it is incorporated into RNA in place of uracil.

Caspofungin (Cancidas) has been introduced more recently for the treatment of serious *Aspergillus* and *Candida* infections. The drug disrupts the integrity of the cell wall by inhibiting the enzyme $\beta(1-3)$-D-glucan synthase and is the first of a new class of antifungals, the echinocandins. It is administered intravenously and is used to treat invasive infections where patients are either unresponsive or intolerant of amphotericin or itraconazole. Anidulafungin can also be used for the treatment of invasive candidiasis.

SUGGESTED FURTHER READING

Enoch, D.A., Ludlam, H.A. & Brown, N.M. (2006) Invasive fungal infections: a review of epidemiology and management options. *J. Med. Micro.* **55**: 809–818.

Hadrich, I., Mary, C., Makni, F. *et al.* (2011) Comparison of PCR-ELISA and Real-Time PCR for invasive aspergillosis diagnosis in patients with haematological malignancies. *Med. Mycol.* **49**: 489–494.

Langan, C., Westbrook, P. & Coulthwaite, L. (2010) Detecting dermatophyte infections in hair, skin and nails. *The Biomedical Scientist*, **11**: 803–804.

Muñoz, P., Guinea, J. & Bouza, E. (2006) Update on invasive aspergillosis: clinical and diagnostic aspects. *Clin. Microbiol. Infect.* **12**: 24–39.

SELF-ASSESSMENT QUESTIONS

1. What is meant by the term dimorphic fungi? Why do they cause such serious infections?
2. Which three genera of dermatophytes are responsible for cutaneous mycoses? Why is the characteristic lesion called a 'ringworm'?
3. Why is it important to know whether a mycology specimen is from an immuno-compromised patient?
4. Which types of specimen are most likely to be sent to the laboratory for the diagnosis of dermatophyte infections?
5. What is the significance of using two culture media for the identification of dermatophytes and non-dermatophytes, one containing cycloheximide and one without?
6. Which cultural and microscopic features enable the identification of fungal pathogens?
7. How would *Cryptococcus neoformans* be identified from a patient specimen?
8. Why is it more difficult to develop antifungal strategies than antibacterial treatments?
9. Outline some of the treatments available for (a) cutaneous mycoses and (b) systemic fungal infection.
10. If a patient has tinea pedis, what are the most likely pathogens?

Answers to self-assessment questions provided at:
www.scionpublishing.com/medmicro

Food and water microbiology

Learning objectives
After studying this chapter you should confidently be able to:

■ **Explain the difference between food spoilage and food-borne disease and describe the principles of food preservation**
Food spoilage occurs when bacteria and fungi, naturally present in or on the food, multiply, either because of the age of the food or poor storage. This then spoils the appearance, texture and flavour. Food-borne disease is the result of the presence of pathogens, either naturally present or introduced by poor hygiene. Bacteria, bacterial toxins, viruses and fungal toxins can all be responsible for the classic symptoms of food poisoning and food-related disease. In contrast to food spoilage organisms, their presence does not alter the appearance, texture and flavour of food. The principles of food preservation are to prevent any pathogens present from multiplying in the food product and to ensure levels of hygiene that prevent pathogens from entering the food.

■ **Outline the ways in which the food industry quality control and test their products**
The quality control system encompasses every ingredient and every step of the process. Quality checks are incorporated at every critical step in an overall system of hazard analysis critical control points (HACCP). Samples of the finished product are also checked; this is known as end point testing. The investigations include total viable counts that give an indication of the microbiological quality, tests for environmental microorganisms and for the food-borne pathogens considered most likely to be present in that specific food product.

■ **Discuss the laboratory methods used to determine the microbiological quality and the presence of pathogens in food samples**
An assessment of the most probable pathogens likely to be present in a particular food sample, dependent on the ingredients, determines the investigations. These can include salmonella, campylobacter, *Staphylococcus aureus*, *Bacillus cereus*, *Escherichia coli* O157, and *Listeria monocytogenes*. An aerobic plate count determines the total number of bacteria present. The acceptable levels and testing methods are guided by national and European legislation.

■ **Discuss the methods used to ensure the quality of drinking water and environmental waters**
Water is tested from a variety of sources including potable (drinking) water and water from pools and cooling towers. Membrane filtration methods and aerobic colony counts are both used to determine the cleanliness and levels of bacterial indicator organisms in the water samples. The acceptable levels and testing methods are guided by UK and European legislation.

Food and water are the major routes of dissemination of a wide range of diseases throughout the world and account for a significant number of deaths worldwide, particularly in countries where clean water is not available. Infections from water can be the result of drinking contaminated water (cholera, for example), or by contaminated water coming into contact with food during crop cultivation, harvesting and food preparation. The World Health Organization (WHO) recognizes that clean drinking water and vaccination are the two most important factors in public health. In areas of the world affected by earthquakes, floods and war, where there are large numbers of displaced people and a breakdown of public health systems, outbreaks of water-borne diseases, such as cholera, typhoid and viral gastroenteritis, are more likely to occur. In the UK, public health systems are well developed and water-borne disease on a large scale is a rare event. Notwithstanding, large scale outbreaks still occur, for example a *Cryptosporidium* outbreak in North Wales in 2005. Microbiological testing of drinking water, sea water, swimming pool waters and water from air conditioning cooling towers (where *Legionella* species could be a problem) is routine and is governed by UK and EU (European Union) legislation.

Raised levels of food-borne disease during the latter half of the 1980s and widespread publicity about the safety of beef, poultry and eggs led to the formation of the Richmond Committee to investigate and advise the government on the microbiological safety of food. A national study into the incidence and risk factors for food-borne disease was set up by the Department of Health and carried out over a three-year period from 1993 to 1996. During this time a cohort controlled study reported on the incidence of infectious diarrhoeal disease in the general population (cases which would not normally be clinically investigated) and cases reported from general practice. The most common pathogens reported by GPs were *Campylobacter* species and viral gastroenteritis. Norovirus was the most common pathogen in the community-acquired cases. The Richmond Committee recommended the introduction of improved reporting systems and a new Government agency to oversee food safety. The Food Standards Agency (FSA) was created in 2000 by an Act of Parliament, and is the independent food watchdog appointed to protect the public's health and consumer interests in relation to food. The FSA was reorganized in July 2010 with a renewed focus on food safety.

Although the overall number of infections has declined in recent years it is estimated that around one million people in the UK suffer from some form of food-borne illness each year, according to the FSA Foodborne Disease Strategy 2010–15. The level of food-borne disease remains an area of concern in the UK, in terms of public health, public confidence in food manufacture and farming practice. The control of food safety throughout the food chain, 'from farm to fork', is complex and is influenced by changes in farming practices and consumer demands. There is constant pressure on producers to deliver 'natural' looking food with long use-by dates, food that requires minimal preparation and cooking, and pressure to supply fresh food throughout the seasons and representing world cuisine. Retail outlets and catering establishments are well regulated and monitored, but once food has been purchased there is only guidance and no control about how consumers store, prepare and cook the products within their own kitchens.

The microbiological safety of food and water and the incidence of food-borne disease are monitored by government laboratories. Routine quality monitoring, together with epidemiology and surveillance of sporadic and outbreak cases, form the remit of the Health Protection Agency (to be subsumed into the Department of Health in England in 2012). Food and water are tested by producers, food manufacturers and water companies, and quality tested on behalf of the consumer by official food control laboratories accredited by the United Kingdom Accreditation Service (UKAS) in accordance with the Food Safety Act of 1990, by public analysts. Consumers are protected by food safety laws and guidelines including Regulation (EC) No. 2073/2005 on microbiological criteria for foodstuffs and the HPA guidelines *Assessing the Microbiological Safety of Ready-to-eat Foods Placed on the Market* (London, November 2009). These not only provide legal protection from unscrupulous practice but set minimum standards for bacterial levels in food. Legal aspects are further monitored by Environmental Health officers, the port authorities who check food imports, and government and European agencies responsible for the quality of sea and river fish and aquaculture (oysters, mussels, etc.).

14.1 FOOD MICROBIOLOGY

Food-borne disease includes both food poisoning and food-related disease. Both are caused by the ingestion of food contaminated with bacteria, bacterial toxins, viruses, fungal toxins or parasites. Food poisoning is associated with a rapid onset of symptoms, usually within 24–48 hours, although this can be up to 11 days for yersiniosis. In contrast, there may be a longer period of time in food-related disease before the patient becomes symptomatic, e.g. hepatitis A, parasitic disease and variant Creutzfeldt–Jakob disease (vCJD). Food-related disease also includes food allergies and syndromes such as Crohn's disease.

Contaminated food is not obvious to the consumer, as there is no loss of appearance or flavour. One exception to this is *Yersinia enterocolitica* which is a food pathogen and food spoilage organism. In food spoilage, microorganisms alter the appearance and taste of food and make it organoleptically unacceptable (e.g. fungi and *Pseudomonas* species).

The microorganisms most often associated with food poisoning and the classic symptoms of infectious gastroenteritis (nausea, vomiting, abdominal pain and diarrhoea) are *Campylobacter* species, *Salmonella* species, *Listeria monocytogenes* (the incidence is low, but it is the most common cause of food-borne mortality in the UK), enteropathogenic *Escherichia coli* including *E. coli* O157, viruses and toxins produced by *Staphylococcus aureus*, *Clostridium perfringens*, *Bacillus cereus* and *Clostridium botulinum*. Less common enteropathogens in the UK include *Vibrio* species (*V. cholerae*, *V. parahaemolyticus* and *V. vulnificus)*, *Yersinia enterocolitica*, *Shigella* species and protozoa (e.g. amoebic dysentery). Other food-borne intoxications include scombroid toxins from fish, toxic mushrooms and mycotoxins from food contaminated with fungal toxins.

It is worth noting that:

■ Some pathogens present in food are associated with the food source itself: salmonella, campylobacter, *Escherichia coli* and *Clostridium perfringens* are present in the animal or bird intestines and can contaminate edible products during slaughter, milking and preparation. Listeria are ubiquitous in food, water and the environment.

- Others are introduced to the food by humans (for example norovirus and *Staphylococcus aureus*), or from the environment (fungi, *Bacillus cereus*, *Clostridium botulinum*).
- Viruses cannot reproduce without an appropriate host; the food is therefore the vehicle of infection (fomite) from one host to the next.
- Toxins can be produced by bacteria or fungi present in the food, but the causative organisms do not need to be present when the food is ingested as the pre-formed toxins cause the symptoms.
- Spores may be present in food and germinate within the human host after ingestion, e.g. *Clostridium perfringens*.

Food preservation

All food has a natural bio-burden of microorganisms, whose sole aim is to feed and reproduce. Food is a rich source of nutrients allowing heterotrophic organisms to break down organic residues into inorganic molecules for growth and reproduction.

There are a number of intrinsic (within the food) and extrinsic (outside the food) parameters that can affect the growth and survival of bacteria in food. The main intrinsic factors are pH, oxidation–reduction potential (*Eh*; aerobic versus anaerobic conditions), water content, nutrient content and antimicrobials (e.g. preservatives and naturally occurring compounds in garlic, onions and some spices). The extrinsic factors are storage temperature, relative humidity and the gaseous environment of the packaging. With pH, for example, many microorganisms grow best at pH 7 (6.6–7.5) but there are some that can grow below pH 4, such as moulds, yeast and lactobacilli. Acidity and alkalinity affect respiration in microorganisms in two main ways; they affect the transport of nutrients into the cell and also affect enzyme function. When organisms are grown in environments above or below their optimum pH there is an increase in the lag phase; the microorganisms may also become more susceptible to antimicrobial agents in the foods. Conversely, microorganisms can also survive outside their 'comfort zone', e.g. salmonella can survive in chocolate because they are protected against desiccation by the fat content and adverse growth conditions. Gram-negative bacteria such as *Escherichia coli* and salmonella survive by inducing a viable non-culturable state, where they exist by expressing the minimal number of gene products and change their shape from rod-like to spherical. When conditions become more favourable they resume growth.

The amount of available water (Aw) in the food is also important. Drying food to preserve it has been a technique used for centuries, because most spoilage bacteria only survive at a minimum water activity of above 0.9 (the water activity scale runs from 0, no water available, to 1, pure water), but this feature is affected by extrinsic factors such as nutrient content and temperature. The ability to survive in dry environments varies across bacterial species: Gram-negative bacteria such as *Escherichia coli* and *Pseudomonas* species, for example, require a minimum water activity of 0.96 and 0.97 respectively, whereas Gram-positive bacteria such as *Staphylococcus aureus* are more resilient to drying, and can survive down to a water activity value of 0.86; yeasts and moulds which cause spoilage can survive at water activity values of 0.88 and 0.80 respectively. Halophilic bacteria and xerophilic (dry-loving) fungi can grow down to 0.75 and 0.61. When the water level (and hence water activity) in the food is lowered it generally increases the lag phase of the bacterial growth cycle.

The principle of food preservation is to extend the lag phase to restrict the growth of microorganisms present in the food. Often two or more methods are combined, providing what is known as the hurdle theory – microorganisms may be able to negotiate one hurdle but are halted by a combination of hurdles, for example

Table 14.1 Food preservation techniques

Method	Inhibitory effect on growth of microorganisms	Application
Fermentation	Sugar converted to alcohol	Bread, alcoholic drinks, cheese
Freezing	Low temperature, reduced available water	Extensive range of meat, vegetables, food products
Blanching and freezing	Rapid heating prior to freezing reduces microorganisms by 99%	Fruit, vegetables
Freeze drying (lyophilization)	Low temperature, no water	Coffee, meat vegetables, milk
Chilling	Reduced temperature	Extensive use to extend shelf life
Pasteurization	Inactivates autolytic enzymes, kills microorganisms	Milk, fruit juice
Canning (appertization)	121°C destroys spores, additives destroy enzymes	Vegetables, meat, fruit
Heat and ultrasound	Disrupts microbial structure	Juices, sauces
Irradiation	Destroys all microorganisms	Meat products, extends life of fruit
Drying, sun drying, vacuum drying	Removes available water	Vegetables, fruit, meat, fish
Smoking	Chemicals in smoke reduce growth	Fish, meat
Salting	Removes water by increased osmotic pressure. 5–10% prevents growth	Vegetables, fish
Sugar	Extracts water, >50% stops growth	Jams, preserved fruits
Acids – citric, acetic, phosphoric	Low pH prevents growth	Pickles, preserves, improves flavour of many products
Sodium nitrate, sodium nitrite, sulphites	Inhibit oxidative processes	Preservatives used in variety of foods
Vacuum packing	Oxygen removed, creates anaerobiasis	Meat, some dried products, preserves in sealed containers, cereals, nuts, salads, coffee
Sous vide – pasteurization under vacuum, sealed pouches, chilled	Heat destroys microorganisms, then kept in vacuum and low temperature	Food can be cooked in the sealed pouches
Controlled atmosphere – 10% carbon dioxide	Slows bacterial growth, prevents spoilage	Apples, pears, salads
Filtration	Filters remove bacteria	Fruit juices and drinks

chilling and vacuum packing, or the addition of salt, vacuum packing and chilling. The methods are deliberately combined to improve the microbial stability, sensory quality and the nutritional and economic properties of the food. A product that was completely microbiologically safe, but looked and tasted unpleasant would be a marketing disaster.

Some of the earliest methods used were fermentation (an excellent way of preserving hops and apples), smoking food over fires, salting and drying. These methods are still in use along with many others, as shown in *Table 14.1*. Predictive computer modelling of the likely flora and potential pathogens is used to design appropriate preservation methods for a wide range of food.

14.2 QUALITY CONTROL OF FOOD PRODUCTS BY MANUFACTURERS

Manufacturers and producers are legally obliged to ensure that their products are safe to eat and consistently of the highest quality before they are released for sale. Retailers and catering establishments then maintain these high standards in the storage, preparation and serving of the products. The food products can be checked at the final stage of their preparation; this is known as end point testing, where a sample is taken and tested. Alternatively, and more usually, they can be checked in combination with an encompassing process from raw materials to end product; this is termed the HACCP (hazard analysis critical control point) system. HACCP evaluates and quality controls every stage of the process, identifying all the potential hazards and their critical control points. This involves careful monitoring, record-keeping, physical measurements, chemical and microbiological testing and a transparent audit trail.

The number of organisms present in food is influenced by several factors, including the general environment from which the food is obtained, the microbiological quality of the food in its raw unprocessed state, the sanitary conditions in which the food is handled and processed, and the effectiveness of processing, handling, packaging and storage conditions.

It is important to keep the numbers of organisms at a low level for reasons of public health and product shelf life. There are also a number of recognized sources of contamination in the food chain; the primary sources are soil, water, plant material, equipment, gastrointestinal tract, food preparation staff, animal feeds and animal housing, and air and dust particles. Each one of these can, to a greater or lesser extent, be involved as sources of bacterial contamination and has to be controlled and monitored as part of the HACCP process. EC regulation No. 852/2004 states that 'food business operators shall ensure that all stages of production and distribution of food under their control satisfy the relevant hygiene requirements laid down in this Regulation'.

The main microbiology evaluations that food manufacturers can be required to test for are as follows:

- Total viable count (TVC) – this gives an overall picture of microbiological quality.
- Enterobacteriaceae – these are hygiene indicator organisms that indicate a failure in hygiene procedures, possibly in manufacturing.
- Coliforms – these are also hygiene indicator organisms.

- Enterococci – these are found in the faeces of most humans and many animals and so can indicate faecal contamination.
- *Escherichia coli* – enteropathogenic strains can cause food poisoning; their presence in ready-to-eat foods is used as a faecal hygiene indicator.
- *Staphylococcus aureus* can cause food poisoning and, if large numbers grow, they leave heat-stable toxins in the product which can be transferred to food products.
- *Campylobacter* species are present in large quantities in chicken carcasses and meat products.
- *Bacillus* species – these are aerobic and spore-bearing; the spores can survive heating and cause food poisoning.
- *Clostridium perfringens* – this is a common anaerobic spore-forming organism which can survive heating and is often associated with food poisoning from meats and meat-based products, and can be found in poorly processed bottled and canned products.
- Lactic acid bacteria – these cause food spoilage in many foods, especially in vacuum or modified atmosphere packaging; they grow at low temperatures and low pH. They form part of the microflora of many cured foods, hams, olives, etc. and levels of up to 10^8/g are quite normal.
- *Pseudomonas* and *Aeromonas* species are found in soil and water, and are mainly associated with spoilage in fish but also in milk and meat.
- Yeasts and moulds – these play an important role in the spoilage of food. Some moulds can also produce mycotoxin, which is harmful to humans.
- *Listeria* species, causing food poisoning in susceptible individuals, are present as contaminants in raw milk, unpasteurized cheese, soft cheese, ice cream, meat and poultry and ready-to-eat meat and poultry. *Listeria monocytogenes* is the only pathogenic species, other *Listeria* species are hygiene indicators.
- *Salmonella* species are major causes of food poisoning and are found in many food ingredients and products.

Microbiological testing is either carried out in appropriately accredited laboratories, which may also monitor retail outlets and catering establishments, etc. or contracted to one of the many private companies (also appropriately accredited) which provide testing facilities. A wide range of methods are used, including specialist culture media, rapid testing kits and automated processes to detect bacteria, fungi and toxins.

It is important to distinguish these tests from the sampling and subsequent testing carried out in selected accredited microbiology laboratories (ISO, UKAS) to monitor food at retail outlets, catering establishments, and imported food controlled by the port authorities, and to investigate cases of food-borne disease. Sampling is carried out by the Local Authority Environmental Health Officers on behalf of the Food Standards Agency. The methods and significance of numbers of microorganisms isolated from food samples described in this chapter are summarized from the National Standard methods produced by the Health Protection Agency as they form the basis for the testing of food, water and environmental samples across the UK, the results of which can form the basis of any legal action. The acceptable levels of different microorganisms are specified by the EC regulations of 2004 and relevant current legislation.

14.3   LABORATORY TESTING FOR PRINCIPAL FOOD-BORNE PATHOGENS AND MICROBIAL CONTAMINATION

Specimen collection and reception

Collection and subsequent audit trails of food samples are carried out according to the code of practice for formal samples in the Food Safety Act 1990 and Local Government Regulation guidance for sampling. Because the results may be used as evidence for enforcement action or prosecution by the Local Authority there has to be a system of documentation and evidence from the time the specimen is collected. It is important that the specimen tested represents the microbiological condition at the time it was taken. Therefore the sampling, transport, storage and examination at all stages must be verified. The temperature must be controlled, cross-contamination prevented by a system of 'bagging and tagging' and accurate documentation must be kept. Food samples taken in the early stages of a food-borne outbreak are not strictly legal action samples, but are treated in the same way because they could form the basis of a prosecution at a later stage. Samples ideally should be at least 100 g, and maintained at an appropriate temperature, with frozen food remaining frozen, chilled and perishable food at 0–8°C and hot food not above 40°C.

On arrival at the laboratory, the samples are received by the designated food examiner, the details checked and the temperature taken. The appearance and condition of the sample are recorded, a unique laboratory number is allocated and the details recorded on to the computer system. The specimen is subsequently tested in accordance with the relevant Standard Operating Procedures.

Preparation prior to testing

Preparation of food samples before testing is important because the bacteria are not evenly distributed throughout the food sample, for example a piece of meat or poultry. Homogenizing the sample before testing releases the bacteria and increases the chance of isolation, as well as making the sample easier to work with. The bacteria may also be stressed within the sample because of the preservation technique, for example, drying, or may just be in small numbers. For this reason enrichment steps, where the sample is incubated in a suitable enrichment broth, are incorporated into the method.

A stomacher bag is used to homogenize the sample. Solid samples, powders and liquids can all be processed in this way and representative samples of complex food, such as sandwiches, are taken. A sample of 25g of the food is added to 225 ml of either maximum recovery diluents (MRD) or buffered peptone water in a stomacher bag and placed into the stomacher machine where it is homogenized for 1 minute. This 1 in 10 dilution can then be further diluted if the sample is expected to contain large numbers of microorganisms. The homogenized samples should be inoculated onto appropriate media within 45 minutes of preparation.

The range of investigations carried out on a particular food type is dependent on the nature of the food, the ingredients and the probability of specific pathogens being present, in much the same way as SOPs for clinical specimens from different body sites are based on knowledge of the most likely pathogens (see *Figure 14.1*).

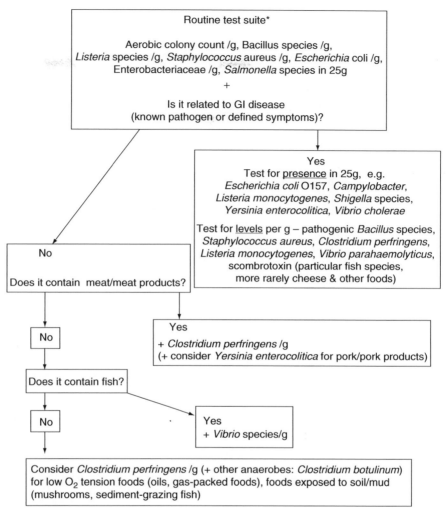

Figure 14.1
Criteria for the investigation of bacteria from food samples.

Aerobic plate counts (total viable count)

The APC or TVC is an indicator of the microbial contamination of a food sample. Half a millilitre of the homogenized sample is inoculated on to the surface of plate count agar and left to absorb into the agar for 15 minutes before the plates are inverted and incubated at 30°C for 48 hours. Further dilutions from the initial 1 in 10 dilution may also be tested.

After incubation the number of colonies is counted, either manually or using an electronic counter. Plates with between 15 and 300 colonies are counted and the number of colony-forming units (CFU)/ml calculated and recorded. The results are reported in CFU per gram or ml. If there is no growth on a 0.5 ml sample at a dilution of 10^{-1} this is reported as 'less than 20 CFU/g'.

The total viable count can be performed at the same time as 0.5 ml quantities are spread onto selective media for a range of target organisms.

Samples of 50 μl can also be inoculated by spiral platers to give a limit of detection of <200 CFU/g.

Escherichia coli

The presence of *Escherichia coli* in food indicates that there has been contamination with bacteria of faecal origin. Levels of greater than 100 CFU/g are unsatisfactory in ready-to-eat food, while for cook–chill products and for commercial ready-to-eat products the cut-off level is 10 CFU/g.

Samples weighing 25 g are prepared by homogenization and 0.5 ml is inoculated on to a chromogenic agar containing a substrate detecting β-glucuronidase activity by the presence of blue colonies. The agar also contains bile salts which are inhibitory to non-faecal bacteria. The plates are incubated at 30°C for 4 hours as a resuscitation step and then at 44°C for a further 18 hours. The higher temperature allows selective growth of *E. coli*. After incubation the number of blue colonies is counted and reported.

Enterobacteriaceae

Enterobacteriaceae may be present in small numbers and in a stressed condition in a variety of foods, including egg, milk and dairy products, dried formula milk, pasteurized milk and meat. They may be present in high levels in raw vegetables, but levels of $>10^8$ CFU/g in a raw salad would indicate that it has probably reached the end of acceptable shelf life. Direct plating onto selective agar (violet red bile glucose agar) is used for most food products, but the most probable number (MPN) method is used where there is a requirement to detect low numbers of bacteria. Dilutions are prepared in buffered peptone water and three tubes of each dilution are incubated for 24 hours at either 30°C for dairy products or 37°C for other foods. They are subcultured to an Enterobacteriaceae enrichment broth for a further 24 hours before subculture to violet red bile glucose agar and further incubation. Enterobacteriaceae produce red–purple colonies and are confirmed by a positive glucose test and negative oxidase reaction. The MPN is calculated from a reference table.

Salmonella species

Dilutions from 25 g samples of food are prepared and incubated first in 225 ml buffered peptone water for 18 hours at 37°C before subculture to two selective enrichment broths: 0.1 ml to Rappaport Vassiliadis soya peptone (RVS) and 1 ml to Muller–Kauffmann tetrathionate novobiocin broth (MKTTn) for serotypes that would be inhibited by RVS broth. If *Salmonella typhi* or *S. paratyphi* are suspected, selenite cystine broth is used. The broths are incubated at 41.5°C and 37°C, respectively, for 24 hours and then inoculated on to two selective culture media, XLD and Brilliant Green agar, for a further 24 hours at 37°C. Confirmation of presumptive *Salmonella* colonies is achieved by serology and biochemical tests. Samples as varied as dog chews, dishcloths and environmental swabs are tested. If the samples tested are part of a salmonella food poisoning investigation, there are additional procedures, including prolonged incubation and retention of the enrichment broths.

The presence of the bacteria is reported as either detected or not detected in 25 g of the sample. Any positive results from live animals or poultry, non-edible products or animal feedstuffs are also reported to the veterinary laboratory association. Their presence is always unacceptable in ready-to-eat food.

Campylobacter species

Because campylobacter are the most frequently isolated bacteria in cases of infectious diarrhoea, the presence of these bacteria in food samples is always significant. A food sample weighing 25 g is homogenized in 225 ml of Bolton broth, a specific pre-enrichment broth for campylobacter. The effect of the broth is to recover the bacteria and resuscitate them from the effect of heating, freezing and chilling of the food. After incubation at 41.5°C for 4–6 hours the broth is subcultured on to specific culture media (CCDA) and incubated in micro-aerophilic conditions at 41.5°C for 44 hours. Campylobacter colonies are then confirmed by a positive oxidase test and culture on blood agar in both aerobic and micro-aerophilic conditions, where no growth is observed on the aerobic plate.

The presence or absence of the bacteria in a 25 g sample is reported. The presence of *Campylobacter* species is always regarded as unacceptable.

Escherichia coli O157

Escherichia coli O157 bacteria have been associated with several serious outbreaks where patients have died or suffered serious illness (haemolytic uraemic syndrome, HUS) from the effect of the bacterial verocytotoxin. The presence of the bacteria in food is therefore significant as the infectious dose is very low. Although associated with undercooked beef and dairy products, *E. coli* O157 infections have originated from a variety of different foods. Because of the highly infectious nature of the bacteria, testing of isolates is carried out at containment level 3.

A sample of the food weighing 25 g is homogenized with 225 ml of pre-warmed modified tryptone soya broth. An automated immuno-magnetic bead separation (AIMS) is then used to remove any bacteria, using beads coated with anti-*E. coli* O157 antibodies. The presence of the bacteria is achieved by subculture to cefixime tellurite sorbitol MacConkey agar, incubated at 37°C for 24 hours. Most strains of *E. coli* O157 are non-sorbitol fermenters and appear as clear colonies. However, there are emergent strains that are sorbitol fermenters. Five colonies are subcultured on to MacConkey agar and nutrient agar. The bacteria grow as lactose-fermenting colonies on the MacConkey agar and confirmation is achieved by latex agglutination tests from nutrient agar plates. Molecular methods have also been used to identify *E. coli* O104:H4 (the cause of the May 2011 outbreak in Germany) from food samples. The presence or absence of the bacteria is reported in 25 g food.

Staphylococcus aureus

Large numbers of *Staphylococcus aureus* in ready-to-eat food suggest that the bacteria could produce toxins and cause food poisoning if consumed, whereas low numbers are indicative of poor handling. The limit for ready-to-eat food is equal to, or greater than 100 CFU/g. A 1 in 10 dilution is prepared in either peptone saline diluents or buffered peptone water from 25 g food, and 0.5 ml is inoculated on to a selective culture medium for *S. aureus*, Baird–Parker. Further dilutions are prepared and inoculated if the numbers are thought to be high. The liquid is left to soak into the agar for 15 minutes, after which the plates are incubated for 48 hours at 37°C. *S. aureus* form colonies on the agar, confirmed as *S. aureus* by the coagulase and DNase tests. The number of CFU/g is calculated and reported. A measurement of <20 CFU/g is satisfactory, between 20 and 10^4 CFU/g is borderline, and >10^4 CFU/g unsatisfactory, perhaps potentially hazardous. At this level the food would be referred to the reference laboratory for testing for enterotoxins and for the presence of toxin-producing genes.

Listeria

Listeria monocytogenes and other *Listeria* species are Gram-positive rods with the ability to grow at low temperatures, and are killed by cooking and pasteurization. The bacteria can be present in unpasteurized cheeses, cold meats, pâté and smoked fish. *L. monocytogenes* causes flu-like symptoms in non-pregnant and immuno-competent individuals and may lead to serious infections in pregnant women; these can lead to miscarriage, premature delivery and severe illness in the neonate. Of just over 200 cases reported to the HPA in 2009, 34 were pregnancy-associated. Provisional figures for 2010 are around 150 cases, with 17 associated with pregnancy. European legislation states that the bacteria must be absent in a 25 g sample or at a level of less

---

Box 14.1 Milk and dairy products

Consumers have a vast choice of milk and milk-based products, including drinks, cheese and cream and, because they are generally considered a healthy option, the fact that they could be a source of food-borne infection is a low priority. However, all these products are subject to routine testing in the same way as other foods. Milk and milk products can be consumed and manufactured from raw, untreated milk from cows, goats or sheep. Generally, milk sold in retail outlets is pasteurized or ultra high temperature (UHT) treated, but it is still possible to buy raw milk. Similarly, cheese, cream and other dairy products state clearly whether they are made from raw or pasteurized milk and from which animal species. All of these milk and dairy products are subject to microbiological testing to ensure that they are safe for the consumer and subject to appropriate regulations.

Raw milk from all species is tested for a total viable count (aerobic colony count) at 30°C, with the acceptable levels dependent on the source of the milk. For example, the acceptable level for raw cow's milk is <100 000 per ml but <1 500 000 for that of other species. If the raw milk is to be made into either heat-treated or non-heat-treated products, the level of *Staphylococcus aureus* is also tested. Raw cream is tested for the presence of salmonella, *Listeria monocytogenes* and *Escherichia coli*. *Listeria monocytogenes* must also be absent in pasteurized milk and cream and levels of Enterobacteriaceae must also be low.

A technique called the most probable number (MPN) method is used to detect the presence of coliforms and *E. coli* in milk and dairy products. The milk samples are diluted in tubes of lauryl tryptone broth containing a chemical, MUG (4 methylumbelliferyl-B-D glucuronide), that fluoresces in the presence of β-glucuronidase produced by *E. coli*. Coliforms are detected by the production of gas before and after subculture to brilliant green bile broth at 30°C. The MPN is ascertained by counting the number of positive tubes and using an interpretation table.

To demonstrate the success of the pasteurization, milk is additionally tested for the enzyme phosphatase, which should be inactivated by the time and temperature used for pasteurization (15–20 seconds at 71.7°C, in a process called high temperature short time – HTST). Alkaline phosphatase activity is measured by a fluorimetric method and recorded as the amount of enzyme present that catabolizes 1 mmol of substrate per minute per litre (mU/l). Levels should be less than 350 mU/l.

than 100 CFU/g at any point in the shelf life of ready-to-eat food. The presence of the bacteria is detected by homogenizing 25g of food into an enrichment broth (in this test, half Fraser broth) and incubating at 30°C for 24 hours. It is then inoculated on to listeria chromogenic agar and Oxford agar for 24 hours at 37°C. A specimen of 0.1 ml from the half Fraser broth is inoculated to Fraser broth for a further 48 hours' enrichment before inoculation on to the solid media. *Listeria* species grow as blue–green colonies on the chromogenic agar, due to β-glucosidase activity, and as grey colonies surrounded by black halos (due to the breakdown of aesculin) on the Oxford agar. The presence of listeria is confirmed by subculture to blood agar, where the presence of haemolysis indicates *L. monocytogenes*, and by API tests. The bacteria can also be enumerated in food samples by plating known quantities of the enrichment broth onto solid agar and calculating the number of bacteria per ml.

Toxin testing

In cases of food poisoning caused by specific toxins (*Staphylococcus aureus, Clostridium botulinum* and *Clostridium perfringens*) specimens are referred to a reference laboratory, where immunoassays, chemiluminescence or molecular methods are used to detect the presence of the toxins and/or enterotoxin-producing genes.

Scombroid toxin poisoning can occur as the result of eating scombroid fish (tuna and mackerel are examples) in which bacterial histidine decarboxylases have converted naturally-occurring histidine into free histamine. The formation of histamine takes place either in the marine environment, when fish is not kept at a sufficiently low temperature after harvest, or as a result of handling of the fish and temperature rises. The histamine can give the fish a sharp peppery taste. The levels of histamine are more toxic than the same dose of pure histamine because biogenic amines also present in the fish may accentuate inhibitory diamine oxidase and histamine methyl transferase, which normally have a detoxifying effect on histamine in the gastrointestinal tract. The symptoms of scombroid toxin poisoning appear very soon after consumption of the food, often within 30 minutes, and can appear similar to an allergic reaction. They include nausea, stomach pain, dizziness, sweating and flushing, headache, increased heart rate and a burning taste in the mouth. Levels of histamine in fishery products associated with high levels of histidine (mackerel, tuna, herrings, sardine, anchovy, mahi-mahi and bluefish) should be 100 mg/kg or less. Nine samples are tested and no more than two can be between 100 and 200 mg; none of the samples must exceed 200 mg/kg.

14.4 WATER MICROBIOLOGY

The scope of microbiological testing of water includes that used for human consumption and food preparation, pool water and cooling tower water. The methods described here are those recommended by the Health Protection Agency in compliance with UK and European legislation.

Drinking (potable) water

The principal sources of drinking water, which includes water used for cooking and food preparation, are the mains supply, water from bowsers or tanks, private water supplies, bottled, spring and mineral waters and the water supplies on ships and aircraft.

Mains water, together with water from bowsers, tanks and private water supplies, is tested by the water companies and must conform to UK and European Drinking Water Directive legislation. Because compliance levels are extremely high, other authorized microbiology laboratories are only involved in testing as the result of complaints or the investigation of an outbreak. The HPA laboratory may be involved in the routine monitoring of private water supplies, for example to a hospital. The water on ships is tested during inspections of the ship by the Port Health Authority using guidelines developed in conjunction with the HPA. Similarly the water supplies on aircraft should conform to the standards required for public water supplies.

Water samples measuring 100 ml are tested for coliforms, *Escherichia coli*, enterococci, indicators of faecal contamination, and an aerobic colony count (total viable count) at 37°C for 48 hours and at 22°C for 72 hours, as shown in *Table 14.2*.

Bottled, spring and mineral waters are also tested for faecal indicators and for *Pseudomonas aeruginosa*, all of which should be absent at the time of bottling, incapable of growth during distribution and absent when the product is consumed. Relevant legal requirements have been implemented by the FSA. Bottled and spring water samples of 250 ml are tested for *Escherichia coli*, enterococci, coliforms and

Table 14.2 Microbiological testing of potable water samples

Source of water	Mains	Bowser/tanker	Private water supplies	Ships	Aircraft	Bottled and spring water, at bottling	Mineral water, at source & during marketing
Test volume	100 ml	100 ml	100 ml	100 ml	100 ml	250 ml	250 ml
Enterococci	√	√	√ *	√	√	√	√
Escherichia coli	√	√	√	√	√	√	√
Coliforms	√	√	√	√	√	√	√
Pseudomonas aeruginosa					√	√	√
ACC 22°C, 72 hrs, 1 ml	√ *	√	√	√	√	√ **	√***
ACC 37°C, 48 hrs, 1 ml	√ *	√	√	√	√	√ **	√***
Clostridium perfringens	√ *		√ *				√ zero spores of sulphite-reducing anaerobes in 50 ml

√ *considered in follow-up of failures/complaints.

√ ** test within 12 hrs of bottling, acceptable levels 100 CFU/ml at 22°C and 20 CFU/ml at 37°C.

√ *** Acceptable level <20 CFU/ml at 22°C, 5 CFU/ml at 37°C at source and only normal increase during marketing.

Action is required if levels exceed zero. Action is also required if there is an abnormal change in the aerobic colony count or counts in excess of 1000 for ships and aircraft water (acceptable levels <100 CFU/ml). Based on data from the HPA guidance on microbiological examination of water samples. Levels are in accordance with council directive 98/83/EC.

Pseudomonas aeruginosa at 37°C for 48 hours and 22°C for 72 hours, as is 1 ml for the aerobic colony count (ACC). Mineral water samples are also tested for spore-forming sulphite-reducing anaerobes, using 50 ml samples.

Pool waters

Pool waters are tested routinely in UKAS-accredited laboratories and include swimming pools, hydrotherapy pools and spa pools (jacuzzis). It is important to test pool water because of the risk of infection if the water is microbiologically contaminated. Contamination can occur from the users of the pool, a failure in the pool filtration system or inadequate chlorination. Testing is carried out monthly and also if any changes occur to the treatment or engineering, if contamination

---

Box 14.2 The significance of the presence of bacterial indicator organisms in potable water and swimming pools

Escherichia coli are used extensively as an indicator of faecal contamination from humans, birds or mammals because they are unable to grow in the environment. In potable waters they are an indication of faecal contamination. The bacteria can be introduced to swimming pools from bathers' skin or from faecal contamination. As they are sensitive to the biocides used, they should not be present. Advice to swimmers to shower before entering pools has a sound microbiological basis, to remove some of the bacterial burden from their skins before swimming. *E. coli* are thermotolerant and will be present after incubation at 44°C as lactose-fermenting, indole-positive bacteria, possessing both β-galactosidase and β-glucuronidase enzymes.

Coliforms can be an indication of faecal contamination but they also provide basic information on water quality. Their presence is investigated in swimming pools and in potable waters. In swimming pools they can be introduced to the water from bathers' shoes, or leaves around an outdoor pool. They are sensitive to the biocides used in swimming pools and so their presence suggests a failure of these biocides. In potable waters their presence also suggests contamination from the environment. Coliforms are Gram-negative rods which are non-sporing, capable of growth in bile salts, oxidase-negative, lactose-fermenting and β-galactosidase positive. They include the genera *Escherichia*, *Citrobacter*, *Enterobacter*, *Klebsiella* and environmental bacteria not found in humans. They multiply at 37°C and, unlike *E. coli*, are not thermotolerant.

Enterococci and faecal streptococci include all Lancefield group D positive streptococci and are of human faecal origin. They are more resistant to stress, chlorination and drying than *Escherichia coli* and are used as indicators of faecal contamination in potable waters. They provide an additional indicator of the efficiency of treatment. They are identified by their growth on selective agar (membrane enterococcus agar) where presumptive enterococci produce red, maroon or pale pink colonies. This is the result of reduction of tetrazolium chloride to formazan, a red dye. The medium also contains sodium azide and glucose. Confirmation is achieved by demonstrating aesculin hydrolysis in the presence of bile salts after 48 hours' incubation.

Pseudomonas aeruginosa can grow in untreated water and in biofilms. It is important to test for their presence in bottled, spring and mineral water and in swimming pools, spa pools and hydrotherapy pools because it can indicate problems with filtration, disinfection and piping. If it is present in swimming pools it can infect humans and cause ear, eye and skin infections and is the cause of swimmers' ear infections if the bacteria enter the ear during a dive. *Pseudomonas aeruginosa* are Gram-negative rods growing with distinctive blue/green, red/brown or fluorescent colonies on selective agar and are oxidase positive.

is suspected or complaints have been made. Hydrotherapy pools are tested more frequently, twice weekly, because the people using them are immersed for longer periods and these patients are more prone to infection.

Samples measuring 100 ml are tested for *Escherichia coli*, coliforms and *Pseudomonas aeruginosa* at 37°C for 48 hours and 22°C for 72 hours, as is 1 ml for the ACC. If there is an outbreak situation, then it may be necessary to test for the presence of *Giardia* or *Cryptosporidia* species in the backwash water or filter material.

Spa pools should be tested at least once a month for faecal indicator organisms and quarterly for *Legionella* species. *Legionella* is a potential problem for spa baths because:

■ The water is at an optimal temperature, 30–40°C, for their growth
■ Jets in the system provide the characteristic bubbles in the pool which create aerosols in which the bacteria can be inhaled
■ The bacteria survive well in the piping and nutrients are available.

Pool closures

The acceptable level for the indicator organisms is shown in *Table 14.3*, along with the levels at which investigations must take place. If the routine test results of pool waters suggest gross contamination, or there has been a failure in the filtration or pumping systems, the pool should be closed to protect the users from infection. Gross contamination is defined as:

■ An *Escherichia coli* count of more than 10/100 ml in conjunction with an unsatisfactory aerobic colony count of >10/ml and or a count of *Pseudomonas aeruginosa* of >10/ml
and
■ A count of *Pseudomonas aeruginosa* >50/100 ml in combination with a high aerobic colony count of >100/ml
■ Greater than 1000 CFU per litre of *Legionella* species.

Table 14.3 Microbiological testing of pool and cooling tower waters

Tests	Swimming pools	Hydrotherapy pools	Spa pools	Cooling towers
Test volume	100 ml	100 ml	100 ml	
Escherichia coli	√	√	√	
Coliform (total coliforms)	√	√	√	
Pseudomonas aeruginosa	√	√	√	
ACC 37°C, 24 hrs, 1 ml	√	√	√	ACC at 30°C/48 hrs must be <10 000/ml
Legionella (1 litre)			√ must be <1000/l	√must be <100/l

Escherichia coli, coliforms and *Pseudomonas aeruginosa* levels should not exceed zero. Action is required for levels of *E. coli* >zero and >10 in 100 ml for coliform and *Ps. aeruginosa* in swimming pools, hydrotherapy and spa pools. *Ps. aeruginosa* must not exceed zero in hydrotherapy pools.

Cooling tower water

Cooling towers are an integral component of air conditioning systems, with tanks usually situated on the roofs of buildings. The water in the tanks cools the hot pipes from the heat exchange system and in the process steam is formed. *Legionella* and other bacteria live and form biofilms in the tanks where the *Legionella* species multiply in the warm water and can be emitted from the tank in the form of aerosols. There have been outbreaks of legionnaires' disease associated with outlets from cooling towers, and for this reason the growth of *Legionella* is kept under control by biocides. The water is tested weekly for ACC, as an indicator of bacterial growth, and quarterly for the presence of *Legionella* species, more frequently when a new plant is being established in compliance with the Health and Safety Commission (2000) Approved Code of Practice and Guidance. Sampling is carried out in accordance with the Standing Committee of Analysts (2005). The results are interpreted as follows:

- ACC ≤ 10 000 bacteria/ml. Acceptable, system is under control.
- ACC 10 000–100 000/ml OR 100–1000 *Legionella*/litre. Control measures reviewed, risk assessment carried out.
- ACC >1 000 000 bacteria/ml OR 1000 *Legionella*/litre. Requires immediate corrective action, disinfection and re-sampling.

Box 14.3 Legionnaires' disease

An unusual name for an atypical pneumonia, but the disease takes its name from the first outbreak and the subsequent discovery of the causative organism. In July 1976 there was a large convention of American legionnaires (ex-servicemen) in a hotel in Philadelphia. Within two days over 200 of them were ill with chest pains and a respiratory disease similar to acute influenza and 34 subsequently died. An investigation into the outbreak lasted several months and in January 1977 a new bacterium was isolated from the air conditioning cooling tower water, later to be called *Legionella pneumophila*. The bacteria are poorly staining Gram-negative bacilli, common inhabitants of water and able to withstand a wide range of temperatures. *L. pneumophila* is not the only species of the genus *Legionella*, but is the one associated with legionnaires' disease and the less serious infection, Pontiac fever. As a result of the first outbreak and realization of the cause, worldwide regulations for climate control systems were introduced. However, there have been significant outbreaks of the disease throughout the world, and they continue to occur: in Merthyr Tydfil, Wales in 2010, nineteen people were ill, and two patients in their 60s and 70s died; the source was thought to be a cooling tower in the town. Other small outbreaks have already occurred in 2011, in the USA and in a hotel in Bali. The largest outbreak in the UK was in 1985 in Stafford hospital, where 28 people died. The source there was the air conditioning cooling tower, shedding aerosols onto an area where clean air was supplied to the outpatient department. In 2002, 172 people were ill, with 7 deaths, in Barrow in Furness after being infected from aerosols from the cooling tower of the Arts centre. The largest outbreak in Europe was in Spain, where there were 800 suspected cases in a hospital in Murcia. Sporadic cases occur all the time after exposure to infected water. The typical patients are elderly and male, but cases of all ages have been reported.

14.5 LABORATORY TESTING PROCEDURES

Table 14.2 summarizes the requirements for the testing of different water samples, acceptable levels and the method used.

Sample requirements

In common with all investigations in microbiology it is important that the sample is representative of the time at which it was taken. Water samples should be tested as soon as possible after arrival at the laboratory and always within 24 hours. They should be protected from sunlight and kept at a temperature between 2 and 8°C. The effect of chlorine, bromine, ozone treatment and hydrogen peroxide is neutralized by the addition of thiosulphate pentahydrate to the bottles prior to collection. A concentration of 18 g/litre neutralizes concentrations of up to 5 mg chlorine/litre. Cooling tower water is heavily chlorinated, with levels up to 50 mg/litre and consequently levels of 180 mg/litre of thiosulphate pentahydrate are used. Samples of pool waters are collected at a depth of 30 cm below the surface of the pool.

Aerobic colony count

The aerobic colony count (ACC) is used as part of a long-term monitoring programme and allows changes in the background level of bacteria to be observed. The ACC is an indicator of cleanliness of the water and any sudden change can be a warning of pollution. Depending on the type of water, bacteria can enter via the soil, vegetation or human sources. The type of water also guides the temperature at which the ACC is carried out because environmental bacteria optimally grow at 22°C, bacteria from human origins at 37°C and *Legionella* at 30–40°C:

- Potable water, including natural mineral water, reservoirs, mains, drinking water in containers, private water supplies, melted ice and water from vending machines, could be contaminated by environmental or human sources. The ACC samples are incubated on yeast extract agar at 22°C for 72 hours and 37°C for 48 hours.
- Pool waters are more likely to be contaminated from human sources if disinfectant levels are inadequate, and are incubated on yeast extract agar at 37°C for 24 hours.
- Cooling systems are tested at 30°C for 48 hours on yeast extract agar to monitor whether the treatment is controlling bacterial growth.
- Purified waters and dialysis fluids require more sensitive testing on tryptone glucose extract agar at 21°C for 7 days.

If the sample is expected to have an ACC of above 300 colonies per ml then a series of ten-fold dilutions is prepared. One millilitre each of neat and all dilutions are pipetted into sterile, labelled Petri dishes. Molten agar is added to each dish and the water mixed in. The plates are incubated at the appropriate temperature and length of time indicated above. After incubation the colonies are counted and the ACC calculated using the formula:

$$\text{ACC (CFU/ml)} = \frac{\text{no. of colonies}}{\text{volume tested}} \times \text{dilution factor}$$

Membrane filtration method

In this method a pre-determined volume of water, dependent on the type of water under investigation (see *Tables 14.2* and *14.3*), is drawn through a filter under vacuum, which speeds up the filtration process. *Figure 14.2* shows an example

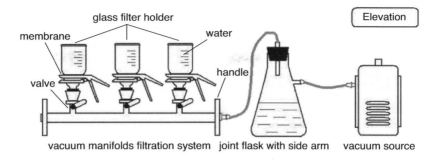

Figure 14.2
Multibranch filtration manifold. When samples of water are filtered, the glass (or plastic) filter holder is lifted and the membrane inserted using sterile forceps. The vacuum pump is switched on. The valve is opened and the water is drawn through the filter and collected in the conical flask. The valve is then closed and the membrane removed, again using sterile forceps, and placed on the surface of the appropriately labelled culture medium or into a small Petri dish containing 2.5 ml lauryl membrane sulphate broth. It is important to keep the whole procedure as sterile as possible.

of a multi-branch vacuum filtration system where three samples can be filtered simultaneously. The pore size of the membrane filters is 0.2 µm and so bacteria are retained on the membrane. Sterile water is run through the membrane before each sample is filtered. By using a new membrane for each 100 ml or 250 ml volume of the sample, the membranes can be incubated on different selective culture media for each bacterium tested. For example, if a water sample is tested for coliforms, *Escherichia coli*, enterococci and *Pseudomonas aeruginosa*, four volumes of the water are filtered onto a new membrane each time; two are placed in appropriately labelled Petri dishes containing 2.5 ml membrane lauryl sulphate broth to test for coliforms and *Escherichia coli*, one is placed on the surface of a selective culture medium for enterococci, and the final membrane is placed on a Petri dish containing selective agar for *Pseudomonas aeruginosa*. After incubation at the requisite temperature and time the plates are examined and confirmatory tests carried out. This is explained further in *Figure 14.3*.

Testing for *Legionella* species in water samples

The presence of *Legionella* species in cooling tower waters and spa pools is tested for either by membrane filtration and centrifugation to concentrate the sample or by centrifugation only, as shown in *Figure 14.4*. Equal quantities (0.2 ml) of the concentrated sample are then treated with heat, with acid and left untreated. This is followed by inoculation on to selective agar (glycine, vancomycin, polymixin cycloheximide agar – GVPC) and incubation for 10 days in a moist chamber at 37°C. Presumptive colonies of legionella are then subcultured to BCYE + and BCYE-ve agar (buffered charcoal yeast extract agar). *Legionella* species have a requirement for L-cysteine and will only grow on BCYE supplemented with L-cysteine (BCYE+) and not on the unsupplemented agar. Confirmation can be achieved by either a specific latex agglutination test or an immunofluorescence test. In the latter the bacteria are incubated on a slide coated with specific fluorescent antibody. After incubation and

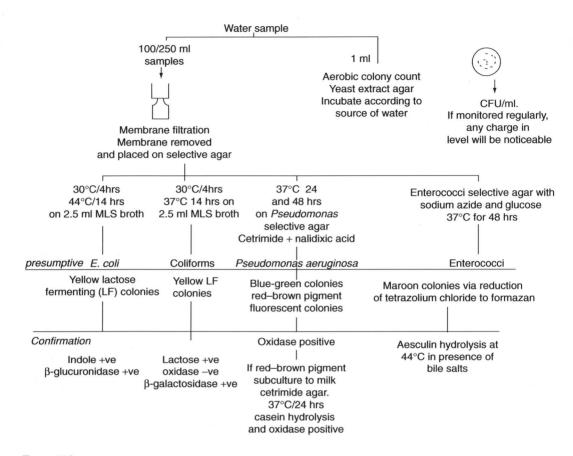

Figure 14.3
Flow diagram to show investigation of water samples and identification of bacteria.

washing, *Legionella* can be observed using the UV microscope as fluorescent green bacteria.

Further bacterial testing can be included as required, for example campylobacter, *Clostridium perfringens* and *Escherichia coli* O157. Water samples for campylobacter and *E. coli* O157 are treated in the same way as food samples to investigate the presence of these bacteria.

Clostridium perfringens

This is tested for by membrane filtration and inoculation onto tryptose sulphite cycloserine agar (TSCA) and incubated at 44°C anaerobically for 24 hours. Characteristic black, grey or yellow colonies of *C. perfringens* are subcultured to two blood agar plates, one incubated aerobically and the other anaerobically at 37°C for 24 hours. *C. perfringens* grows anaerobically with clear zones of haemolysis. Confirmation is achieved by stab inoculation of these colonies to a buffered nitrate motility agar for 24 hours at 37°C. The motile bacteria demonstrate diffuse growth along the stab line.

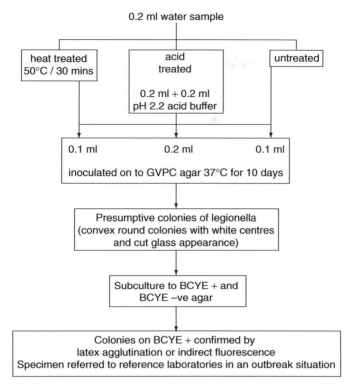

Figure 14.4
The isolation and identification of *Legionella* species from water samples. Water samples are either
filtered and then centrifuged prior to testing, or centrifuged only. Heating and acid treating the
samples reduces the burden of non-*Legionella* bacteria in the water samples, because *Legionella*
species are resistant to lower pH levels and heat exposure. GVPC, glycine vancomycin polymixin
cycloheximide agar; BCYE, buffered charcoal yeast extract agar with (+) and without (-) L-cysteine.

SUGGESTED FURTHER READING

Amar, C.F.L., East, C.L., Gray, J. *et al.* (2007) Detection by PCR of eight groups
of enteric pathogens in 4,627 faecal samples: re-examination of the English
case-control Infectious Intestinal Disease Study (1993–1996). *Eur. J. Clin.
Micro. and Infect. Dis.* **26:** 311–323.

Batt, C.A. (2007) Materials science: food pathogen detection. *Science,* **316:**
1579–1580.

Brehm-Stecher, B.F. & Johnson, E.A. (2004) Single-cell microbiology: tools,
technologies, and applications. *Microbiol. Mol. Biol. Rev.* **68:** 538–559.

Cabral, J.P.S. (2010) Water microbiology. Bacterial pathogens and water. *Int. J.
Environ. Res. Public Health,* **7:** 3657–3703 (can be accessed online at
http://mdpi.com/journal/ijerph).

Hrudey, S.E. & Hrudey, E.J. (2004) *Safe drinking water: Lessons from recent
outbreaks in affluent nations.* International Water Association Publishing.

Hunter, P.R. (2010) Drinking water safety and weather extremes. *Microbiologist,*
11: 34–36.

Hurst, C.J., Crawford, R.L., Garland, J.L. *et al.* (2007) *Manual of Environmental Microbiology*, 3rd edn. American Society for Microbiology.

Kennedy, S. (2008) Epidemiology: why can't we test our way to absolute food safety? *Science*, **322:** 1641–1643.

Kümmerer, K. (2004) Resistance in the environment. *J. Antimicrob. Chemother.* **54:** 311–320.

Lipp, E.K., Huq, A. & Colwell, R.R. (2002) Effects of global climate on infectious disease: the cholera model. *Clin. Microbiol. Rev.* **15:** 757–770.

Molmeret, M., Horn, M., Wagner, M. *et al.* (2005) Amoebae as training grounds for intracellular bacterial pathogens. *Appl. Environ. Microbiol.* **71:** 20–28.

Petry, F. (ed.) (2000) *Cryptosporidiosis and Microsporidiosis.* Karger.

Phillips, I., Casewell, M., Cox, T. *et al.* (2004) Does the use of antibiotics in food animals pose a risk to human health? A critical review of published data. *J. Antimicrob. Chemother.* **53:** 28–52.

Qadri, F., Svennerholm, A.-M., Faruque, A.S.G. & Sack, R.B. (2005) Enterotoxigenic *Escherichia coli* in developing countries: epidemiology, microbiology, clinical features, treatment, and prevention. *Clin. Microbiol. Rev.* **18:** 465–483.

Rangdale, R. (2009) Sewage borne pathogens associated with bivalve shellfish. *Microbiologist*, **10:** 29–32.

Tannock, G.W. (2004) A special fondness for Lactobacilli. *Appl. Environ. Microbiol.* **70:** 3189–3194.

The Food Standards Agency website has current information on food-related issues in the UK: www.food.gov.uk

SELF-ASSESSMENT QUESTIONS

1. Freezing is a common method used for preserving food. Explain how this method affects the normal growth cycle of bacteria.
2. Explain the difference between HACCP and end point testing.
3. Why is it important to homogenize food samples before testing them?
4. A resuscitation step is included in many of the food testing methods. Why is this necessary?
5. Different tests are carried out on mains drinking water than on drinking water used on aircraft. What is the reason for this?
6. A spa pool is tested for the presence of *Legionella* whereas the adjacent swimming pool is not. Suggest reasons for this and outline other sources of these bacteria monitored by laboratories.
7. A swimming pool is closed because the levels of *Pseudomonas aeruginosa* were high. What could be the source of these bacteria and how could they affect healthy bathers? (See also *Section 10.6*)
8. Explain why aerobic colony counts (ACCs) are most beneficial if they are performed routinely over an extended period of time.
9. Explain the value of performing total viable counts on food samples.
10. How would the presence of *Escherichia coli* O157 be detected in a sample of food? Why is it important to identify these bacteria in food?

Answers to self-assessment questions provided at:
www.scionpublishing.com/medmicro

Index